Adult Nurse Practitioner Intensive Review

Fast Facts & Practice Questions

About the Author

Maria T. Codina Leik [MSN, ARNP, BC, NP-C (GNP, ANP, FNP)], designed and developed materials for the nurse practitioner review courses that she has presented nationally since 1997 through her company, National ARNP Services, Inc. (www.npreview.com). She is board-certified as an Adult Nurse Practitioner (ANP) and Gerontological Nurse Practitioner (GNP) with the American Nurses Credentialing Center (ANCC). She is board-certified by the American Academy of Nurse Practitioners (AANP) as Family Nurse Practitioner (FNP). She has been in the field of nursing for the past 23 years and has been in active practice as a nurse practitioner since 1991 in the South Florida area. Maria is also a speaker and is a twice published chapter author.

Adult Nurse Practitioner Intensive Review

Fast Facts & Practice Questions

Maria T. Codina Leik, MSN, ARNP, BC, FNP-C

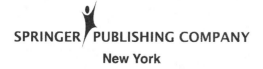

SPRINGER PUBLISHING COMPANY

New York

Springer Publishing Company, LLC
11 West 42nd Street
New York, NY 10036–8002
www.springerpub.com

Acquisitions Editor: Sally J. Barhydt
Managing Editor: Mary Ann McLaughlin
Production Editor: Matthew Byrd
Cover Design: Joanne E. Honigman
Composition: Aptara, Inc.

07   08   09   10/   5   4   3   2   1

Library of Congress Cataloging-in-Publication Data

Codina Leik, Maria T.
  Adult nurse practitioner intensive review : fast facts & practice questions / Maria T. Codina-Leik.
      p.   ;   cm.
    Includes bibliographical references and index.
    ISBN 978-0-8261-0295-9
  1. Nurse practitioners—Examinations, questions, etc.   I. Title.
[DNLM: 1. Nurse Practitioners—Examination Questions.   2. Nursing Care—Examination Questions. WY 18.2 C669a 2007]

RT82.8.C62   2007
610.73076–dc22

                                                              2007029922

Printed in the United States of America by Victor Graphics.

Preface

This Adult Nurse Practitioner (ANP) review guide has been designed to save you valuable study time reviewing for the ANP board-certification examinations.

The content of this review book is applicable to the board-certification exams given by the American Nurses Credentialing Center (ANCC) and the American Academy of Nurse Practitioners (AANP). This review guide covers the lifetime periods ranging from adolescence, adulthood, and into geriatrics. Non-clinical content such as the nurse practitioner role, medico-legal issues, reimbursement and others are also included.

This book, a "Mega Review" study guide, combines five different resources into one: (1) specific certification exam information that includes instructions on speeding up the application process, (2) test-taking techniques that are highly relevant for both the ANCC and AANP exam, (3) a question dissection and analysis section where you learn to pick out the "Best Clues" to solve problems along with the necessary clinical knowledge, (4) a review of primary care disorders including specific "Exam Tips" with advise on some current exam topics, and finally (5) a total of 500 sample questions and answers to practice your new skills.

Included in this review guide are many pictures and tables. Physical exam maneuvers (i.e., the Drawer sign, McMurrays sign, etc.) are beautifully illustrated by photographs and notes. This review guide will not only help to cut down your total review time, but will also give you a more productive and less frustrating experience. A special effort has been made to cut down as much extraneous information as possible without sacrificing the quality of the book's contents.

If you have comments and suggestions for this book or are interested in having an intensive NP Review Course held in your school or local area, please contact me by email from my company's web site, National ARNP Services, Inc., at *www.NPreview.com*.

Writing this book taught me many things.
Most importantly, how blessed and lucky I am,
to have E.J.L., my wonderful husband,
and daughters Maryfaye and Christina.
I am truly grateful for your love and support.
A smart and talented editor like Sally Barhydt,
and Springer Publishing Company
Can help make a dream into solid reality
Thank You All.

Contents

Certification Exam Information

American Nurses Credentialing Center (ANCC)

www.nursecredentialing.org

Phone: 1-800-284-2378

Local & International: 301-628-5250

Prometric Contacts

Web site: http://www.prometric.com/ANCC/

Phone (ANCC only): 1-800-350-7076

The ANCC is the credentialing body of the American Nurses Association (ANA). The credentialing exams that are currently being offered to nurse practitioners are for the following specialties: adult, family, pediatric, gerontologic, acute care, adult or family psychiatric and mental health, and advanced diabetes management. The entire application packet can be downloaded from their Web site.

American Academy of Nurse Practitioners (AANP)

www.aanp.org

Phone: (512) 442-5202

Fax : (512) 442-5221

Email: certification@aanp.org

Prometric Contacts

Web site: http://www.prometric.com/AANP/

Phone (AANP only): 1-888-680-5327

The AANP is a specialty organization that serves only nurse practitioners. It is currently offering three specialty exams: adult, family, and geriatric nurse practitioner. The entire application packet can be downloaded from their Web site.

Thomson Prometric Computer Testing Centers

Prometric Calling Center Hours: 8:00 AM to 8:00 PM Eastern Standard Time (EST)

Both the ANCC and the AANP use this company to administer their computer-based certification exams. All testing centers are open from Monday to Friday with many centers open on evenings and weekends.

There are three methods available for locating, scheduling, or rescheduling yourself for the exam. In addition, you may also cancel or confirm an appointment this way.

You can do all these online (open 24/7), by phone, or onsite (not all centers have this option). But first, you must have your candidate eligibility number to do so. The number is assigned to you directly by Prometric and is mailed within 2 weeks after you receive your acceptance to test letter from either the ANCC or the AANP.

Qualifications

Graduate of an approved master's, postmaster's, or doctor of nursing practice (DNP) adult nurse practitioner program and hold an active RN (registered nurse) license.

Background Information

ANCC and AANP

Generally, the ANCC updates their nurse practitioner exams every 2 to 3 years. The time period that the AANP updates their exams is unknown. The questions for both exams are referenced from major nursing textbooks, national treatment guidelines, papers, and official governmental reports. Do not assume that because both exams are for nurse practitioners, the references used are written mostly by nurses. The opposite is true. A large number of the references used for both the exams are derived from major medical textbooks.

Exam Format

Both are computer-based tests (CBTs) designed in a multiple-choice format. Each question has four answer choices with only one answer per option.

Total Number of Questions

ANCC

The ANCC exam has 175 total questions. Of these, 25 sample questions are not scored (for statistical evaluation only). Therefore, only 150 of the questions are graded.

AANP

The AANP exam has a total of 150 questions.

Total Time

ANCC and AANP

The actual testing time allowed for both exams is 3.5 hours. Before the actual exam starts, a computer tutorial "free" time of 30 minutes is given. This is when the instructions and the computer commands are discussed. When the tutorial period expires, the computer automatically starts the exam. Therefore, the total time for the entire test is 4 hours.

The computer will automatically shut down the exam when the 3.5 hours of allotted time expires. There is no extra time allotted for a break. If you need a break during the counted time of 3.5 hours, then you will be using actual test time.

Fast Facts Certification Exam Questions

Because the AANP certification exam has fewer questions, there is more time allotted to solve their questions compared with the ANCC exam. Each question (ANCC exam only) is worth one point no matter how easy or difficult it is to solve.

ANCC: 1.2 minutes per question (total 175 questions)
AANP: 1.4 minutes per question (total 150 questions)

Fast Facts Comparing the ANCC Versus the AANP Exam

1) Which board certification is better?

Both are equally recognized as national specialty certifying bodies and are acceptable to governmental entities such as Medicare and Medicaid; as well as to local state agencies such as the state boards of nursing (BON). If you are a new graduate, it is a good idea to speak to nurse practitioners in your area as well as faculty to find out whether one certification is preferred over the other in your area of practice.

2) What is an "official" transcript?

A transcript is considered "official" only if it remains inside the sealed envelope in which it was mailed from your college registrar's office. Preferably, have your transcripts mailed directly to your residence. Another option is to have the school registrar mail the transcript directly to the certifying organization. Order at least three to four copies of your final transcripts and keep the extras unopened to keep it official. Open one copy (yours) and check it for accuracy.

3) What is the ANCC's "Form E" used for?

Form E is part of the application packet from the ANCC. It is also known as the "Nurse Practitioner Educational Preparation" form. It must be signed off by the current director of your school's nurse practitioner program even if you are not a recent graduate.

If you are a new graduate, make sure that you have the form signed off before leaving school. Even if you plan to take the AANP's test, it is still a good idea to get a copy of Form E. If you ever need to take the ANCC test in the future or change your mind, it will help save time during the application process.

4) What is the difference between the testing dates for the AANP and those for the ANCC?

ANCC

ANCC exams can be taken at almost any time of the year (except for major holidays) whenever the Thomson Prometric Testing Centers are open. The ANCC does not have any application deadlines.

AANP

AANP exams can only be taken three times a year during a specified 10-week time period known as the testing "window". Each window has its own application deadline. Therefore, there are three deadlines per year to watch for when applying for the AANP exam. If you miss the regular deadline for your window, there is also a "late deadline" (you are charged a late fee). To get the most current AANP schedule, check their Web site at www.aanp.org.

AANP Exam Schedule

Window 1: January to April
The application deadline is usually in the last week of December
Late deadline is in January

Window 2: May to August
The application deadline is usually in the 3rd week of April
Late deadline is in May

Window 3: September to December
The application deadline is usually in the 3rd week of July
Late deadline is in August

5) When can I apply for the certification exams?

ANCC

You are allowed to apply as early as during the last semester/quarter before you graduate. If you apply early, you must include an official copy of your current transcript (even if it is not the final one). As soon as the final transcripts are available, mail the official copy to complete your application. According to the ANCC staff I have spoken with (by phone), their organization prefers that test takers apply only when the final transcripts are available. They apparently prefer that the entire application along with the final transcript and test fee be sent in together as one package instead of separately.

Within 2 to 3 weeks, a notice that they received the application along with the General Testing Information Booklet will be mailed to you. The ANCC takes from 4 to 8 weeks to process an application. If you are deemed eligible, the authorization-to-test (ATT) form letter is mailed directly to you from the testing agency within 4 to 8 weeks. If you are deemed not eligible, you can appeal an application to the ANCC. A letter regarding the appeal process will be mailed to you within a few weeks.

AANP

The AANP also allows test takers to apply as early as during the last semester/quarter before graduation. Because each of the AANP testing windows has a deadline, I suggest that you apply early a few weeks before you graduate.

This is especially important for those planning to graduate during December. If you decide to wait until your final transcripts are released, you can easily miss the December deadline or possibly the late deadline (January). Test takers who miss both deadlines for the 1st AANP testing window of the year have to wait until the next one opens in June. If you are a new graduate, this translates into a wait of at least 6 months after you have graduated and results in big delay in your ability to practice as a nurse practitioner.

Note:

For both exams, do not forget to photocopy all the contents in your application before mailing it in a large envelope.

6) Special instructions for AANP applications

Be careful when you are filling out the AANP applications. Do not leave any of the questions unanswered or leave any blanks on the application forms. It will delay your application by several weeks since it can not be fully processed until all the required documentation is correctly completed. Also, do not answer *"refer to enclosed transcript"* (or the equivalent) on any question asking you for the number of credits or course numbers. You must fill in the required course numbers, credit hours, and dates by hand.

7) After receiving an acceptance letter, how much time do I have before it expires?

ANCC

You have up to 90 days from the date stamped in the acceptance letter to take your exam.

AANP

The AANP's acceptance letter is valid only for one 10-week testing window. If you do not take your exam within the dates assigned for the window, then your acceptance letter will expire and is no longer valid. A memo must be faxed to the AANP certification department with a request to sit for another testing window. For more information and instructions, call their office in Texas at (512) 442-4262.

8) What is the Prometric candidate eligibility number?

ANCC and AANP

This is the number that is assigned to you directly by Prometric that allows you to schedule an appointment for the exam. Your candidate eligibility number is mailed directly from Prometric within two weeks after you receive your acceptance to test letter.

9) How do I schedule myself for the exam?

ANCC and AANP

There are three methods available. They are listed under the Thomson Prometric information on the first page. Do not forget that you will need your candidate eligibility number which is assigned to you directly by Thomson Prometric. It is mailed to you within 2 weeks after you receive your acceptance letter.

You must give a minimum of 48 hours notice to cancel an appointment. If you have less than 48 hours left, the testing center must be called directly and informed about the cancellation. When you reschedule, you will be charged a rescheduling fee.

Note:

Avoid scheduling yourself at the time of the day when you tend to get tired or sleepy. For most, this is usually after lunchtime. Simply picking the wrong time can cause you to fail the exam, sometimes by as little as two points.

10) What should I do if the time slot I want is no longer available?

If the testing center you chose does not have the time or date you want available, then look for another testing center as soon as possible. This is a good idea if your acceptance letter or testing window is about to expire. For some, it may mean a long drive to another city, but it may well be worth the extra time and effort to avoid the extra paperwork needed if you miss your designated deadline.

Note:

Morning time slots tend to get filled quickly. If you are unable to find one, some testing centers do have a waiting list. Unfortunately, this option is not available online; you must call the local testing center to find out if a waiting list is available.

11) When do I receive my test scores?

ANCC

A new change with the ANCC computer-based nurse practitioner exams was implemented this year. You will learn right away whether you have passed or failed. After you complete the test or when the 3.5 hour time limit expires, your results will be shown to you on the computer. Your official test scores are mailed to you within 1 to 2 weeks after taking the exam.

AANP

For the last few years, AANP test takers have been shown their unofficial test result in the computer after they have completed the exam (or when the 3.5-hour time limit expires).

This is known as the unofficial score. The official scores are mailed to you within the next few weeks.

12) What are the passing scores?

ANCC

The passing score is 350 points or higher. ANCC scores range from 100 to 500 points.

AANP

The passing score is 500 points or higher. AANP scores range from 100 to 800 points.

13) What are the passing rates for each exam?

ANCC

The latest passing rate for the ANCC ANP exam is 80% (2006). The passing rates for the exam over the years have ranged from between the mid-70th to the low 80th percentile.

AANP

Currently, the passing rates for the AANP exams are not released to the public.

14) How are scores listed?

ANCC and AANP

The scores for each domain (ANCC term) or category (AANP term) are listed individually in addition to the total score. The highest score is listed first and the lowest score is last.

The lower scores indicate your weakest areas; devote more study time into these areas if you do not pass. If you did not take a review course, I recommend that you find one or buy their tapes. My review courses are listed in my Web site at www.npreview.com.

15) How do I inform the BON of my certification status?

Both the AANC and the AANP can give your scores to your state's BON with your permission. A special form must be filled out and is available for download at their Web sites.

16) What happens if I do not pass the exam?

ANCC

A few weeks after you receive your official score letter, the "permission to retest" letter with application is automatically mailed to you by the ANCC along with a re-test fee charge. There is a time requirement of a minimum of 90 days after the date of taking the last exam before you are allowed to retest. Unlike the AANP, the ANCC does not require any continuing education credits (CEUs) in order to be allowed to retest.

AANP

Although there is no 90 day time requirement required, the AANP requires test-takers to take 15 CEUs in their area(s) with the weakest score. Choose courses that address the area(s), if in doubt, call the AANP. The CEUs taken before taking your certification exam are not eligible. After completing this requirement, you can mail or fax your certificates of completion as proof. Call the AANP certification office first before faxing any documents. After your CEUs have been approved, an "application to retest" form is mailed to you along with the charge for a retest fee.

17) If you fail the AANP or ANCC exam the second time:

You must resubmit a full application (like the first time) along with all the required documentation and pay the full test fee.

18) What is the professional designation used by each organization?

ANCC

The initials "APRN,BC" (Advanced Practice Registered Nurse, Board Certified) are used. No periods or spaces are necessary when writing these initials.

AANP

The designation "NP-C" (Nurse Practitioner-Certified) is used. Do not use a comma before the "C" (certified). Use only a dash.

19) How long is my certification valid?

Board certification from both the ANCC and AANP is valid for 5 years. It can be renewed by the following methods or by retaking the certification exam. A grace period is available for both, but after the grace period expires, you must retake the exam again.

ANCC

Recertification for adult nurse practitioners (ANPs) and family nurse practitioners (FNPs) no longer requires the mandatory 1,000 hours of clinical practice (over a 5-year period) as before. These are the only two NP specialties that are exempted from the clinical practice requirement.

You must complete at least 75 contact hours of continuing education (at least 50% of credits must come from ANCC-approved providers) plus fulfill any one of the ANCC designated professional development categories below. Examples of some of the methods acceptable for recertification are the following:

a) Continuing education credits
b) Presentations and lectures
c) Publications and research
d) Development of education materials such as CD ROM, videotape, or other media presentation
e) Preceptorship

You can also choose to retake and pass the certification exam to renew your board certification. This is mandatory if you let your certification expire and do not renew it within the allowed grace period.

Note:

Full-time nursing faculty are not allowed to used didactic lecture time that is part of their job requirements as continuing education credits.

Adapted from the ANCC at http://www.nursecredentialing.org/cert/recert/

AANP

A minimum of 1,000 hours of clinical practice as a nurse practitioner in your area of specialty is mandatory along with 75 contact hours of continuing education credits.

20) Is there any reciprocity between the ANCC and AANP?

Family and adult nurse practitioners who are certified by an approved national certification body (i.e., ANCC, AANP, etc.) who meet criteria are eligible to apply. To request for information and applications, contact the AANP certification department by the following methods:

1) Email: certification@aanp.org

Table 1.1 ANCC Domains of Practice

Adult Nurse Practitioner Exam	Percent
I. Health Promotion and Disease Prevention	19%
	29 Questions
II. Assessment of Acute and Chronic Illness	22%
	33 Questions
III. Clinical Management	32%
	48 Questions
IV. Nurse Practitioner and Patient Relationship	12%
	18 Questions
V. Professional Role and Policy	9%
	13 Questions
VI. Research	6%
	9 Questions
Total	100%

Note.   Adapted from the ANCC Adult Nurse Practitioner Board Certification Exam Content Outline; retrieved July 5, 2007, from http://www.nursecredentialing.org/cert/

2) Fax: (512) 442-5221
3) Phone: (512) 442-5221

The ANCC can be contacted by calling their Customer Care Center at 1-800-284-2378.

Test Question Classification

American Nurses Credentialing Center

Classification
Table 1.1 shows a breakdown of the domains used in the ANCC exam. These numbers are not static and they have changed over time. For example, the percentage makeup of the test questions that I consider the "non-clinical" domains (NP and patient relationships, professional role and policy, and research) have increased to 27%. This means that 40 out of the 150 total questions are from the non-clinical domains.

Summary
1) These are the top three domains in the ANCC ANP certification exam:
   - Clinical management (32%)
   - Assessment of acute and chronic illness (22%)
   - Health promotion and disease prevention (19%)
2) Test takers who score low in any two of the domains just listed will usually fail the exam because these domains account for 110 out of the 150 total questions in the ANP ANCC exam.

3) The percentage of nonclinical questions has recently increased from 19% to 27%.
   - Nurse practitioner and patient relationship (12%)
   - Professional role and policy (9%)
   - Research (6%)

American Academy of Nurse Practitioners Scoring System

Classification

Currently, the AANP does not release its statistics. The percentage makeup of their exam questions for each of the categories listed below is not public knowledge.

   I. Health promotion
  II. Disease prevention
 III. Diagnosis
  IV. Management of acute disease
   V. Management of chronic disease

Summary

A larger number of questions on this exam are clinically based. This conclusion is drawn not only from my personal experience, but also from feedback from former review course students.

Fast Facts | ANCC and AANP Exams

A. The most current treatment guidelines and protocols are those that were probably released about 3 years (or longer) before the current exam you will be taking. The more recent guidelines will not be in the exams.

B. The nurse practitioner certification tests are national exams concentrating on primary care disorders. These are not tests on specialty disorders. Keep this in mind when you are reading the answer options. In general, avoid picking exotic diseases as answers.

C. AANP exams list the normal lab results of the pertinent lab in a test question. Remember, normal lab results are shown only once on the exam. Write them down on your scratch paper. The ANCC does not do this.

D. No asymptomatic or "borderline" cases of disease states are presented in the test.

   Example: In real life, most patients with iron-deficiency anemia are asymptomatic and do not have either pica or spoon-shaped nails. In the exam, they will probably have these clinical findings.

E. Disease states are presented in their "classic" textbook presentation.

Example: If a case of acute mononucleosis is being presented, the patient will most likely be a teen presenting with the classic triad of sore throat, fatigue, and enlarged cervical nodes.

F. Learn the disorders for which maneuvers are used.

Example: Tinel's or Phalen's is used to assess for carpal tunnel syndrome.

G. Learn what a positive result means for a physical exam maneuver.

Example: A positive anterior or posterior drawer test means that a knee is unstable.

H. Be knowledgeable about physical exam "normals." There are very few questions on benign variants.

Example: Torus palatinus, fishtail uvula (listed under the head, eye, ear, nose, and throat [HEENT] system review).

I. Learn what a lab result means and the follow-up needed to further evaluate the patient. It is very rare to get a question asking for actual number values.

J. Medications are listed in both generic and brand-name forms, or they may be listed only as a drug class.

Example: The drug class *macrolide* is used instead of *erythromycin or azithromycin* as the answer option.

K. Most of the drugs mentioned in the exam are the older, well-recognized drugs.

Example:
Macrolide: erythromycin or clarithromycin (Biaxin)
Cephalosporins: first-generation (Keflex), second-generation (Ceftin/ Cefzil), third-generation (Rocephin)
Quinolones: ciprofloxacin (Cipro) ; ofloxacin (Floxin)
Quinolones with gram-positive coverage levofloxacin (Levaquin)
Sulfa: trimethoprim/sulfamethazole (Bactrim, Septra)
Tetracyclines: tetracycline ; doxycycline (Vibramycin)
Nonsteroidal anti-inflammatory (NSAID): ibuprofen ; naproxen (Anaprox)
Cough suppressant: dextromorphan (Robitussin)
Other examples are listed in both Chapter 2 and Chapter 3 sections.

L. Some Category B that are allowed for pregnant or lactating women may be included in the ANP exam

Example: For pain relief, pick acetaminophen (Tylenol) instead of NSAIDs such as ibuprofen (Advil) or naproxen (Aleve, Anaprox DS).

M. When memorizing drugs, you do not have to memorize every side effect. Instead, learn about a drug's common side effects, dangerous side effects, contraindications, and drug interactions. There is no need to memorize drug doses.

Example: ACE inhibitors: a common side effect is a dry cough (up to 10%). A well-known side effect is a dry cough. A serious side effect is hyperkalemia (rarely angioedema). Do not mix this drug class with potassium-sparing diuretics (i.e., triamterene). It is the preferred drug to treat hypertension in diabetics because of its renal-protective properties.

N. The ANCC exam is more likely to have answer options written as verbal statements with questions addressing mental health topics. Keep these good communication rules in mind: Ask open-ended questions, avoid judgmental statements, do not reassure, do not give abrupt responses, respect the patient's culture, and do not confront the patient.

O. One to two questions on bioterrorism topics have appeared in the exam. Remember that the best method for spreading viruses or bacteria is to make them airborne or nebulized. Anthrax is treated with ciprofloxacin.

P. Questions about nursing theory have not been seen on either exam for several years.

Q. Other health theorists (not nurses) who have been included on the exams in the past are (not inclusive): Erickson, Freud, Piaget, systems theory, Elizabeth Kübler-Ross's theory on bereavement, Health Belief Model, Self-Efficacy Model.

R. ANCC has increased the number of questions on nonclinical issues (27%).

Example: Nursing practice, health policy, Nurse Practice Act, nurse practitioner role, living will, durable power of attorney, advance directives, privacy laws, documentation, quality assurance, risk management, reimbursement issues, Medicare, research. These are discussed in Chapter 3.

S. Keep in mind that the majority of questions in the AANP and 73% of the questions (2006 statistics) on the ANCC exams are clinically based.

T. Follow national treatment guidelines for certain disorders. The following is a list of treatment guidelines used as references by the ANCC.

National Treatment Guidelines

Hypertension
Joint National Committee on Prevention, Detection, and Treatment of High Blood Pressure (JNC) 7th Report

Community-Acquired Pneumonia (CAP)
American Thoracic Society (ATS) Treatment Guidelines for Outpatient Community-acquired Pneumonia

Hyperlipidemia
National Cholesterol Education Panel (2002). Third Report of the Expert Panel on Detection, Evaluation, and Treatment of High Cholesterol in Adults

Asthma
Guidelines for the Diagnosis and Management of Asthma. Expert Panel Report. National Asthma Education and Prevention Program (2003)

Sexually Transmitted Diseases (or sexually transmitted infections)
Sexually Transmitted Disease Treatment Guidelines (2002). Centers for Disease Control and Prevention

Healthy People 2010
U.S. Department of Health and Human Services. Healthy People 2010, 2nd edition.

Health Prevention
The Guide to Clinical Preventative Services (2002). U.S. Preventative Task Force

Links to the national treatment guidelines are available at www.npreview.com

Fast Facts Maximizing Your Scores

1) There is no penalty for guessing. If you run out of time, quickly fill out the remaining questions at random. Never leave any question unanswered.
2) "Mark" questions that you want to review later after you have completed your exam. This is a special command that you will learn how to use during the 30 minute computer tutorial period. Marking a question allows you to return to it later or to change the answer. To save yourself more time, learn how to use the computer's commands before taking the exam. Go to the ANCC Web site at www.nursingworld/ancc/ and click the "Computer Tutorial" link to practice.
3) Plan ahead what you want on the scratch paper before the test by making one at home. Practice writing it down and memorize the notes so that you do not waste time trying to remember it when you are taking the exam.
4) Save yourself time (and mental strain) by reading the last sentence (or stem) of long questions and case scenarios *first*. Then read the question again from the beginning.
5) The advantage of this "backward reading" technique is that you know ahead of time what the question is asking for. When you read it again "normally," it becomes easier to recognize important clues that will help you answer the question.
6) To avoid making careless errors, do not read the questions too rapidly. You will go into "autopilot" mode. Remind yourself to read slowly and carefully throughout the test.
7) If you are having problems choosing or understanding the answer options, try to read them from the bottom up (from option D to A).
8) One method of guessing is to look for a pattern. Pick the one answer that does not fit the pattern. Another is to pick the answer that you are most "attracted"

to. Go with your gut feeling and do not change the answer unless you are very sure of the answer.

9) In general, it is not a good idea to change too many answers on an exam.

10) The first few questions are usually harder to solve. This is a common test design. Do not let it shake your confidence. Guess the answer and mark it. All questions are worth only one point.

11) If you spend more than 1 minute on a question, you are wasting time. Answer it at random and mark it so that you can return to it later after you finish the entire test. Never leave any question unanswered. You can loose one point (or more) because there is a one in four chance of guessing correctly.

12) Wear a watch with a second hand. It makes it easier to see if you are spending too much time on a question.

13) In general, each question is allotted about 60 seconds to solve. Most test takers finish the exam within 2.5 to 3 hours.

14) If you have failed the test before, try not to memorize what you did on the previous exam you took. The answers you remember may be wrong.

15) Pretend that you have never seen the test before so that you can start out fresh mentally (for repeat test takers).

16) Consider a quick break (if you have enough time) if you get too mentally fatigued. Go to the bathroom and get a drink of water, and splash cold water on your face. This can take less than 5 minutes.

17) Eat some hard candy. Hard candies are allowed inside the testing area as long as they are unwrapped.

18) Dress in comfortable clothes and shoes. Dress in layers.

19) The countdown clock in the computer does not stop for breaks. Do not use more than 5 minutes for your quick bathroom break.

20) Do not forget that the testing areas are monitored by both video cameras and microphones.

Fast Facts Review Timeline

1) The amount of time you need to study depends on how well prepared you are. The minimum time it takes is about 6 weeks.

2) Look over the table of contents of your primary care textbook and plan the time you want to allocate to each organ system. Do not forget to review the normal findings as well.

3) Plan and write down your study schedule. Post it in a visible area.

4) Start reviewing your weakest areas first and assign more time to them. Save the areas you know well for the last. Do not get fixated on memorizing too much rote information at once (i.e., cranial nerves). Use a mnemonic or make up your own.

5) Besides reading books, also use tapes or CDs, especially if you learn best by listening. The more of senses you use (reading and listening), the easier it is to remember facts.

6) Use a new notebook to write yourself reminders during your review. When reading on a topic, write down brief notes. Write yourself reminders and tips.

7) Read your notes at the end of the study session and several times a day.

8) Pick an area to study where you will not be disturbed. For some with small children, this may mean studying outside the home (i.e., library, bookstore).

9) If you learn better in a group, organize one. Decide ahead of time what to cover so that you do not waste time.

10) Try to study daily even if you can only afford 10 to 15 minutes of time. Consistency is important. You can break up your study sessions over the day. You will retain information better this way than by doing one large cram session per week.

11) Take some notes or photocopy material that you want to learn and place it in your purse or wallet.

Fast Facts Other Test-Taking Issues

A. Emotional Readiness

Your internal beliefs about how well you will do in the exam are very important and should not be minimized. Try the following exercises if you are feeling too anxious.

This is a good exercise for test takers who have failed the exam before. Of course, you must also devote enough time and effort into your review studies.

Instructions: Programming Your Subconscious Mind

Make a tape/CD or write down positive affirmations. Post them on your bathroom mirror and the dashboard of your car. Keep repeating the phrases to yourself.

Examples:

"I feel confident that I will pass my certification exam and do very well."
"I always do well in multiple-choice tests."
"I feel secure in myself and am confident that I will pass the exam."

1) Imagine vividly, believe, and feel yourself passing the exam.

2) Do this exercise as much as you can, especially during the two weeks before the exam.

B. Your Panic Button

If you find yourself starting to panic, try the following calming technique:

1) Close your eyes. Tell yourself very firmly to *stop*. Keep repeating it until you calm down and your heart rate slows down.

2) Concentrate hard to consciously slow down your breathing.

3) Take three deep breaths and exhale slowly through pursed lips.

4) Tell yourself "I am breathing in 'self-confidence' and exhaling out my 'fear'."

C. Testing Center Details

1) Call the testing center a few days before to verify your appointment.
2) Locate and drive to the testing center before taking the exam.
3) Arrive at least 20 minutes before your scheduled time to get checked in.
4) Required documentation:
   - Authorization to test (ATT) letter and two types of positive identification.
   - You will NOT be allowed to take the exam without both these documents Your primary ID should contain both your picture and signature (driver's license, passport, or a U.S. government ID). Expired IDs are not acceptable.Your second ID must have your signature on it such as a valid credit/debit card, check cashing card or citizenship ID (permanent resident/green card). The following are not acceptable ID: social security card, draft registration card, or student ID cards.
5) The only things you can bring inside a testing area are scratch paper and pencils given to you by the testing center staff. Ask for extra paper if you tend to write a lot.
6) Each test taker is assigned one small cubicle with one computer. If you are having problems with visualizing the computer screen, bring it to the proctor's attention as soon as possible.
7) You can request ear plugs; consider this option if you are sensitive to noise.
8) Do not forget your computer glasses if you need them to read text on the computer.
9) The test-taking room is monitored closely by videotape and microphones.

D. The Night Before the Exam

1) Briefly go over your notes for a quick review.
2) Avoid eating a heavy meal or consuming alcoholic drinks.
3) Get enough sleep. Aim for 7 to 8 hours. Lack of sleep affects memory.
4) Set two alarms to wake you up on time the next morning.

E. The Day of the Exam

1) Avoid a heavy or fatty breakfast. The best meals are a combination of protein with a complex carbohydrate.
2) Do not forget to bring some small hard candy (without the wrappers) with you. You may need to eat some, especially after the second hour of testing.
3) Wear comfortable clothing and dress in layers.
4) Consider limiting the amount of fluid you drink 1 to 2 hours before the test.
5) Do not forget to empty your bladder before starting your exam.

Question Dissection and Analysis

LAB RESULTS AND DIAGNOSTIC TESTS

I. Discussion

The ANCC exam does not list the normal results of laboratory tests in their certification exams. Therefore, it is necessary to memorize some of the normal results of commonly used laboratory tests.

Unfortunately, the normal lab values are shown only once. Therefore, whenever a normal laboratory test result is shown on the AANP exam (i.e., CBC, creatinine, WBC), copy it down in your scratch paper so that you can refer to it again for a future question. Be aware that lab norms may differ slightly, base your "diagnosis" on the norms given to you by the AANP.

Learn the significance of common abnormal lab results and the follow-up tests that are needed in order to evaluate the result further. Be warned that lab results are also used as distractors; the labs may not be necessary to solve the exam question correctly.

II. Example

An elderly male of Mediterranean descent has a routine CBC (complete blood count) done for an annual physical. The following are his lab test results: hemoglobin of 12.5 g/dL, a hematocrit of 38%, and an MCV (mean corpuscular volume) of 72 fL. His PSA (prostate specific antigen) result is 3.2 ng/mL. The urinalysis (UA) shows no leukocytes and a few epithelial cells. Which of the following laboratory tests are indicated next:

a) Serum B12 and folate level and a peripheral smear
b) Complete blood count (CBC) with white cell differential and urinalysis

| Table 2.1 | List of Laboratory Norms |

Complete Blood Count	Reference Ranges
Hemoglobin	
Males	13.5 to 17.5 g/dL
Females	12.0 to 15.5 g/dL
Hematocrit	
Males	41% to 53%
Females	36% to 46%
MCV (size) Mean Corpuscular Volume	80 to 100 fL
Platelet count	150,000 to 400,000/mm^3
Reticulocytes	0.5% to 1.5% of red cells (↑ acute bleeds, starting tx for vitamin deficiencies (iron, B12, folate), acute hemolytic episodes
Total WBC count	4,500 to 11,000/mm^3 (↑ bacterial infections)
Neutrophils (or Segs)	56% to 62% (↑ bacterial infections)
Band forms	3% to 5% (↑ severe bacterial infections) Also called "shift to the left"
Eosinophils	1% to 3% (↑ allergies, some parasites)

c) A peripheral smear and urine for culture and sensitivity

d) Serum iron, serum ferritin, and TIBC (total iron binding capacity)

III. Correct Answer: Option D

d) Serum iron, serum ferritin, and TIBC (total iron binding capacity)

IV. Question Dissection

Best Clues

1) Low hemoglobin and hematocrit indicate anemia (lab result).
2) An MCV of 72 fL is indicative of microcytic anemia (lab result).
3) The ethnic background of the patient (demographics).

Notes

1) You must go through three steps to answer this question correctly:

   1st step: A hemoglobin of less than 13.5g/dL in males (but not in females) is indicative of anemia.

   2nd step: An MCV of 72 fL is indicative of microcytic anemia (norm 80–100 fL).

   3rd step: The work-up is determined by the differential diagnosis for microcytic anemia. These are iron deficiency and alpha/beta thalassemia trait/minor for the exams.

2) In iron-deficiency anemia, the following results are found:
   Low (serum ferritin and serum iron levels)
   Elevated (TIBC/transferrin levels)
3) In alpha or beta thalassemia trait or minor, the following results are found:
   Normal to high (ferritin/iron levels)
   Normal (TIBC/transferrin levels)
4) The gold standard test to diagnose thalassemia (or any anemia with abnormal hemoglobin, such as sickle cell) is the hemoglobin electrophoresis.
5) Ignore the urinalysis and PSA tests (distractors) since they are not necessary to solve the problem.

QUESTIONS ABOUT FOOD

I. Discussion

There are basically three kinds of food-related questions on the exam. You may be asked to pick the foods that have high levels of certain minerals such as sodium, calcium, or magnesium. Other questions about food address food and drug interactions or the types of foods that are contraindicated (or indicated) for a particular disease process.

   Certain foods are recommended for certain diseases (i.e., hypertension, hyperlipidemia) because of their favorable effect. In contrast, certain foods are contraindicated for some conditions because of adverse or dangerous effects.

II. Example

Which of the following foods are known to have high potassium content:

a) Yogurt, banana, red meat
b) Aged cheese, red wine, chocolate
c) Most fruits and vegetables
d) Low-fat ice cream, orange juice, banana

III. Correct Answer: Option C

c) Most fruits and vegetables

IV. Question Dissection

Best Clues
1) First, look at the answer option pairs for inconsistencies in the list of foods.
2) Rule out option D because of low-fat ice cream on the list (dairy).
3) Rule out option A because of yogurt (dairy) and red meat (protein, iron, amino acids).

4) If options A, B, and D are incorrect, then the only one left is option C (most fruits and vegetables are rich in potassium).

Notes
1) If one of the food choices in an answer option is incorrect, rule out this answer option because all of the foods on the list have to be correlated.
2) As this example has shown, foods from different groups are mixed into one answer.
3) The two diseases where a food question might be found are migraine headache and hypertension.

Examples of Food Groups:
1) High sodium content
   Cold cuts, pickles, preserved foods, canned foods, hot dogs, chips, and so forth
2) Calcium
   Low-fat dairy, yogurt, cheeses
3) Potassium
   Most fruits, most vegetables, orange juice, banana
4) Magnesium
   Whole grains, whole wheat bread, some nuts
5) Folate
   Green leafy vegetables (i.e., spinach), liver
6) Unsaturated fats
   Olive oil, canola oil, walnut oil
7) Saturated fats
   Animal fats, coconut oil
8) Iron
   Red meat, black beans, liver
9) Vitamin K
   Green leafy vegetables

Common Disorders Associated With Certain Foods
1) Hypertension
   Avoid high-sodium foods: Cold cuts, pickles, preserved foods, canned foods, hot dogs
   Maintain an adequate intake of calcium, magnesium, and potassium
   Calcium: low fat dairy, yogurt, cheeses
   Magnesium: whole grains, whole wheat bread, some nuts
   Potassium: most fruits, most vegetables, orange juice, banana
2) Migraine headaches
   Avoid chocolate, aged cheese, red wine, MSG (monosodium glutamate)
3) Patient on a monoamine oxidase inhibitor (MAOI) drug (Parnate or Nardil)
   Avoid high-tyramine foods: red wine, aged cheese, chocolate, beer or any fermented foods

4) Anticoagulation therapy (ie: warfaring sodium or Coumadin)
   Avoid foods with high Vitamin K content such as green leafy vegetables

MEDICATIONS

I. Discussion

Questions regarding drugs or pharmacotherapeutic agents are listed in two ways. It is either listed by name (generic and brand) or by the drug classification. Therefore, it is necessary to learn both. When picking a drug to memorize, pick out the most commonly used drugs in the class. These are usually the older versions of the drug.

A good example is the macrolides (drug class). Erythromycin is the oldest and most common form of the drug. It is also seen more often in the exams compared with the newer versions of the drug; azithromycin (Zithromax) and clarithromycin (Biaxin). An important area to study is the drug "safety" issues such as major drug and/or food interactions, contraindications and well-known side effects. In addition, it is helpful to memorize the names of FDA Category X drugs (listed in this section under "notes").

II. Examples

Example A
Using the drug class as the answer option:
   Which of the following classes of drugs is preferred treatment for community-acquired pneumonia in patients below the age of 60 with no comorbidity:

a) Macrolides
b) Beta lactams
c) Cephalosporins
d) Fluoroquinolones

Example B
Which of the following drugs is preferred treatment for community-acquired pneumonia for patients below the age of 60 with no comorbidity:

a) Erythromycin (Ery-Tab) 500 mg po BID for 10 days
b) Amoxicillin (Amoxil) 500 mg po TID for 14 days
c) Cephalexin (Keflex) 500 mg po QID × 12 days
d) Levaquinolone (Levaquin) 500 mg po daily × 7 days

Example C
The following is an example of a question of a common side effect:
   A side effect that may be seen in a patient who is being treated with captoril (Capoten) for hypertension is which of the following:

a) dry cough
b) swollen ankles
c) hyperuricemia
d) hypotension

III. Correct Answers

Example A: Option A
a) Macrolides

Example B: Option A
a) Erythromycin (Ery-tab) 500 mg po BID for 10 days

Example C: Option C
a) dry cough

IV. Question Dissection

Best Clues
1) There are no obvious clues in any of these sample questions.
2) Picking the correct answer for examples A and B is dependent on your knowledge of the American Thoracic Society (ATS) treatment guidelines for community-acquired (CAP) pneumonia (covered in the Chapter 3 Pulmonary review).
3) For example C, picking the answer is based on memorization of a side effect of ACE inhibitors, a drug-induced cough that is not associated with cold-like symptoms such as a runny nose, nasal congestion and sore throat.

Notes
1) The age and lack of co-morbidity in the patient is an important criteria. According to ATS guidelines; the preferred drug class for this group of patients are the macrolides.
2) ACE inhibitors (ie: captoril, lisinopril, etc.) are associated with about a 10% risk of new onset of a drug-induced dry cough. Angiotensin II receptor blockers (ARBs) are associated with a lower risk of cough (ie: losartan, valsartan).
3) Category B antibiotics for pregnant women: penicillins, macrolides (except Biaxin, a category C macrolide), cephalosporins, and sulfas (avoid in the 3rd trimester).
4) For pain in pregnant women, acetaminophen (Tylenol) is the preferred treatment. Avoid NSAIDs in these patients (blocks prostaglandins).

5) Avoid Category D drugs in patients suspected of being pregnant: quinolones, tetracyclines, ARBs, ACE inhibitors, etc.

DESCRIBING A FINDING VERSUS USING THE NAME

I. Discussion

A clinical finding, sign and/or symptom may be described in detail instead of using its name. Be aware of this method when you see a description or clinical finding that you do not recognize.

In the following example, instead of using the common name *clue cell*, it is instead described as "squamous epithelial cells with numerous bacteria on the cells' surface."

II. Example

A 20-year-old female patient who is sexually active complains of a large amount of light gray-colored vaginal discharge with milklike consistency after she had finished a prescription of antibiotics. She denies itch or redness of the external vagina. A microscopy slide reveals squamous epithelial cells with numerous bacteria on the cells' surface. The vaginal pH is at 6.0. Which of the following is most likely:

a) Trichomoniasis
b) Bacterial vaginosis
c) Candidal infection
d) Normal finding

III. Correct Answer: Option B

b) Bacterial vaginosis

IV. Question Dissection

Best Clues
1) The pH is alkaline (pH 6.0). BV is the only vaginal condition with an alkaline pH for the exam.
2) Rule out candida because it is classified as a yeast organism (process of elimination).
3) Rule out trichomonas because it is a protozoan or unicellular organism (process of elimination).

Notes

1) Bacterial vaginosis (BV) is caused by bacterial overgrowth. The exact mechanism for the condition is unknown.

2) BV has an alkaline pH of 6.0 (vagina normally has an acidic pH of 4.0). Since the bacteria inside the vagina does not cause inflammation, BV is known as a vaginosis (not vaginitis) and is not considered a sexually transmitted infection. The sex partner does need treatment.

3) The vaginal discharge in candidal infection is a white color with a thick and curdlike consistency. Candidal infection of the vulvovaginal area causes redness and itching due to irritation and inflammation. Candida yeast is normal flora of the gastrointestinal (GI) tract and in some women's vagina. Frequent vaginal candidal infections may be a sign of immunodeficiency such as HIV infection. It can also be a result of antibiotic treatments.

4) Trichomonas infection (or trichomoniasis) vaginal discharge is copious, bubbly, and green in color. It causes a lot of inflammation resulting in itching and redness of the vulvovagina. It is considered a sexually transmitted infection. The sex partner also needs treatment.

COMORBID CONDITIONS

I. Discussion

Test-takers will find that some of the questions in the exam involve several disease processes presented in one problem. These type of questions are usually written in case scenario format and involve from two or more pre-existing medical conditions (comorbidity) in addition to the primary disease process being presented.

These type of questions contain many pieces of information that need to be analyzed along with distractors. A distractor is simply any type of extraneous information that is included which is not necessary to solve the test question correctly. The following presents an example of a patient with a complicated medical history.

II. Example

A 55-year-old type 2 diabetic Hispanic male presents to the community health clinic for a follow-up visit. The patient's diabetes has been well-controlled with two oral antidiabetic medications and lifestyle changes for the past 7 years. Recently, his blood glucose levels have ranged between 180 to 250 mg/dL over the past few weeks. The patient's chart indicates a long-term history of schizophrenia complicated with depression which is being treated with an oral antipsychotics and flouxetine (Prozac). The urinalysis result is negative for leukocytes, blood, ketones, and ntirites. Which of the following is the best intervention regarding the management of this patient's type 2 diabetes?

a) Discontinue both the oral antidiabetic medications
b) Start the patient on insulin and continue the oral antidiabetic medcations
c) Start the patient on insulin and discontinue both oral antidiabetic medications
d) Discontinue the patient's antipsychotic medication but continue the oral antidiabetic medications and the flouxetine (Prozac)

III. Correct Answer: Option B

b) Start the patient on insulin and continue the oral antidiabetic medications

IV. Question Dissection

Best Clues
1) The patient has been on oral antidiabetics for 7 years. Total pancreatic failure in type 2 diabetics generally occurs about 7 years after diagnosis.
2) The majority of antipsychotic drugs causes weight gain with chronic use.

Notes
1) The combination of weight gain plus total pancreatic failure has exacerbated the patient's type 2 diabetes in this case scenario.
2) Insulin is recommended for type 2 diabetics whose blood glucose levels are not well-controlled by multiple oral antidiabetic medications and lifestyle changes.
3) Since peripheral tissue resistance plays such a large role in type 2 diabetes, oral antidiabetics combined with insulin injections is the best treatment choice.
4) Flouxetine (Prozac) is being used as a distractor. SSRI's have no effect on blood sugar levels.
5) The urinalysis result is normal. It is also used as a distractor in this question.

EMERGENT CASES

I. Discussion

The ability to recognize and initially manage emergent conditions that may present in the primary care arena is a skill that is expected of all nurse practitioners. It is important to memorize not only the presenting signs and symptoms of a given condition, but also its initial management in primary care.

Learn how these conditions present so that you can recognize them in the exam. The following is a list of emergent conditions. They are discussed in detail under each "Danger Signals" section under the appropriate organ system under the Systems Review section in the next chapter (Chapter 3).

Cardiovascular Section
Acute myocardial infarction
Deep vein thrombosis (DVT)
Dermatological Section
Stevens-Johnson syndrome
Meningococcemia
Rocky Mountain spotted fever
Gastrointestinal (GI) Section
Acute abdomen
Acute appendicitis
Acute pancreatitis
Men's Health
Testicular torsion
Prostate cancer
Neurology Section
Cauda equina syndrome
Temporal arteritis headache
Dangerous headache signals
Pulmonary Section
Anaphylaxis
Severe asthmatic exacerbation
Pulmonary emboli
Women's Health
Dominant breast mass
Ruptured tubal ectopic pregnancy

II. Example

During an episodic visit, an asthmatic middle-aged male complains of a sudden onset of itching and coughing after taking two aspirin tablets for a headache in the waiting room. The patient's lips are starting to swell. Which of the following is the best initial intervention to follow:

a) Initiate a prescription of a potent topical steroid and Medrol Dose Pack
b) Ask the patient whether he wants to lie down on an examining table until he feels much better before being examined by the nurse practitioner
c) Give an injection of epinephrine 1:10,000 subcutaneously immediately
d) Administer intramuscular injections of both prednisone and cimetidine (Tagamet) immediately.

III. Correct Answer: Option C

c) Give an injection of epinephrine 1:10,000 subcutaneously immediately

IV. Question Dissection

Best Clues
1) Signs and symptoms are classic for anaphylaxis
2) The quick onset of symptoms after taking aspirin. Severe anaphylactic episodes occur almost immediately or within 1 hour after exposure

Notes
1) Treatment of Anaphylaxis:

   If only one clinician present:
   - Give an injection of epinephrine 1:10,000 stat (immediately) and then call 911.

   If two clinicians are present:
   - One gives the epinephrine and the other clinician calls 911.
2) Emergency room (ER) treatment: intravenous epinephrine; an antihistamine, diphenhydramine (Benadryl); a B2 agonist cimetidine (Tagamet); a short-acting B2 agonist and bronchodilator, albuterol (Ventolin); systemic steroids such as prednisone; and 100% oxygen.
3) Look carefully at the "time factor" involved in this question. A quick onset of symptoms or sudden change in symptoms signals a possible emergent condition.
4) There is a higher risk of aspirin and NSAID allergies among asthmatics.

PRIORITIZING OTHER EMERGENT CASES

I. Discussion

During life-threatening situations, managing the airway, breathing, and circulation (the ABCs) is always the top priority. If the question does not describe conditions requiring the ABCs, then the next level of priority is listed below. One of the most important clues in these type of problems is the acute timing or a recent change from baseline. The mnemonic device to use if the ABCs do not apply is AMPICILLIN.

     A: Acute
    M: Mental status changes
     P: Pain
      I: Infection
CILLIN: No meaning. Makes mnemonic easier to remember.

II. Example

The grandmother of a 17-year-old male presents to a community clinic with the teen. She complains that her grandson fell down on the street during a bicycle ride that morning. She denies that the child lost consciousness. The health history is uneventful. The vital signs are within normal range. Which of the following statements is indicative of an emergent condition:

a) The teen denies syncope and injuries, but seems to be very anxious.
b) The teen complains of a headache, but took acetaminophen (Tylenol) with relief obtained from the headache.
c) Teenagers commonly used acetaminophen (Tylenol) when committing suicide in an attempt to overdose on the medicine.
d) An alert patient who is starting to develop problems following normal conversation and answering questions.

III. Correct Answer: Option D

d) An alert patient who is starting to develop problems following normal conversation and answering questions.

IV. Question Dissection

Best Clues
1) Acute and recent change in the level of conciousness.

Notes
1) Any recent changes in level of consciousness, even one as subtle as difficulty with normal conversation, should ring a bell in your head and remind you of the AMPICILLIN mnemonic.
2) Notice the word *normal* conversation. Do not overread the question and ask yourself what they mean by "normal conversation." Take it at face value.
3) The question is not asking directly about the teen's condition. It is asking about an emergent condition. Do not automatically assume that the stem relates directly to the patient discussed in the case scenario. Therefore, this rules out Option A and Option B.
4) Option C does not indicate an emergent condition.
5) Changes in level of consciousness on the test are usually subtle changes. Words to watch for are difficulty answering questions, slurred speech, seems confused, not understanding instructions/conversation, stuporous, lethargic, combative, and so forth.
6) Acute change can mean from seconds to hours. The most important clue to look for is the change from baseline in the patient's condition.

COMPLEX SENTENCES

I. Discussion

Complex sentences are written with two or more topics in one statement. It is not uncommon for the sentence to contain both negatively and positively oriented points. When answer options are written in this style, it makes them more time-consuming to solve because they are harder to comprehend. Design a note-writing system to use for the exam. Use symbols and abbreviations to save time. For example, if you are not sure of an answer, write down a question mark (?) or a "T" for true or "F" for false.

If you find yourself spending more than 3 minutes on one question, you are wasting time. Answer the question at random and "mark" it. This special command is taught during the computer tutorial and allows you to return to the question and change the answer at a later time in the exam.

There is no penalty for guessing. Never leave any exam question unanswered. If you run out of time and leave blank questions, you can lose points and fail the test. Many students who fail the exam do so by missing as few as from two to three more points.

II. Example

A female elderly patient, who is 92 years of age, has recently been diagnosed with community-acquired bacterial pneumonia. During the follow-up visit, the son reports that the patient seems to be getting better. Which of the following statements about the patient is not indicative of a serious condition?

a) The patient is sleeping more in the daytime, <u>but</u> *is alert when awakened* (negative/positive).
b) The patient developed aphasia 2 days ago (negative) <u>and</u> is also sleeping more and drinking less fluids in the daytime (negative/negative).
c) The patient's appetite is much better, <u>but</u> she has lost 10% of her previous body weight (positive/negative).
d) The patient has become more agitated <u>and</u> confused at night and is sleeping more in the daytime (negative/negative).

III. Correct Answer: Option A

a) The patient is sleeping more in the daytime, <u>but</u> *is alert when awakened.*

IV. Question Dissection

Best Clues
1) The patient's level of conciousness (LOC) is "alert when awakened."

Notes
1) When reading the first half of the question in Option A, note that even though the first half of the sentence is a negative situation (sleeping more), the patient's LOC is normal (alert) when she is awakened.
2) Elderly patients who lose weight are at higher risk of complications and death. An unintentional weight loss of 10% is considered as pathologic in any age group.

3) An elderly patient who becomes agitated and confused at night is experiencing "sundowning." Sundowning is seen in patients who have dementia and delirium.

4) If you have problems with complex sentences, write notes on your scratch paper to help figure it out.

CHOOSING THE BEST INITIAL INTERVENTION

I. Discussion

Numerous questions on the exam will ask test takers about the best initial intervention to perform in a given case scenario. The question may ask you to pick out the best initial evaluation, treatment, or statement to say to a patient.

One of the reasons why some test takers answer these questions incorrectly is because they skip a step in the "SOAPE" process (Subjective, Objective, Assessment, Planning, and Evaluation). The first step of the patient evaluation is to find "subjective" information such as asking about the patient's symptoms or current medications. The next step is to find "objective" information. Start with the low-tech maneuvers. For example, in a case of peripheral vascular disease (PVD), it makes sense to check the pulse and blood pressure first before ordering an expensive test such as a doppler flow study. The following are examples of actions that can be done using the "SOAPE" as a guide.

S: Look for subjective evidence (S)
    1) Interview the patient and/or family member
    2) Ask about the current medications, signs and symptoms, duration of illness, past medical history, diet, lifestyle, and so forth
O: Look for objective evidence (O)
    1) Perform a physical exam (general or targeted)
    2) In general, perform a physical maneuver first (check pulse, if applicable) before ordering laboratory tests or other exams/procedures
A: Diagnosis or Assessment (A)
    1) What is the most likely diagnosis?
    2) Is the condition emergent or not?
P: Treatment Plan (P)
    1) Initiate or prescribe medications
    2) Patient education
    3) Lifestyle recommendations such as diet and exercise
E: Evaluate response to the treatment/intervention or evaluate the situation (E)
    1) Poor or no response to treatment (or worsens), refer out
    2) If emergent, refer to emergency room

II. Example

A 30-year-old woman with a history of mild intermittent asthma complains of a new onset of cough that has been waking her up very early in the morning for the past 2 weeks. She reports a history of a viral upper respiratory infection 1 week before the onset of her current symptoms. Her last office visit was 8 months ago. Which of the following is the best initial course of action:

a) Initiate a prescription of a short-acting B2 agonist
b) Refer the patient for a scratch test
c) Interview the patient and find out more about her symptoms
d) Perform a thorough physical examination

III. Correct Answer: Option C

c) Interview the patient and find out more about her symptoms

IV. Question Dissection

Best Clues
1) Complaint of new signs/symptoms
2) Patient has not been seen for 8 months (needs follow-up)

Notes
The correct order of actions to follow in this case scenario is the following:

1) Interview the patient to find out more about her symptoms (correct answer)
2) Perform a thorough physical examination
3) Initiate a prescription of a short-acting B2 agonist
4) Refer the patient to an allergist for a scratch test (if necessary)
5) The case scenario is describing an asthmatic exacerbation. If it is not treated, it can worsen and may progress into status asthmaticus and respiratory failure, a life-threatening condition.
6) The differential diagnosis for an early morning cough includes postnasal drip, sinusitis, allergic rhinitis, GERD (gastroesophageal reflux disease), and so forth.

QUESTIONS ASKING FOR A DIAGNOSIS

I. Discussion

There are numerous questions asking for the diagnosis. According to recent ANCC data, this area accounts for up to 26% of the total questions in the ANCC family nurse practitioner exam. Test takers who are weak in this area are more likely to fail the certification exam from both the ANCC or the AANP because the area makes up a large number of the questions.

These questions commonly will ask for the diagnosis based on the description of the disease's history along with the signs and/or symptoms. A more complicated question design is to ask you for the correct intervention, laboratory test, or the medication without mentioning the diagnosis. You must first figure out the diagnosis "in your head" in order to answer the question correctly.

Another word of advice is to pick the most specific answer if a question is asking about the most common findings for a certain diagnosis or disease. When reviewing for the exam, learn the unique or the most specific signs/symptoms that is mainly associated with the disease. The following is a good example of this concept.

II. Example

Which of the following is most likely to be found in patients with a long-standing case of iron deficiency anemia:

a) Pica
b) Fatigue
c) Pallor
d) Irritability

III. Correct Answer: Option A

a) Pica

IV. Question Dissection

Best Clues
1) The diagnosis (iron deficiency anemia).
2) Memorization that pica is associated with iron-deficiency anemia.

Notes
1) If you are guessing, use common sense. Fatigue and irritability are found in many conditions, including in healthy persons (i.e., lack of sleep).
2) Using common sense, pallor is also seen in many disorders such as shock, illness, and anemia.
3) By process of elimination, you are left with option A, the correct choice.
4) Pica is also found in pregnancy, but compared with the other options given in this question, it is the best answer choice.
5) Another specific clinical finding in iron-deficiency anemia is spoon-shaped nails (or koilonychia). Do not confuse this finding with pitted nails seen in psoriasis.

HISTORY AND PRESENTATION

I. Discussion

Arriving at the correct diagnosis is dependent upon a good and thorough history. Be alert for the historical findings in the questions on the exam because these are important clues that help point to the correct diagnosis (or differential diagnosis).

Only the classic historical findings are used as described in the major medical and nursing textbooks.

II. Example

A male nursing assistant who works in a nursing home is complaining of multiple pruritic rashes which have been disturbing his sleep at night for the past several weeks. He reports that several members of his family are starting to complain of pruritic rashes. On physical examination, the family nurse practitioner (FNP) notices several excoriated rashes on the axilla, waistline and the penis. They are also present on the interdigital webs of both hands. Which of the following conditions is most likely:

a) Scarlatina
b) Impetigo
c) Erythema migrans
d) Scabies

III. Correct Answer: Option D

d) Scabies

IV. Question Dissection

Best Clues
1) The history (pruritic rashes disturbs sleep at night, several family members with same symptoms, and works in a higher risk area such as nursing homes).
2) Classic clinical finding (pruritic rashes located in the interdigital webs).

Notes
1) Assume that a patient has scabies if excoriated pruritic rashes are located in the fingerwebs and the penis until proven otherwise. Higher risk groups are health care givers or any person working with large populations such as schools, nursing homes, group homes, or prisons.
2) The rash of scarlatina has a sandpaper-like texture and accompanied by a strawberry tongue and skin desquamation (peeling) of the palms and soles. It is not pruritic.
3) Impetigo rashes are pruritic and contagious. They appear as papules, and bullae shich rupture easily becoming superficial bright weeping rashes with honey-colored exudate that becomes crusted as it dries. The rashes are located on areas that are easily traumatized such as the face, arms, or legs. Insect bites, acne lesions, and varicella lesions can become secondarily infected, resulting in impetigo.
4) Erythema migrans rashes are very pruritic, but are shaped like raised wavy lines (serpinginous or snakelike) and are alone or few. It is caused by hookworm

larva moving under the skin. The areas of the body that are exposed directly to contaminated soil or sand, such as the soles of the feet or the buttocks, are common locations. Treatment is with mebendazole (Vermox) applied topically over the rash.

CHOOSING THE CORRECT DRUG

I. Discussion

Test takers are expected to know not only the drug's generic and/or brand name, but also its drug class. If you are only familiar with the drug's brand name or generic form, you will still be able to recognize the drug on the test because both names will be listed.

In addition, the drug's action, indication(s), common side effects, drug interactions, and contraindications are important to learn. Drugs may only be listed as a drug class.

II. Examples

Example A
Which of the following drugs is indicated as first-line treatment for community-acquired atypical pneumonia in patients younger than 60 years of age with no comorbidity:

a) Macrolides
b) Penicillins
c) Fluoroquinolones
d) Sulfas

III. Correct Answer: Option A

a) Macrolides

IV. Question Dissection A

Best Clues
1) The diagnosis (community-acquired atypical pneumonia)
2) The demographic (age younger than 60 years)
3) Lack of a comorbid condition (lacking a risk factor)

Notes
1) Be familiar with the guidelines for community-acquired pneumonia from the American Thoracic Society (ATS). It is listed in Chapter 3 in the Pulmonary section.

2) This is a rote type of question. Answering the question is dependent on your memorization of information.

3) The treatment guidelines used for the exams are listed under the certification exam information section (Chapter 1), and also under the pertinent organ system (Chapter 3).

Example B

A 14-year-old female student complains of pain and fullness in her left ear that is getting steadily worse. She has a history of allergic rhinitis and is allergic to dust mites. On physical exam, the left tympanic membrane is red with cloudy fluid inside. The landmarks are displaced in the same ear. The student denies frequent ear infections, and the last antibiotic she took was 8 months ago for a urinary tract infection. She is allergic to sulfa and tells the nurse practitioner that she will not take any erythromycin because it makes her very nauseated. Which of the following is the best choice of treatment for this patient:

a) Amoxicillin/clavulanic acid (Augmentin) 875 mg one tablet po (by mouth) twice a day for 14 days
b) Pseudoephedrine (Sudafed) 20 mg po as needed every 4 to 6 hours
c) Amoxicillin 500 mg one tablet po three times a day for 14 days
d) Biaxin (clarithromycin) 500 mg po two times a day for 10 days

V. Correct Answer: Option C

c) Amoxicillin 500 mg one tablet po three times a day for 14 days

VI. Question Dissection B

Best Clues

1) Red TM with cloudy fluid inside and displaced landmarks (classic sign of acute otitis media [AOM])
2) Last antibiotic taken was 8 months ago and infrequent ear infections (lack of risk factors for beta-lactamase resistant bacteria)
3) Complaints of erythromycin making her nauseated (rule out Biaxin)

Notes

1) This question is more complicated compared to the first example. Although the question is regarding the correct drug treatment, it also lists the signs/symptoms of the disease. In order to answer this question correctly, you must first arrive at the correct diagnosis, which is AOM.
2) Amoxicillin is the preferred first-line antibiotic for both AOM and acute sinusitis in certain patient populations.

3) The ideal patient is someone who has not been on any antibiotics in the previous 3 months and/or does not live in an area with high rates of beta-lactam resistant bacteria.

4) If the patient is a treatment failure, or was on an antibiotic in the previous 3 months, then a second-line antibiotic such as Augmentin, Ceftin, or Rocephin injection (up to three separate injections) is indicated.

5) Biaxin is a good choice for penicillin-allergic patients, but this patient's adverse reaction of severe nausea to erythromycins is problematic.

6) Pseudoephedrine (Sudafed) is useful for symptoms only. It is not used to eradicate the infecting bacteria. Avoid this drug in patients with hypertension and pheochromocytoma.

DIAGRAMS

I. Discussion

Currently, neither chest x-ray (CXR) films nor electrocardiogram (EKG) strips have been seen on the NP certification exams. The only diagram seen on the test at the moment is one of a chest with the four cardiac auscultory areas (aortic, pulmonic, tricuspid, and mitral) marked. The diagram is used for questions on either cardiac murmurs or the heart sounds.

II. Example

In which of the following areas is the best location to auscultate for the S3 heart sound:

a) Aortic area
b) Pulmonic area
c) Tricuspid area
d) Mitral area

III. Correct Answer: Option B

b) Pulmonic area

IV. Question Dissection

Best Clues
1) There are no clues to this question.

Notes
1) The best place to listen for the S3 heart sound is the pulmonic area.
2) The answer to this question is based on rote memory.

"GOLD STANDARD" TESTS

I. Discussion

Learn to distinguish between a screening test and a diagnostic test (the "gold standard"). Diagnostic tests are more specific and/or sensitive than screening tests. They give objective proof that a disease process or abnormal condition is present. Some examples of diagnostic tests are tissue biopsies, cultures, and CT or MRI scans.

In contrast, screening tests are usually less specific but are more available and cost effective. Some examples of screening tests are the hemoglobin and/or hematocrit (anemia), blood pressure (hypertension), Mantoux test (tuberculosis) and the fasting blood glucose for diabetes.

Although hundreds of laboratory and other diagnostic tests are available, there are still many diseases that do not have any screening tests. This is because the ideal screening test is one that can detect disease at its earliest stages when it is potentially curable.

A good example of a disease with no approved screening test for the general population is ovarian cancer. Although the CEA 125 and pelvic ultrasounds are currently available, they are not sensitive enough to be useful as screening tests. Usually by the time the CEA 125 is elevated, the disease has already metastasized. Another good example is lung cancer. The chest x-ray is currently not recommended as a screening test because it cannot pick up the disease at an early stage.

II. Example

A middle-aged male nurse is having his PPD (purified protein derivative or Mantoux test) result checked. A reddened area of 10.5 millimeters is present. It is smooth and soft and does not appear to be indurated. During the interview, the patient denies fever, cough, and weight loss. He is a nonsmoker. Which of the following is a true statement:

1) The PPD result is negative
2) It is a positive result and a sputum culture and chest x-ray is necessary
3) The PPD should be repeated in 2 weeks
4) Only a chest x-ray is indicated

III. Correct Answer: Option A

a) The PPD result is negative

IV. Question Dissection

Best Clues
1) The test result (PPD result is negative).
2) The patient does not have the signs or symptoms of TB.

Notes

1) Test takers who read too fast or answer the question too rapidly are more likely to make errors with this type of question. When some test takers see the 10.5 millimeter size, they will assume automatically that it is a positive result, especially with the erythema on the site. The induration and not the redness is what counts.

2) When the question is read carefully, you realize that the PPD result is negative because of the description of the soft and smooth skin that is not indurated.

3) The PPD result must be indurated to be valid. Erythema alone is not an important criterion.

4) For pulmonary TB, a sputum culture is the gold standard. Treatment is started with at least three antitubercular drugs because of high rates of resistance. When the sputum culture and sensitivity result is available, the treatment can be narrowed down to the more specific drug(s).

5) TB is a reportable disease.

6) For someone who is less than 35 years of age with a negative CXR who is asymptomatic with no active liver disease or elevation in the LFTs (liver function tests), prophylaxis with INH (isoniazid) is recommended by the CDC (Centers for Disease Control).

7) A baseline LFT level and follow-up testing is recommended for this patients.

ARE TWO NAMES BETTER THAN ONE?

I. Discussion

Some diseases and conditions are known by two different names that are used interchangeably in both the clinical area and literature. Sometimes, the alternate name is the one being used in the exam questions in the exam. This can fool the test taker who is familiar with the disease but only recognizes it under its other name.

II. Examples

1) Degenerative joint disease (DJD) or osteoarthritis
2) Atopic dermatitis or eczema
3) Senile arcus or arcus senilis
4) Purulent otitis media or acute otitis media
5) Group A beta streptococcus or strep pyogenes
6) Tinea corporis or ringworm
7) Enterobiasis or pinworms
8) Vitamin B12 or cobalamin or cyanocobalamin (chemical name)
9) Scarlet fever or scarlatina
10) Otitis externa or swimmer's ear
11) Condyloma acuminata or genital warts
12) Tic douloureux or trigeminal neuralgia

13) Tinea cruris or jock itch
14) Thalassemia minor or thalassemia trait (either alpha or beta; it does not matter)
15) Giant cell arteritis or temporal arteritis headache
16) Asthma or reactive airway disease (infants and children)
17) Psoas sign or ilipsoas muscle sign
18) Tinea capitis or ringworm of the scalp
19) Light reflex or the Hirschsprung test
20) Sentinel nodes or Virchow's nodes
21) PPD or the Mantoux test
22) Erythema migrans or early Lyme's disease

MAJOR DEPRESSION (UNIPOLAR DEPRESSION)

I. Discussion

All depressed patients should be screened for suicidal and/or homicidal ideation. This is true in the clinical arena as well as in the exam. Avoid picking statements that do not directly address the issue or are too generalized.

Incorrect answers are statements that are judgmental, reassuring to the patient, vague, disrespectful, or do not address the issue of suicide (or homicide) in a direct manner.

Risk Factors for Suicide

1) History of previous suicide attempt
2) Acute suicidal ideation
3) Positive family history of suicide
4) Plan to use a gun or other lethal methods (60% of successful suicide deaths due to use of a firearm)
5) Major loss or separations (relational, financial, social, work)
6) History of mental disease
7) Feelings of hopelessness

Although females make more suicide attempts, males have a higher rate of death. Also Whites are more likely to commit suicide compared to other ethnic groups (CDC 2004).

II. Example

A nurse practitioner working in a school health clinic is evaluating a new patient who has been referred to him by a teacher. David is an 18-year-old male with a history of attention deficit disorder (ADD). He complains that his parents are always fighting and he thinks that they are getting divorced. During the interview, he is staring at the floor and avoiding eye contact. He reports that he is having problems falling asleep at night and has stopped seeing friends, including his girlfriend. Which of the following statements is the best choice to ask this teen:

a) "Do you want me to call your parents after we talk?"
b) "Do you have any plans of killing yourself or hurting other people?"
c) "Do you have any close friends?"
d) "Do you want to wait to tell me about your plans until you feel better?"

III. Correct Answer: Option B

b) "Do you have any plans of killing yourself or hurting other people?"

IV. Question Dissection

Best Clues
1) Classic behavioral cues (avoidance eye contact, insomnia, social isolation).
2) Parents getting divorced (risk factor).

Notes
1) Option B is the most specific approach in the evaluation for suicide in this case.
2) Although option C ("Do you have any close friends?") is a question commonly asked of teenagers, it is incorrect because it does not give specific information about suicidal ideation or specific plans of suicide.
3) Always avoid picking answer choices in which an intervention is delayed. The statement "Do you want to wait to tell me about your plans until you feel better?" is a good example. This advice is applicable to all areas of the test.
4) Teenagers are separating from their parents emotionally and value their privacy highly. When interviewing a teen, do it privately (without parents) and with the parent(s) present.

OTHER PSYCHIATRIC DISORDERS

I. Discussion

Other psychiatric disorders such as obsessive compulsive disorder (OCD), anxiety, panic disorder, alcohol addiction, attention deficit hyperactivity disorder (ADHD) or attention deficit disorder (ADD) may be included in the exams. Not all of these disorders are usually seen together in one exam. The most common psychiatric conditions on the exam are major depression, alcohol abuse, and suicide risk. The question may be as straightforward as querying about the correct drug treatment for the condition as illustrated in this example.

II. Example

Which of the following drug classes is indicated as first-line treatment of both major depression and obsessive compulsive disorder (OCD):

a) Selective serotonin reuptake inhibitors (SSRIs)
b) Tricyclic antidepressants (TCAs)
c) Mood stabilizers
d) Benzodiazepines

III. Correct Answer: Option A

a) Selective serotonin reuptake inhibitors (SSRIs)

IV. Question Dissection

Best Clues

1) Rule out benzodiazepines, which are used to treat anxiety or insomnia (process of elimination).
2) Mood stabilizers such as lithium salts are used to treat bipolar disorder (process of elimination).
3) The stem is asking for the "first-line treatment," which are the SSRIs.

Notes

1) Tricyclic antidepressants are now considered second-line treatment for depression.
2) TCAs are also used as prophylactic treatment of migraine headaches, chronic pain, and neuropathic pain (i.e., tingling, burning) such as post-herpetic neuralgia.

   Example of TCA: amitriptyline (Elavil)

3) Ideally, do not give suicidal patients a prescription of TCAs because of increased risk of hoarding the drug and overdosing. Overdose of TCAs can be fatal (development of fatal heart arrhythmias)
4) SSRIs are also first-line treatment for OCD, generalized anxiety disorder (GAD), panic disorder, social anxiety disorder (extreme shyness), and premenstrual mood disorder (fluoxetine or Prozac).

   Examples of SSRIs: fluoxetine (Prozac), sertraline (Zoloft), paroxetine (Paxil)

5) Anticonvulsants such as carbamazepine (Tegretol) are also used for chronic pain.

ABUSIVE SITUATIONS

I. Discussion

Health care workers by law are required to report suspected and actual child abuse to the proper authorities. Abuse-related topics may include domestic violence, physical abuse, child abuse, elderly abuse, and sexual abuse.

II. Example

A 16-year-old teenager with a history of ADHD is brought in to the emergency room by his mother. She does not want her son to be alone in the room. The NP doing the intake notes several burns on the teen's trunk. Some of the burns appear infected. The NP documents the burns as mostly round in shape and about 0.5 cm (centimeter) in size. Which of the following questions is most appropriate to ask the child's mother:

a) "Your son's back looks terrible. What happened to him?"
b) "Does your son have more friends outside of school?"
c) "Did you burn his back with a cigarette?"
d) "Can you please tell me what happened to your son?"

III. Correct Answer: Option D

d) "Can you please tell me what happened to your son?"

IV. Question Dissection

Best Clues
1) Option D is the only open-ended question in the group.
2) In addition, it is not a judgmental statement.

Notes
1) In general, open-ended questions are usually the correct answer in cases where an NP is trying to elicit the history in an interview.
2) "Your son's back looks terrible. What happened to him?" and "Did you burn his back with a cigarette?"
   - Both are considered judgmental questions
   - Judgmental questions are always the wrong choice
   - These types of questions are more likely to make people defensive or hostile
3) "Does your son have more friends outside of school?"
   - This question does not elicit specific information
   - It does not address the immediate issue of the burn marks on the boy's back
4) *Communication Tips*
   Questions on abuse: If a history is being taken, pick the open-ended question
   Questions on depression:

Pick the statement that is the most specific to find out if the patient is suicidal or homicidal

Any answer considered judgmental is wrong

Do not pick answers that "reassure" patients about their issues, because this discourages them from verbalizing more about it

In addition, do not ignore cultural beliefs. Integrate them into the treatment plan if they are not harmful to the health of the patient

THE "CAGE" MNEMONIC

I. Discussion

The CAGE is a screening tool used to screen patients for possible alcohol abuse. Scoring two out of four questions is highly suggestive of alcohol abuse. In the exam, you are expected to use higher level cognitive skills and apply the concepts of CAGE. One example of this concept are questions that ask you to pick the patient who is most likely (or least likely) to abuse alcohol.

CAGE Screening Tool (a score ≥ 2 positive answers is suggestive of alcoholism)

C: Do you feel the need to cut down?
A: Are you annoyed when your friend/spouse's comments about your drinking?
G: Do you feel guilty about your drinking?
E: Do you need to drink early in the morning? (eye-opener)

II. Example

Which of the following individuals is least likely to become an alcohol abuser:

a) A housewife who gets annoyed if her best friend talks to her about her drinking habit
b) A carpenter who drinks one can of beer nightly when playing cards with friends
c) A nurse who feels shaky when she wakes up, which is relieved by drinking wine
d) A college student who tells his friend that he drinks only on weekends but feels that he should be drinking less

III. Correct Answer: Option B

b) A carpenter who drinks one can of beer nightly when playing cards with friends

IV. Question Dissection

Best Clues
1) Lack of risk factor (one drink of beer at night is considered normal consumption).

2) There is no description of any negative effects on the carpenter's daily function, social environment, or mental state.

Notes

Any person who feels compelled to drink (or use drugs) no matter what the consequences are to their health, finances, career, friends, and family is addicted to the substance.

1) "A housewife who gets annoyed if her best friend talks to her about her drinking habit." This is the "A" in CAGE ("Annoyed"). A good example of an alcohol abuser getting annoyed when someone close remarks about her drinking problem.
2) "A nurse who feels shaky when she wakes up, which is relieved by drinking wine." This is the "E" in CAGE ("Eye-opener"). The patient is having withdrawal symptoms and must drink in order to feel better.
3) "A college student who tells his friend that he drinks only on weekends but feels that he should be drinking less." This fits the "C" in CAGE ("Cut down"). This student is aware that he is drinking too much.

"FACTOID" QUESTIONS

I. Discussion

Questions that simply ask for facts are what I call "factoid" questions. Some of my review course students in the past have remarked about these types of questions that "you either know the answer or you don't." Unfortunately, this statement is applicable in these types of questions. The correct answer is either based on your memorization of the facts (rote memory) or from a lucky guess. No reasoning or higher level thinking is required.

II. Example

Which of the following drugs is the latest recommendation as first-line treatment for an uncomplicated case of hypertension by the Joint National Commission on the Evaluation, Management, and Treatment of High Blood Pressure (JNC 7):

a) Angiotensin-converting enzyme (ACE) inhibitors
b) Thiazide diuretics
c) Calcium channel blockers
d) Beta blockers

III. Correct Answer: Option B

b) Thiazide diuretics

IV. Question Dissection

Best Clues
1) There are no clues in the question.

Notes
1) ACE inhibitors are first-line drugs except for patients with comorbidity such as diabetes mellitus (DM). This is the drug of choice for diabetics due to their renal protective properties.
2) Beta blockers are for patients with both hypertension and migraine.
3) Beta blockers are contraindicated in asthmatics or patients with chronic lung diseases such as asthma, chronic obstructive pulmonary disease (COPD), emphysema or chronic bronchitis.

PHYSICAL ASSESSMENT FINDINGS

I. Discussion

Questions about physical exam findings are plentiful. Learn the classic presentation of disease and emergent conditions. The knowledge of normal findings, as well as some variants, will be on the exam. In addition, if the question style used is negatively worded, careful reading is essential.

II. Example

An older woman complains of a new onset of severe pain over her left ear after taking swimming classes for 2 weeks. On physical exam, the right ear canal is red and swollen. Purulent green exudate is seen inside. Which of the following is not a true statement:

a) Pulling on the tragus is painful
b) The tympanic membrane is translucent with intact landmarks
c) Most adults have tinnitus associated with the condition
d) She is at higher risk of acute mastoiditis

III. Correct Answer: Option C

c) Most adults have tinnitus associated with the condition

IV. Question Dissection

Best Clues
1) Positive risk factor (history of swimming).
2) Classic signs (reddened and swollen ear canal with green exudate).

Notes

1) Acute otitis externa is a superficial infection of the skin in the ear canal. It is more common during warm and humid conditions such as swimming and summertime.
2) The most common bacterial pathogen is pseudomonas (bright green pus).
3) Otitis externa does not involve the middle ear nor the tympanic membrane
4) Acute otitis externa does not cause tinnitus (seen in Meniere's disease).
5) Meniere's disease is associated with a triad of: acute vertigo, tinnitus, and hearing loss.

GRADING MURMURS

I. Discussion

Expect at least one question about grading heart murmurs. It is helpful if you have a system for remembering this type of information. This topic is essentially based on memorization skills.

Grading System for Murmurs
Grade I: A very soft murmur that is difficult to hear
Grade II: A soft murmur that is heard more easily than a grade I
Grade III: A loud murmur that is easy to hear
Grade IV: First time a thrill is palpated
Grade V: The murmur can be heard with the stethoscope partly off the chest
Grade VI: The murmur is so loud that it can be heard with the stethoscope off the chest

II. Example

A loud heart murmur that is easily heard when the stethoscope is placed on the chest is which of the following:

a) Grade II
b) Grade III
c) Grade IV
d) Grade V

III. Correct Answer: Option B

b) Grade III

IV. Question Dissection

Best Clues
1) No thrill is present (the murmur is less than a Grade IV).

2) The only answer options left are Grade II or Grade III.
3) The description of an "easily heard" murmur that is not accompanied by a thrill best describes a Grade III murmur.

Notes

1) A good system of remembering heart murmurs is to remember that the first time a thrill is palpable is at Grade IV.
2) Therefore, any murmur that is less than Grade IV has no thrill.

NEGATIVE POLARITY QUESTIONS

I. Discussion

Many test takers have problems solving negatively oriented questions. These questions use negative words (sometimes two) together in the same sentence, which may sometimes be confusing.

One technique that helps in solving these questions is to simply drop the negative word in the sentence and make it into a positive one. If it has two negative words (a double negative), one of the negative words can be dropped; this makes it easier to understand what the question is asking. Examples of some negatively oriented words are *not, except, never, least, false,* and so forth.

II. Examples

Example A

All of the following are *false* statements *except*: (double negative):

To make it easier to understand this sentence (the stem), drop one of the negative words such as *except*. Now, you understand that there are three false statements to avoid. The true statement is the correct answer.

Example B

All of the following are false statements about colonic diverticula except:

a) Diverticulitis is more common in young adults
b) It is associated with chronic low dietary intake of fiber
c) All diverticula are infected with gram-negative bacteria
d) Supplementing with fiber such as psyllium (Metamucil) is not recommended

Drop the second negative term *except*. This makes the question easier to understand.

All of the following are false statements about colonic diverticula except:

a) Diverticulitis is more common in young adults
b) It is associated with chronic low dietary intake of fiber
c) All diverticula are infected with gram-negative bacteria
d) Supplementing with fiber such as psyllium (Metamucil) is never recommended

III. Correct Answer for Both Examples: Option B

b) It is associated with chronic low dietary intake of fiber

IV. Question Dissection

Best Clues
1) Process of elimination.
2) Careful reading of negative polarity words.

Notes
1) Rule out answers that have "all-inclusive" words (i.e., *all*, *not*, *never*), such as seen under option C "*All* diverticuli are . . . " (process of elimination). This narrows your choices down to three options.
2) Supplementing with fiber is never (an all-inclusive word) recommended. This helps to rule out option D. Eliminating patently wrong options helps increase your chances of answering correctly, especially if you are guessing.
3) Diverticulitis are infected diverticula. Diverticula is the name for these abnormal small pouches in the colon. It is asymptomatic except during exacerbations and is treated with fiber supplements such as psyllium (Metamucil), which is taken two to three times a day.
4) Diverticulitis infections can be life-threatening. If the infected diverticula ruptures, it can cause an acute or surgical abdomen

TWO-PART QUESTIONS

I. Discussion

Fortunately, there are usually only one to two questions of this type per exam. These questions are problematic because the two questions are dependent on each other.

To solve both correctly, the test taker must answer the first portion by figuring out the diagnosis in order to solve the second question correctly.

II. Example

Part One
A patient reports of returning home from a camping trip in Massachusetts 2 weeks before without any apparent health problems. Now, the patient complains of a

bad headache for the past 2 days along with high fever and chills. He denies a stiff neck. A rash that started on both his wrist and ankles is starting to spread towards his trunk. Some of the lesions are a dark red to purple color with some which are tender to palpation. Which of the following conditions is most likely:

a) Thrombocytopenia
b) Rocky Mountain spotted fever
c) Idiopathic thrombocytopenic purpura (ITP)
d) Lyme's disease

Part Two
Which of the following is the best treatment plan to follow:

a) Refer the patient to an infectious disease specialist
b) Refer the patient to a hematologist
c) Order a CAT scan of the head
d) Treat the patient with antiviral medication as soon as possible

III. Correct Answers

Part One: Option B
b) Rocky Mountain spotted fever

Part Two: Option A
a) Refer the patient to an infectious disease specialist

IV. Question Dissection

Best Clues

Part One:
1) Positive risk factor (history of a camping trip in a higher-risk area).
2) Classic sign (rash that starts on the wrist and ankles spreading centrally).
3) Clinical finding (rash which is a dark red to purple color).

Part Two:
1) No clues; picking the correct answer depends on correctly answering part one of the question (option B or Rocky Mountain spotted fever).

Notes
1) Rocky Mountain spotted fever (5% mortality)
   Tick bite: spirochete called *Rickettsia rickettsii*
   Treatment: Doxycycline or chloramphenicol
2) Early Lyme's disease (erythema migrans rash stage):
   Ixodes tick (deer tick) bite; spirochete called *Borrelia burgdorferi*
   Treat with doxycycline × 21 days

Majority of the cases are in the Northeast and mid-Atlantic states (i.e., CT, MA, NY, NJ, PA)

3) Thrombocytopenia and ITP:

ITP is an autoimmune disorder. Platelets are broken down by the spleen, causing thrombocytopenia.

NORMAL PHYSICAL EXAM FINDINGS

I. Discussion

A good review of normal physical exam findings and some benign variants is necessary. Pertinent physical exam findings are discussed at the beginning of each organ system review.

A good resource to use in your review is the advanced physical assessment textbook that was used in your program. Keep in mind that sometimes questions about normal physical findings are written as if it is a pathological process. Keep this in mind when you encounter these type of questions.

II. Example

A 13-year-old girl complains of an irregular menstrual cycle. She started menarche 6 months ago. Her last menstrual period was 2 months ago. She denies being sexually active. Her urine pregnancy test is negative. Which of the following would you advise the child's mother:

a) Consult with a pediatric endocrinologist to rule out problems with the hypothalamus, pituitary, and adrenal (HPA) axis

b) Advise the mother that irregular menstrual cycles are common during the first year after menarche

c) Advise the mother that her child is starting menarche early and has precocious puberty

d) Ask the medical assistant to get labs drawn for TSH (thyroid stimulating hormone), FSH (follicle stimulating hormone), and estradiol levels

III. Correct Answer: Option B

b) Advise the mother that irregular menstrual cycles are common during the first year after menarche

IV. Question Dissection

Best Clues

1) Patient recently started menarche 6 months ago (knowledge of pubertal changes).

2) The teen is not sexually active (rule out pertinent negative such as the negative pregnancy test).

Notes
1) This question describes normal growth and development in adolescents.
2) Irregular menstrual cycles are common during the first year after menarche.
3) When girls start menarche, their periods may be very irregular from several months up to 2 years.

ADOLESCENCE

I. Discussion

During this period of life, numerous changes are occurring, both physically and emotionally. Adolescents are thinking in more abstract ways and are psychologically separating from their parents. The opinions of peers are more important than those of the parents. Privacy is a big issue in this age group and should be respected.

II. Example

Which of the following is one of the highest causes of mortality among adolescents in this country:

a) Suicide
b) Smoking
c) Congenital heart disease
d) Illicit drug use

III. Correct Answer: Option A

a) Suicide

IV. Question Dissection

Best Clues
1) Rote memory (suicide is the second cause of mortality among adolescents).

Notes
1) The number one cause of mortality in this age group is motor vehicle accidents.
2) The second most common cause of mortality for this age is death from suicide.
3) Screening for depression in all adolescents is recommended. Signs of a depressed teen include falling grades, acting out, avoiding socializing, moodiness, so forth.
4) Smoking is ruled out because its health effects take decades.

5) Most deaths from congenital heart disease are during infancy. Mortality from illicit drug use is more common among adults.

LEGAL RIGHTS OF MINORS

I. Discussion

Certain legal issues exist in this age group that are not seen in pediatric and adult patients. These are the issues of confidentiality and right to consent without parental involvement.

II. Example

All of the following can be considered as emancipated minors except:

a) A 15-year-old who is married
b) A 14-year-old single mother who has one child
c) A 17-year-old who is enlisted in the U.S. Army
d) A 16-year-old who wants to be treated for dysmenorrhea

III. Correct Answer: Option D

d) A 16-year-old who wants to be treated for dysmenorrhea

IV. Question Dissection

Best Clues
1) This is the only option with a clinical answer (dysmenorrhea)

Notes
1) Emancipated minors: These are kids who are younger than 18 years of age. They have the same legal rights as adults.
2) Emancipated minors can give full consent, sign contracts and other legal documents as an adult would.
3) Criteria for an emancipated minor (United States)
   ■ Any minor who is married
   ■ Any minor who is a parent
   ■ Any minor who is enlisted in the U.S. military

DIFFERENTIAL DIAGNOSIS

I. Discussion

Differential diagnoses are conditions whose presentations share many similarities.

The signs and/or symptoms can be challenging to tell apart clinically. The other similar diseases must be ruled out of the picture in order to avoid mistakes with the diagnosis.

II. Example

A 57-year-old male executive with a history of asthma walks into an urgent care center. The patient complains of an episode of chest pain on his upper sternum, which is relieved after he stops the offending activity. He has had several episodes of the chest pain before. A fasting total lipid profile is ordered. The result reveals total cholesterol of 245 mg/dL, an LDL (low-density lipoprotein) of 165 mg/dL, and an HDL (high-density lipoprotein) of 25 mg/dL. Which of the following is most likely:

a) Acute esophagitis
b) Myocardial infarction (MI)
c) Gastroesophageal reflux disease (GERD)
d) Angina

III. Correct Answer: Option D

d) Angina

IV. Question Dissection

Best Clues
1) Classic presentation (chest pain that is precipitated by exertion and is relieved by rest).
2) History (several episodes of the same chest pain).
3) Positive risk factors (elevated lipid levels, age and male gender).

Notes
All four answer options are some of the differential diagnoses for chest pain. The differences and similarities must be compared for all four options, and the best fit is the correct answer (option D or angina).

1) Aggravated by meals (*angina*, acute esophagitis, MI, GERD)
2) Pain is relieved by rest (*angina*).
3) Pain is not relieved by rest (esophagitis, GERD)
4) Presence of risk factors for heart disease (*angina*, MI)
5) Description of the history, signs and symptoms fits (*angina*)
6) Description of the signs and symptoms does not fit angina
7) Male over age 50 (*angina*, MI)
8) Physical activity aggravates condition (*angina*, MI)

CLASSIC PRESENTATION

I. Discussion

Since certification exams are administered all over the country, the questions are written to conform to the classic "textbook presentation." This allows the test to be valid and statistically sound. All of the questions on the exam are referenced by at least two to three reliable sources. For both exams, a large number of clinical questions are referenced by popular medical textbooks.

The disease process is described in its height, although in real life practice, the signs and/or symptoms are dependent upon the stage of the illness. For example, for the majority of disease processes, usually the prodromal period or the early phase is usually asymptomatic or mildly symptomatic while during the height of the illness, it is usually when the full signs and symptoms are present. Unfortunately, there are many exceptions to this rule such as certain cancers like ovarian cancer, melanoma, lung cancers, etc. Luckily, in the certification exam, almost all of the diseases presented are fully symptomatic.

II. Example

While performing a routine physical exam on a 60-year-old male, the NP palpates a pulsatile mass in the patient's mid-abdominal area. A loud bruit is auscultated over the soft mass. Which of the following conditions is most likely:

a) This clinical finding is considered a normal variant
b) A stool impaction in the lower segment of the colon
c) Aortic abdominal aneurysm
d) Adenocarcinoma of the colon

III. Correct Answer: Option C

c) Aortic abdominal aneurysm

IV. Question Dissection

Best Clues
1) Pulsatile mass located in the middle of the abdomen (classic sign)
2) The presence of a bruit (classic sign)

Notes
1) This question describes the classic case of an aortic abdominal aneurysm (AAA) which is more common in older patients. Mild cases are observed with serial abdominal ultrasounds. Severe cases are fixed surgically. In these patients, it is imperative that the blood pressure is controlled tightly.
2) Stool impaction and colon cancer do not pulsate or have bruits. These masses are harder in texture.

3) Colon cancer screening by colonoscopy is recommended for persons from the age of 50 years or older or in younger patients with risk factors (i.e., positive family history, Crohn's disease).

UNCOMMON DISEASES

I. Discussion

Although this exam is on primary care disorders (both normals and disease), it is possible to be questioned about unusual disorders that sometimes initially present in the primary care area.

II. Example

An elderly Hispanic woman is complaining of a painful swollen area in her left lower leg on the shin area. The NP notes a large, indurated bright red skin lesion that has very distinct edges. It looks like a raised plateau and is warm to touch. The patient's history includes a long drive of 6 hours in the previous day. During the physical exam, the nurse practitioner notes that the Homan's sign is negative. The skin does not have bullae or dark necrotic areas. The circumferences of both calves are equal. Which of the following conditions is most likely:

a) Deep vein thrombosis (DVT)
b) Necrotizing fasciitis
c) Erysipelas
d) Inflamed psoriatic plaque

III. Correct Answer: Option C

c) Erysipelas

IV. Question Dissection

Best Clues
1) Homan's sign is negative and both the legs are equal in circumference (negative findings for DVT).
2) Distinct edges in a plateau-like lesion with no silvery scales (a negative finding for psoriasis).
3) No necrotic areas or bullae present; patient has no systemic symptoms and is not toxic (negative finding for necrotizing fasciitis).

Notes
1) Erysipelas:
   ▪ A subtype of cellulitis where the infection goes deeper down the fascial plane. It can spread to local lymphatic channels (looks like red streaks)
   ▪ Caused by Group A beta strep (gram positive)

57

- Usual locations are the face or the lower leg
- Treatment: Penicillin G injection or penicillin V orally (po) for at least 10 days

2) Deep vein thrombosis (DVT):
   - On the exam, DVT is associated with a positive Homan's sign
   - In real life, Homan's sign is not considered a reliable indicator for DVT
   - The swelling in DVT usually involves the whole limb, not just a localized area

3) Necrotizing fasciitis ("flesh-eating bacteria"):
   - An aggressive and serious infection
   - Early phase: Appears as a round red papule; may have necrosis on the center
   - Patient complains of pain that is out of proportion to the size of the wound
   - During the height of the infection, larger necrotic areas and bullae are seen along with severe systemic symptoms
   - Treatment: Hospitalize; high-dose antibiotics intravenously (IV) and aggressive surgical debridement of the infected tissue

ETHNIC BACKGROUND

I. Discussion

Ethnic background is an important clue for certain genetic disorders. For example, people affected by thalassemia have a background of being either of Mediterranean (i.e., Italians, Greeks, etc.) or of Asian descent (i.e., Chinese). A question on thalassemia minor/trait can include the ethnic background. Sometimes, only labs are given with no information on ethnicity. A warning about ethnic background: It can also be used as a distractor. One's ethnic background in the majority of medical conditions does not usually affect the treatment plan or the patient's response to treatment. The next question is an example of this concept.

II. Example

Which of the following laboratory tests is a sensitive indicator of renal function in people of African descent:

a) Serum blood urea nitrogen (BUN)
b) Serum creatinine
c) Serum albumin
d) Serum BUN-to-creatinine ratio

The question in this example can also be phrased as:
Which of the following laboratory tests is a sensitive indicator of renal function in people of Hispanic or Asian or ___ descent?

III. Correct Answer: Option B

b) Serum creatinine

IV. Question Dissection

Best Clues

1) It is asking for a "sensitive indicator" of renal function.
2) The ethnic background does matter in this question.

Notes

1) Ethnic background has no effect on the creatinine level, but gender, age, certain medications, and preexisting disease do.
2) The other three renal tests are not as specific as the serum creatinine.
3) If results are abnormal, the next step in the work-up is a 24-hour urine collection for protein and creatinine level.

ASKING THE SAME QUESTION TWICE

I. Discussion

A question can be used twice on the exam with some minor variations. It is unknown whether these questions are both valid or are sample questions that are being evaluated statistically. Unfortunately, there is no way to distinguish between the two.

When you see two questions that appear very similar, do not automatically assume that both questions are the same. Slowly read each question so that you are able to pick out the differences between the two. The changes may seem minor, but they can completely change the meaning and answer to the question. In the following example, notice that the diagnosis is different for each question, although most of the wording is similar.

II. Examples

Example A

The nurse practitioner suspects that an older patient who is complaining of a headache in the right temple may have *giant cell arteritis*. A sedimentation rate is ordered. Which of the following is the expected result:

a) Normal
b) Borderline
c) Markedly elevated
d) Below normal

Example B

The nurse practitioner suspects that an older patient who is complaining of a headache in the right temple may have *trigeminal neuralgia*. A sedimentation rate is ordered. Which of the following is the expected result:

a) Normal
b) Borderline
c) Markedly elevated
d) Below normal

III. Correct Answers

Example A: Option C
c) Markedly elevated

Example B: Option A
a) Normal

IV. Question Dissection

Best Clues
1) Notice that the diagnosis in each question is different (careful reading).
2) The type of headache (trigeminal neuralgia vs. temporal arteritis) is the best clue.

Notes
1) When reading these two "similar" questions, the mind automatically assumes that it is the same question used twice. Therefore, the same answer is picked for both.
2) Get out of "autopilot" mode; read and compare both questions carefully.
3) Temporal arteritis is a systemic inflammatory process that primarily affects the medium to large-sized arteries (a vasculitis). It often involves the temporal arteries and if untreated, results in blindness in up to 50%. The screening test: sedimentation rate (markedly elevated). The diagnosis of choice is a temporal artery biopsy.
4) Trigeminal neuralgia is not a systemic illness. Therefore, the sedimentation rate is normal. It is caused by the local irritation, inflammation, or compression of cranial nerve V (CN 5 or the trigeminal nerve).

BENIGN PHYSIOLOGIC VARIANTS

I. Discussion

A benign variant is a physiological abnormality that does not interfere with bodily process or function. There are only very few questions on benign variants. Some examples of the benign variants that have been seen on the exams include the geographic tongue, torus palatinus, and a split or fishtail uvula (listed in

HEENT section). Benign variants are listed on under the appropriate organ system (Chapter 3).

II. Example

A 45-year-old patient complains of a sore throat. Upon examination, the NP notices a bony growth midline at the hard palate of the mouth. The patient denies any changes or pain. It is not red, tender, or swollen. She reports a history of the same growth for many years without any change. Which of the following conditions is most likely:

a) Torus palatinus
b) Geographic tongue
c) Acute glossitis
d) Leukoplakia

III. Correct Answer: Option A

a) Torus palatinus

IV. Question Dissection

Best Clues
1) A good clue is the presence of the growth for many years without any changes.
2) Rule out glossitis, geographic tongue, and hairy leukoplakia because they are all located on the tongue and not on the hard palate (roof of the mouth).

Notes
1) A torus palatinus is a benign growth of bone (an exostoses) located midline on the hard palate and covered with normal oral skin. It is painless and does not interfere with function.
2) A geographic tongue has multiple fissures and irregular smoother areas on its surface that makes it look like a topographic map. The patient may complain of soreness on the tongue after eating or drinking acidic or hot foods.
3) Leukoplakia is not a benign variant. It appears as a slow growing white plaque that has a firm to hard surface that is slightly raised. It is considered a precancerous lesion (i.e., cancer of the tongue) and is due to chronic irritation of the skin on the tongue and inside the cheeks. Its causes include poorly fitting dentures, chewing tobacco (snuff), and using other types of tobacco. If present, refer the patient for a biopsy.
4) Hairy leukoplakia
   Oral hairy leukoplakia (OHL) of the tongue is frequently seen in HIV and AIDs. It is caused by the Epstein-Barr virus (EBV) infection.

ALL QUESTIONS HAVE ENOUGH INFORMATION

I. Discussion Only

Assume that all the questions on the exams contain enough information to answer them correctly. Do not read too much into a question or assume that it is missing some vital information. As far as the ANCC and AANP are concerned, all questions contain enough information to allow you to solve them correctly. Unless it is indicated, consider a patient as in good health unless a disease or other health conditions are mentioned in the test question.

Health Screening and Systems Review 3

UNITED STATES HEALTH STATISTICS

MORTALITY STATISTICS

Leading Cause of Death (all ages/gender)

1) Heart disease

Leading Cause of Death (adolescents)

1) Motor vehicle crashes

CANCER STATISTICS

Leading Cause of Cancer Deaths

1) Lung cancer

Most Common Cause of Cancer Deaths: By Gender Only

Males
1) Lung cancer
2) Prostate cancer

Females
1) Lung cancer
2) Breast cancer

Most Common Skin Cancer

1) Basal cell cancer is the most common of all skin cancers, but melanoma causes 75% deaths from skin cancers.

*Adapted from the CDC (Centers for Disease Control). Retrieved January 10, 2007, from http://www. cdc.gov/cancer/.

SCREENING TESTS

Specificity:
   ▪ These screening tests detect individuals who *do not* have the disease
Sensitivity:
   ▪ These screening test detect individuals who *have the disease*

HEALTH PREVENTION: HEALTH SCREENING RECOMMENDATIONS FROM THE U.S. PREVENTATIVE TASK FORCE

Primary Prevention (prevention of disease/injury)

Immunizations, seatbelts, airbags, bicycle helmets
Habitat for Humanity (shelter)
Education for a healthy population
If preexisting disease: tertiary prevention (i.e., exercise class for diabetics)

Secondary Prevention (detect disease early to minimize bodily damage)

All screening laboratory tests are secondary prevention.

Mammography with Clinical Breast Exam
Baseline mammogram between ages 35 to 40 years.
Age 40 or older: annual mammogram recommended
Higher Risk
   ▪ Older age: >50 (most common risk factor)
   ▪ Previous history breast cancer, first-degree relative breast cancer (mother, sister)
   ▪ Early menarche, late menopause, nulliparity (longer exposure to estrogen)
   ▪ Obesity (adipose tissue can synthesize small amounts of estrogen)

Pap Smears
All Sexually Active Girls and Women
   ▪ Start at any age when sexually active
   ▪ Virgins can start at 21 years of age

▓ Women age 70 years (or older) with 3 or more normal paps in a row and no abnormal pap in the last 10 years can choose to stop having pap smears (American Cancer Society, 2007).

Higher Risk

▓ Multiple sex partners (defined as >4 lifetime partners)

▓ Younger age onset of sex (immature cervix easier to infect)

▓ Immunosuppression and smokers

PSA (prostate specific antigen) with Digital Rectal Exam (DRE)

All males at age 50 except those with higher risk, start younger at age 40

Higher Risk: start at age 40 years

▓ All black males start at age 40 years

▓ If first-degree relative (father or brothers) with prostate cancer

Colon Cancer

Fecal occult blood test (FOBT) and digital rectal exam: start at 40 years of age

Colonoscopy: start at age 50 years (highest risk factor is older age), repeat every 10 years.

Flexible sigmoidoscopy every 5 years

Higher Risk (refer to gastroenterologist/GI)

▓ Screening started at younger ages

▓ History of familial polyposis (multiple polyps on colon)

▓ First-degree relative with colon cancer, Crohn's disease

STD (Sexually Transmitted Disease) Testing

The CDC (Centers for Disease Control) recommends screening all women between the ages of 20 and 24 years for STDs or STIs (sexually transmitted infections).

Higher Risk

▓ Multiple sexual partners

▓ Earlier age onset of sex

▓ New partners (defined as <3 months)

▓ History of STD

▓ Homeless

Tuberculosis (TB)

PPD (purified protein derivative) or Mantoux test

Sputum cultures or chest x-rays: not for screening; they are for diagnosis

Tertiary Prevention (rehabilitate and avoid further bodily damage)

Any type of rehabilitation: cardiac rehab, physical therapy or speech therapy

Support groups (or a group of people meeting to deal with a common problem):
    Alcoholics Anonymous, Al-Anon (for families of alcoholics)

Education for patients with preexisting disease (i.e., diabetics, hypertension): avoidance of drug interactions, proper use of wheelchair or medical equipment, and so forth

Exam Tips

1) Self breast examination is commonly mistaken as primary prevention (it is secondary).
2) Chest x-ray is not a screening test for TB or lung cancer. Screening is not currently recommended for lung cancer because no test can detect it at an early stage.
3) Read questions asking for mortality stats carefully. Is it asking for the most common cause of death overall, or is it asking for it by gender? Most common cancer in males, or overall?

ORGAN SYSTEM REVIEW

DERMATOLOGY

Fast Facts Danger Signals

Actinic Keratosis

Older to elderly adult complains of numerous dry round and red-colored lesions with a rough texture that do not heal. Lesions slow growing. Most common locations are sun-exposed areas such as the cheeks, nose, face, neck, arms, and back. Highest risk if light-colored skin, hair, and/or eyes. A precancerous lesion of squamous cell carcinoma.

Early childhood history of frequent sunburns at higher risk.

Meningococcemia

Sudden onset of sore throat, cough, fever, headache, stiff neck, photophobia, changes in LOC (drowsiness, lethargy to coma). Toxic appearance. Petechial to hemorrhagic rashes (pink to purple-colored) in the axillae, flanks, wrist, and ankles (50% to 80% of cases). Rapid progession in fulminant cases which results in death within 48 hours. Higher risk in college students residing in dormitories (the CDC recommends vaccination for this higher risk group). Spread by aerosol droplets.

Erythema Migrans (early Lyme's disease)

Lesion starts as a small red papule (usually located on the lower leg). Areas of central clearing appear as it grows larger. The lesions starts to resemble a target

(target lesion). Lesions have a rough texture and are red in color (maculopapular) and spontaneously resolves within a few weeks. Most common in the southeastern regions of this country.

Rocky Mountain Spotted Fever (RMSF)

Acute onset of high fever (103 to 105 degrees) and myalgia accompanied by a severe headache, fatigue, myalgia, nausea/vomitting, and rash. By the second to third day, a petechial rash (looks like small spots) appears starting on the wrist and ankles (including soles and palms) that spreads rapidly toward the trunk and the face. Mortality rate up to 25% if untreated. Highest incidence in the southeastern/south central areas of the United States.

Stevens-Johnson Syndrome (SJS)

The classic lesions appears like a two-colored target. Multiple lesions start erupting abruptly and can range from hives, blisters (bullae), petechiae, or other hemorrhagic lesions. Extensive mucosal surface involvement with blistering of the eyes, nose, mouth, esophagus and bronchial tree.

A severe hypersensitivity reaction due to many causes such as medications, viral, bacterial, or fungal infections, and malignancies. The most common drug class associated with SJS are the penicillins, sulfas, and phenytoin (Dilantin). Mortality rate up to 25% to 35%. Also known as erythema multiforme major. Related to toxic epidermal necrolysis.

Shingles Infection of the Trigeminal Nerve (ophthalmic branch)

If herpetic rash seen on tip of nose, assume it is shingles until proven otherwise. Herpetic lesions (small vesicles in groups, ruptures and crusts) follow the ophthalmic branch of the trigeminal nerve and erupt only on one side of forehead, tip of nose. More common in elderly patients. If not treated, can result in corneal blindness.

Melanoma

Dark-colored moles with uneven texture, mixed colors, and irregular borders. May be pruritic. If melanoma is in the nailbeds (ungal melanoma), it may be more aggressive. Lesions can be located anywhere in the body including in the retina. Highest incidence in patients with family history of melanoma.

Fast Facts | Normal Findings

Anatomy of the Skin

Three layers: epidermis, dermis, and the subcutaneous layer
Epidermis: no blood vessels; gets nourishment from the dermis
Epidermis (two layers)

- Topmost layer are keratinized cells (dead squamous epithelial cells)
- Bottom layer is where melanocytes reside and vitamin D synthesis occurs

Dermis: blood vessels, sebaceous glands, and hair follicles
Subcutaneous layer: fat, sweat glands, and hair follicles

Vitamin D Synthesis

People with darker skin require longer periods of sun exposure to produce vitamin D. A deficiency in pregnancy results in infantile rickets (brittle bones, skeletal abnormalities).

Skin Lesion Review

Bulla: elevated superficial blister filled with serous fluid and >1 cm in size

Example: impetigo, second-degree burn with blisters, Stevens-Johnson syndrome lesions

Vesicle: elevated superficial skin lesion <1 cm in diameter and filled with serous fluid

Example: herpetic lesions

Pustule: elevated superficial skin lesion <1 cm in diameter filled with purulent fluid

Example: acne pustules

Macule: flat nonpalpable lesion <1 cm diameter

Example: freckles, lentigenes, small cherry angiomas

Papule: palpable solid lesion up to 0.5 cm

Example: nevi (mole), acne

Plaque: flattened elevated lesions with variable shape that is >1 cm in diameter

Example: psoriatic lesions

Fast Facts | Benign Variants

Seborrheic Keratoses

Soft and round wartlike fleshy growths in the trunk that are located mostly on the back. Lesions on the same person can range in color from light tan to black. Asymptomatic.

Xanthelasma

Raised and yellow-colored soft plaques that are located under the brow, upper and/or lower lids of the eyes in the nasal side. May be a sign of hyperlipidemia if present in persons younger than 40 years of age.

Melasma (mask of pregnancy)

Brown to tan colored stains located on the upper cheeks and forehead in some women who have been or are pregnant or on oral contraceptive pills. More common in darker skinned women. Stains are usually permanent and can lighten over time.

Vitiligo

Hypopigmented patches of skin with irregular shapes. Progressive and can involve large areas. Can be located anywhere on the body. More visible in darker skin.

Cherry Angioma

Benign small and smooth round papules that are a bright cherry red color. The sizes range from 1 to 4 mm. Lesions are due to a nest of malformed arterioles. Asymptomatic.

Lipoma

Soft fatty cystic tumors located in the subcutaneous layer of the skin. Round to oval shape. Can be large in size and located mostly on the neck, trunk, legs, and arms. Painless unless they become too large, are irritated, or rupture.

Nevi (moles)

Round macules to papules (junctional nevi) in colors ranging from light tan to dark brown. Borders may be distinct or slightly irregular.

Xerosis

Inherited skin disorder resulting in extremely dry skin. May involve mucosal surfaces such as the mouth (xerostomia) or the conjunctiva of the eye (xerophthalmia).

Fast Facts | Topical Steroids

1) Avoid steroids if suspected viral etiology because it will worsen the infection.
2) Infants, child, and facial skin (thin skin): do not use fluorinated topical steroids
   - Use 0.5% to 1% hydrocortisone

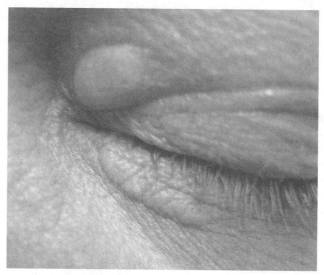

Figure 3.1. Xanthelesma

3) Topical steroids: HPA (hypothalamus, pituitary, adrenal) axis suppression, striae, skin atrophy, telangiectasia, acne, and hypopigmentation.

Fast Facts Disease Review

PSORIASIS

An inherited skin disorder in which squamous epithelial cells undergo rapid mitotic division and abnormal maturation. The rapid turnover of skin produces the classic psoriatic plaque.

Special Findings

Koebner phenomenon: new psoriatic plaques form over areas of skin trauma
Auspitz sign: pinpoint areas of bleeding remain in the skin when a plaque is removed

Classic Case

Complains of pruritic erythematous plaques covered with fine silvery white scales along with pitted fingernails and toenails. The plaques are distributed in the scalp, elbows, knees, sacrum, and in the intergluteal folds. Patients with psoriatic arthritis will complain of painful red, warm, and swollen joints (migratory arthritis) in addition to the skin plaques.

Medications

Topical steroids and tar preparations (psoralen drug class).

Antimetabolites (i.e., methotrexate) are used for severe forms of the disease. Goeckerman regimen (UVB light and tar-derived topicals) may induce remission in severe cases.

Complications

Guttate psoriasis (drop shaped lesions): severe form of psoriasis resulting from a beta-hemolytic streptococcus Group A infection (usually due to strep throat).

ACTINIC KERATOSES

Precancerous precursors to squamous cell carcinoma.

Classic Case

Older to elderly adult complains of numerous dry round and red-colored lesions with a rough texture that do not heal. Lesions slow growing. Most common locations are sun-exposed areas such as the cheeks, nose, face, neck, arms, and back. Highest risk if light-colored skin, hair, and/or eyes. A precancerous lesion of squamous cell carcinoma.

Early childhood history of frequent sunburns at higher risk.

Medications

If only small number of lesions, can be treated with cryotherapy. If larger numbers, fluorouracil cream 5% (5-FU cream), a topical antineoplastic agent, is used over several weeks.

TINEA VERSICOLOR

A superficial skin infection caused by yeasts *Pityrosporum orbiculare* or *Pityrosporum ovale*.

Classic Case

Complains of multiple hypopigmented round macules in the chest, shoulders, and/or back that "appear" after skin becomes tan from sun exposure. Asymptomatic.

Labs

Potassium hydroxide (KOH) slide: hyphae and spores ("spaghetti and meatballs").

Medications

Topical selenium sulfide or ketoconazole (Nizoral) shampoo or cream BID × 2 weeks.

ECZEMA (ATOPIC DERMATITIS)

A chronic inherited skin disorder marked by extremely pruritic rashes that are located in the hands, flexural folds, and the neck (older child to adults). The rashes are exacerbated by stress and environmental factors (i.e., winter). The disorder is associated with atopic disorders such as asthma, allergic rhinitis, and multiple allergies (family history).

Classic Case

Infants up to age 2 years have a larger area of rash distribution compared to teens and adults. The rashes are typically found on the cheeks, entire trunk, knees, and elbows.

Older children and adults have rashes in the hands, neck, antecubital and popliteal space (flexural folds). The classic rash starts as multiple small vesicles that rupture, leaving painful, bright red, weepy lesions. The lesions become lichenified from chronic itching and can persists for months. Fissures form that can be secondarily infected with bacteria.

Medications

Topical steroids, systemic oral antihistamines, skin lubricants (Eucerin, Keri Lotion, baby oil). Avoid drying skin (i.e., hot water baths, harsh detergents, chemicals, wool clothing).

CONTACT DERMATITIS

An inflammatory skin reaction due to contact from an irritating external substance.

Can be a single lesion or generalized rash (i.e., sea-bather's itch). Common offenders are poison ivy (rhus dermatitis), nickel. Onset can occur within minutes to several hours after skin contact.

Classic Case

Acute onset of one to multiple bright red and pruritic rashes that evolve into bullous or vesicular lesions. Easily ruptures, leaving bright red moist areas that are painful. When rash dries, becomes crusted. Very pruritic and gets lichenified from chronic itching. The shape may follow a pattern (i.e., a ring around a finger). Asymmetric distribution.

Medications

Wet compresses for weeping lesions. Topical steroids. Oatmeal baths. Calamine lotion. Generalized severe rash: oral prednisone for 12 to 14 days (wean). Avoid reexposure.

CANDIDIASIS

Superficial skin infection from the yeast *Candida albicans*. Environmental factors promoting overgrowth are increased warmth and humidity and decreased immunity.

Classic Case

Obese adult or women with pendulous breasts complain of bright red and shiny lesions that itch or burn. Usually located in skin fold areas such as under the breast and in the groin area. May have been present from weeks to months.

If oral thrush, complains of a severe sore throat with white adherent plaques with a red base that are hard to dislodge on the pharynx. Thrush in adults may signal immunodeficient condition.

Treatment Plan

1) Nystatin powder in skin folds (intertriginous areas) BID.
2) Nystatin oral suspension for oral thrush.
3) Keep skin dry and aerated.

ACUTE CELLULITIS

An acute skin infection caused by gram-positive bacteria (rarely gram negatives).
   Points of entry are skin breaks, insect bites or abrasions, surgical wounds
Infections range from local superficial infections to more serious or deeper skin
   infections that may be life-threatening
Gram-positive bacteria: *Staphylococcus aureus* and strep pyogenes/beta strep
   group A.
Dog and cat bites: *Pasteurella multicida* (gram negative)

Classic Case

Acute onset of diffused pink to red colored skin on the site and periphery of a wound or skin trauma (i.e., scratch) that becomes indurated, swollen, and tender. Deeper infection of the skin is manifested by red streaks radiating from infected area under the skin.

Labs

Skin culture and sensitivity (C&S)
CBC (complete blood count) if fever

Treatment Plan

1) Dicloxacillin po (orally) TID × 10 days (good choice if high rate of beta-lactam resistance).
2) Cephalexin (Keflex) po × 10 days (not active against beta-lactamase resistant bacteria).
3) Penicillin-allergic: erythromycins (macrolides), cephalosporins, clindamycin.
4) Td booster if last dose was more than 5 years ago.

Complications

1) Osteomyelitis.
2) Tendon and fascial extension.
3) Sepsis.

ERYSIPELAS

A subtype of cellulitis involving deeper tissue involvement caused by beta strep.

Classic Case

Complaints of acne or insect bite that became infected and now appears like a raised indurated plaque with distinct edges. The plaque is a bright pink color and is located on the cheeks (or on the shins of the legs).

BITES: HUMAN AND ANIMAL

Human Bites

The "dirtiest" bite of all. Watch for closed-fist injuries of the hands (may involve joint capsule and tendon damage).

Dog and Cat Bites

Pasteurella multicoda (gram negative). Cat bites higher risk of infection than dog bites.

Bat, Raccoon, or Skunk Bites

Do not forget to rule out rabies infection. Call local public health department for advice.

Treatment (both human and animal bites)

1) Amoxicillin/clavulanic (Augmentin) po × 10 days (penicillin allergy, use clindamycin plus fluoroquinolone).
2) All bites need wound cultures with sensitivity testing (C&S).
3) Do not suture infected wounds of the hand and puncture wounds.
4) Tetanus prophylaxis (if last booster >5 years, needs booster).
5) Certain animal bites (dog, cat, bat, raccoon, skunk) require rabies immune globulin plus rabies vaccine if animal suspected rabid. An option is to quarantine the animal and watch for signs and symptoms of rabies.
6) Follow up patient within 24 to 48 hours after treatment.

HIDRADENITIS SUPPURATIVA

A bacterial infection of the sebaceous glands of the axilla (or groin) by *Staphylococcus aureus* (gram positive) that frequently becomes chronic. Marked by flareups and resolution. Usually both axillae are involved. Chronic episodic infection eventually leaves sinus tracts and heavy scarring.

Classic Case

Patient complains of an acute onset of painful large dark red nodules and papules under one or both axillae that become abscessed. Ruptured lesions drain purulent green-colored discharge. Pain resolves when the abscess drains and heals. History of recurrent episodes on the same areas in the axilla resulting in sinus tracts and multiple scars.

Labs

Culture and sensitivity (C&S) of purulent discharge.

Treatment Plan

1) Amoxicillin/clavulanate (Augmentin) po BID or dicloxacillin TID × 10 days.
2) Muciprocin ointment to lower third of nares and under fingernails BID × 2 weeks.
3) Use antibacterial soap (i.e., Dial), especially on axilla and groin areas.
4) Avoid underarm deodorants during acute phase.

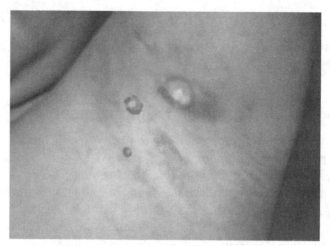

Figure 3.2. Hidradenitis Suppurativa

IMPETIGO

Acute superficial skin infection caused by gram-positive bacteria such as strep pyogenes (beta strep) or *Staphylococcus aureus*. Very contagious and pruritic. More common in warm and humid weather. Two types: bullous and nonbullous forms.

Classic Case

More common in children and teens. Acute onset of itchy pink to red lesions that become bullous, then crusty and maculopapular. The bulla are thin-roofed and easily ruptured.

After rupture, lesions covered with honey-colored crusts (dried serous fluid).

Labs

C&S of crusts/wound.

Treatment Plan

1) Cephalexin (Keflex) QID, dicloxacillin QID × 10 days.
2) PCN allergic: Azithromycin 250 mg × 5 days (macrolides), clindamycin × 10 days.
3) If very few lesions with no bulla, may use topical 2% Mupirocin ointment (bacitracin) × 10 days.
4) Frequent handwashing, shower/bath daily to remove crusts.

MENINGOCOCCEMIA

A serious life-threatening Infection caused by *Neisseria meningitides* (gram-negative diplococci) that are spread by respiratory droplets. Associated with 20% mortality rate.

College students living in dormitories are at higher risk. If treated early, mortality is less than 5%. The bodily damage is due to endotoxin's effects on the endothelium of blood vessels.

Classic Case

Described earlier under "Danger Signals."

Prophylaxis

Close contacts must be given oral antibiotic rifampin
Meningococcal vaccination recommended for all college students living in dormitories

Labs

Lumbar punctures: culture CSF (cerebrospinal fluid)
Blood cultures, throat cultures, etc. CT or MRI of the brain

Treatment Plan

1) Systemic penicillin (PCN) × 10 days; ceftriaxone (Rocephin) × 5 days if penicillin allergic.
2) Hospital; isolation precautions; supportive treatment.

Complications

1) Tissue infarction and necrosis (i.e., gangrene of the toes, foot, fingers, etc.) causing amputation.
2) Death.

EARLY LYME'S DISEASE

Erythema migrans is a skin lesion caused by the bite of an infected *Ixodes* tick with *Borrelia burgdorferi*. If untreated, infection becomes systemic and affects multiple organ systems.

Classic Case

Described earlier under "Danger Signals."

Labs

Serum antibody titers IgM (early) and IgG (late)

Treatment Plan

1) Early Lyme's only: doxycycline BID (twice daily) or tetracycline × 14 days (amoxicillin if pregnant).

Complications

1) Neurological system problems such as Guillain-Barré syndrome.
2) Migratory arthritis, chronic fatigue, and so forth.

ROCKY MOUNTAIN SPOTTED FEVER (RMSF)

Caused by the bite of a tick that is infected with the parasite *Rickettsia rickettsii*. The mortality rate ranges from 1% to 7% if untreated.

Classic Case

Described earlier under "Danger Signals."

Labs

Complete blood count (CBC) with white cell count, liver function test, CSF (cerebrospinal fluid), antibody titers, skin biopsy of lesion.

Medications

Doxycycline BID or tetracycline QID (4 times daily) × 21 days.

Complications

1) Death.

HERPES ZOSTER (SHINGLES)

Reactivation of the varicella zoster virus (or herpes zoster virus). After an initial varicella/chickenpox infection, the virus becomes latent in a dermatome and is kept under control by an intact immune system. The elderly and immunocompromised are at higher risk for shingle breakouts and post-herpetic neuralgia.

Classic Case

Complains of sudden onset of groups of small vesicles on a red base following linear pattern (dermatomal) on one side of the body. If prodrome present, may have been preceded by severe pain or itching or burning sensation on the site of the breakout. The vesicles rupture and become crusty and dry.

Labs

Serum antibody titers IgM and IgG if not sure of diagnosis.

Medications

Acyclovir (Zovirax) five times a day or valacyclovir (Valtrex) BID × 10 days for initial breakouts and 7 days for flare-ups.

Complications

1) Post-herpetic neuralgia: more common on elderly and immunocompromised patients.
2) Treat with tricyclic antidepressants (i.e., low-dose amitriptyline) or anticonvulsants (i.e., Depakote) at HS (bedtime).
3) Infection on CN 5 (trigeminal nerve ophthalmic branch): can result in corneal blindness. Refer immediately to ophthalmologist or ER (described under the "Danger Signals" section).

PITYRIASIS ROSEA

Cause unknown. Self-limiting illness (4 to 5 weeks) and asymptomatic.

Classic Case

Complains of oval rashes with fine scales that follow skin lines (cleavage lines) of the trunk or a "Christmas tree" pattern of papulosquamous rashes.

"Herald rash": first rash to appear and largest in size. Appears 2 weeks before full breakout.

Medications

No medications. Advise patient lesions will take about 4 weeks to resolve
If high-risk sexually active adolescent or adults, check rapid plasma reagin (RPR) to rule out secondary syphilis

SCABIES

An infestation of the skin by the *Sarcoptes scabiei* mite. The female mite burrows under the skin to lay her eggs. Transmitted by close contact.

Classic Case

Complains of pruritic rashes located in the interdigital webs, axillae, buttock folds, waist, and penis. The itching is worse at nighttime and interferes with sleep. Other family members may also have the same symptoms.

Objective

The rash appears as serpinginous (snakelike) or linear burrows. Lesions can be papular, vesicular, or crusted. Higher incidence in crowded conditions (i.e., nursing homes, etc.) and the homeless.

Labs

Scrape burrow or scales with glass slide, use coverslip. Look for mites or eggs.

Medications

Permethrin 5% (Elimite) apply cream entire body and head; wash off at 8 to 14 hours
Must treat entire household. Wash linens and clothes in hot water
Alternative: lindane (Kwell); remove in 8 to 12 hours (contraindicated pregnancy, infants, toddlers, seizure disorder). Out of favor as treatment due to neurotoxicity

TINEA INFECTIONS (DERMATOPHYTOSES)

An infection of superficial keratinized tissue (skin, hair, nails) by tinea yeast organisms.

Labs

KOH slide of scales, hair, nails (look for hyphae and spores)
Fungal cultures of scales, hair, and/or nails

Medications

Topical azoles: OTC (over the counter) clotrimazole, miconazole. Terconazole (Terazol) is a prescription topical antifungal

| Table 3.1 | Common Skin Rashes |

Disease	Description
Impetigo	"Honey-colored" crusts. Fragile bullae
Measles	Koplik's spot. Pink morbilliform rash
Scabies	Very pruritic especially at night Serpenginous rash Interdigital webs, waist, axilla, penis
Scarlet Fever	"Sandpaper" rash with sore throat (strep throat)
Tinea Versicolor	Hypopigmented round to oval shape macular rashes Located on the upper shoulders and the back Not pruritic
Pityriasis Rosea	"Christmas tree" pattern rash (rash on cleavage lines) "Herald lesion" largest rash, appears initially
Molluscum Contagiosum	Smooth papules 5-mm size that are dome-shaped with central umbilication with a white "plug"
Erythema Migrans	Red maculopapular target-like lesions that grow in size Some central clearing. Early stage of Lyme disease
Meningococcemia	*Purple-colored to dark red painful skin lesions all over body. Reportable disease Rifampin prophylaxis close contacts*
Rocky Mountain Spotted Fever Rickettsia ricketsii From Tick Bite	*Round red rashes with petechiae, maculopapular Headache. Fever. Myalgias. Reportable disease*

Note. Rashes in italics are life-threatening

Systemic oral antifungals: ketoconazole, fluconazole (Diflucan) weekly for 6 months (pulse therapy). Antifungals have numerous drug interactions (warfarin, anticonvulsants, etc). Hepatotoxic. Baseline liver function tests. Avoid hepatotoxic substances (alcohol, statins)

Tinea Capitis (scalp)

More common in black children. Patchy alopecia with "black dots" (broken hair shaft) and fragile hair shaft. Fine scales on scalp.

Medications
Treat only with oral antifungals such as griseofulvin (Fulvicin) × several weeks.

Complications
1) Kerion: inflammatory and indurated lesions that permanently damage hair follicles causing patchy alopecia.

Tinea Pedis (athlete's foot)

Two types: scaly and dry form or moist type (strong odor). Moist lesions between toe webs which are white-colored with strong unpleasant odor. Dry type with fine scales only.

Tinea Corporis or Tinea Circinata (ringworm of the body)

Ringlike pruritic rashes with a collarette of fine scales that slowly enlarges with some central clearing. Large numbers or severe cases can also be treated with oral antifungals.

Tinea Cruris ("jock itch")

Perineal and groin area with pruritic red rashes with fine scales. May be mistaken for candidal infection (bright red rashes with satellite lesions) or intertrigo (bright red diffused rash due to bacterial infection).

Tinea Manuum (hands)

Pruritic round rashes with fine scales on the hands. Usually infected from chronic scratching of foot that is also infected with tinea (athlete's foot).

Tinea Barbae (beard area)

Beard area affected. Scaling with pruritic red rashes.

Onychomycosis (nails)

Nail becomes yellowed, thickened, and opaque with debris. Nail may separate from nailbed (onycholysis). Great toe is the most common location.

Labs
Fungal cultures.

Medications
Oral itraconazole or terbinafine (Lamisil) × several weeks
Mild cases: Penlac nail lacquer × several weeks. Works best in mild cases of the fingernails

ACNE VULGARIS (COMMON ACNE)

Inflammation and infection of the sebaceous glands. Multifactorial cause such as high androgen levels, bacterial infection, and genetic influences. Found mostly on the face, shoulders, chest, and back. Highest incidence in puberty and adolescence.

Mild Acne

Open comedones (blackheads), closed comedones with small papules. Treat using topicals only. Benzoyl peroxide, erythromycin solution, retinoic acid (Retin-A) gel or cream.

Retin-A: photosensitivity reaction possible (use sunscreen)

Moderate Acne

As for mild acne plus large numbers of papules and pustules. Treat with topicals plus oral tetracycline (category D) or minocycline (Minocin).

Tetracyclines: permanent discoloration of growing tooth enamel. Do not use if younger than age 18. Tetracycline decreases effectiveness of oral contraceptives (use additional method).

Severe Cystic Acne

All of the preceding findings plus painful indurated nodules and cysts over face, shoulders, chest.

Medications

Isotretinoin (Accutane) is a category X (extremely teratogenic). Need to sign special consent forms. Females must use two forms of reliable contraception and show two negative pregnancy tests before starting drug. Prescribe 1-month supply only. Monthly pregnancy testing and show results to pharmacist before refills. Pregnancy test 1 month after discontinued. Discontinue if the following are present:

- Severe depression, visual disturbance, hearing loss, tinnitus, GI pain, rectal bleeding, uncontrolled hypertriglyceremia, pancreatitis, hepatitis

ROSACEA (ACNE ROSACEA)

Cause is unknown.

Classic Case

Light-skinned adult to older patient with Celtic background (i.e., Irish, Scottish, English) complains of chronic and small acnelike papules and pustules around the nose, mouth, and chin. Patient blushes easily. Patient usually is blond to red haired and has blue eyes.

Medications

Metronidazole gel and/or oral tetracycline for several months.

Complications

1) Rhinophyma: hyperplasia of tissue at the tip of the nose from chronic severe disease.

BURNS

First Degree (superficial thickness)

Erythema only (no blisters). Painful. Cleanse with mild soap and water (or saline) Cold packs for 24 to 48 hours. Topical OTC anesthetics such as benzocaine if desired.

Second Degree (partial thickness)

Red-colored skin with superficial blisters (bullae). Painful. Use water with mild soap or normal saline to clean broken skin (not hydrogen peroxide or full-strength Betadine). Do not rupture blisters. Treat with silver sulfadiazine cream (Silvadene) and apply dressings.

Third Degree (full thickness)

Initial assessment: Rule out airway and breathing compromise. Smoke inhalation injury is a medical emergency. Painless. Entire skin layer, subcutaneous area and soft tissue fascia may be destroyed.

Refer: facial burns, electrical burns, third-degree burns, cartilaginous areas such as the nose and ears (cartilage will not regenerate). Burns greater than 10% of body.

SMALLPOX (VARIOLA VIRUS)

Infects respiratory and oropharyngeal mucosal surfaces. Eliminated in 1977? Incubation period: 2 weeks

Classic Case

Fever, headaches, photophobia, myalgia, and fatigue. Characteristic rash is large nodules that appear mostly in the central area of the face, arms, and legs. Treatment is symptomatic. Mortality rate (variola major) is from 20% to 50%.

Treatment Plan

If vaccine given within 3 to 4 days post exposure, can lessen severity of illness
Vaccinia immune globulin available (pregnant, immunosuppressed, etc.)

DERMATOLOGY EXAM TIPS

1) Differentiate between contact dermatitis and atopic dermatitis. The best clue is the unilateral location and the shape of the lesions in contact dermatitis.
2) Rashes that are very pruritic at night and located on the interdigital webs and/or penis are scabies until proven otherwise.
3) The dirtiest bite wound is the human bite.
4) If allergic to penicillin, may also be allergic to cephalosporins (cross-reactivity of 10%). Instead, use macrolides such as azithromycin (Zithromax) or erythromycin.
5) Do not confuse actinic keratosis (precursor to squamous cell cancer) with seborrheic keratoses (benign).
6) Learn definition of bullae.
7) Diagnosing hidradenitis suppurativa, psoriasis, Rocky Mountain spotted fever, meningococcemia, Stevens-Johnson, contact dermatitis, rosacea.
8) Instead of silvery scales, may see "covered with fine scales" with psoriasis.
9) Psoralens (tar-derived topicals) used to treat psoriasis, antimetabolite (methotrexate).
10) Working in oily environments (i.e., fast food cook) does not cause acne.
11) Mild acne is treated only with topicals.
12) Accutane in females: use two forms of reliable birth control, and so forth.
13) "Herald patch" or a "Christmas tree pattern" is found in pityriasis rosea.
14) Post-herpetic neuralgia prophylaxis: tricyclic antidepressants (TCA) amitriptyline (Elavil).
15) A clue in a case scenario on cellulitis may be of a patient walking barefoot.
16) If beta strep. Group B infection in cellulitis, also at risk for developing post-glomerular nephritis as seen in strep throat. Treat for 10 days with a penicillin or macrolide.

CLINICAL TIPS

1) Use ophthalmic grade/sterile cream/ointments for rashes near the eyes.
2) Pruritis may persist up to 2 weeks even after successful treatment of scabies.
3) Human and cat bites are more likely to become infected compared with dog bites.
4) On thin skin such as the facial and intertriginous areas (skin folds), use low-potency topical steroids (i.e., hydrocortisone 1%). On thicker skin such as the scalp, back, or soles, may use higher potency steroids.
5) Elavil is very sedating; give at HS (bedtime).
6) Antivirals are most effective (i.e., Zovirax) if given within 72 hours after onset.

ENDOCRINE SYSTEM

Fast Facts | Danger Signals

Severe Hypoglycemia

Blood glucose is <50 mg/dL. Complains of weakness, "feel like passing out," headache, clammy hands, and anxiety. Difficulty in concentration and thinking. If severe hypoglycemia is uncorrected, it will progress to coma.

Type 1 Diabetes Mellitus

School-aged child with recent history of viral illness complains of excessive hunger and thirst. Urinating more than normal (polyuria). Starts losing weight despite eating a large amount of food. Breath has a "fruity" odor. Large amount of ketones in urine.

Thyroid Cancer

A single large nodule (>2.5 cm) on one lobe of the thyroid gland, size >2.5 cm. Positive family history of thyroid cancer. History of facial, neck, or chest radiation therapy.

Pheochromocytoma

Random episodes of severe hypertension (systolic >200 mm Hg or diastolic > 110 mm Hg) associated with abrupt onset of severe headache, tachycardia, and anxiety. Episodes resolve spontaneously, but occur at random. In between the attacks, patient's vital signs are normal.

Hyperprolactinemia

Can be a sign of a pituitary adenoma. Slow onset. When tumor is large enough to cause a mass effect, the patient will complain of headaches.

Fast Facts | Normal Findings

1) The endocrine system works in a "negative feedback" system. If a low level of "active" hormone occurs, it stimulates production. Inversely, high levels of hormones stop production.
2) The hypothalamus stimulates the anterior pituitary gland into producing the "stimulating hormones" (such as FSH).
3) These "stimulating hormones" tell the target organs (ovaries, thyroid, etc.) to produce "active" hormones (estrogen, thyroid hormone, etc.).

4) High levels of these "active" hormones work in reverse. The hypothalamus directs the anterior pituitary into stopping production of the stimulating hormones (TSH, LH, FSH, etc).

ENDOCRINE GLANDS

Hypothalamus ("Master Gland")

Directs the anterior pituitary gland. Directly produces oxytocin, the hormone responsible for uterine stimulation in labor and milk production.

Pituitary Gland

Located at the sella turcica (base of the brain). Stimulated by the hypothalamus into producing the "stimulating hormones" that turn on the "switch" of the target organs (i.e., ovaries, etc.). The target organ then synthesizes the active hormones (i.e., estrogen).

Anterior Pituitary Gland

Produces hormones that regulate the target organs (ovary, thyroid, etc.).

1) FSH (follicle-stimulating hormone)
   - Stimulates the ovaries enabling growth of follicles (or eggs)
   - Production of estrogen
2) LH (luteinizing hormone)
   - Stimulates the ovaries to ovulate
   - Production of progesterone (by corpus lutea)
3) TSH (thyroid stimulating hormone)
   - Stimulates thyroid gland
   - Production of thyroid hormone
4) Growth hormone
   - Stimulates somatic growth of body
5) ACTH (adrenocorticotropin hormone)
   - Stimulates the adrenal glands (two portions of gland—medulla and cortex)
   - Production of glucocorticoids

Posterior Pituitary Gland

Vasopressin (antidiuretic hormone or ADH) and oxytocin are made by the hypothalamus but stored and secreted by the posterior pituitary.

Parathyroid Gland

Located behind the thyroid gland and produces antidiuretic hormone.

| Table 3.2 | Endocrine System |

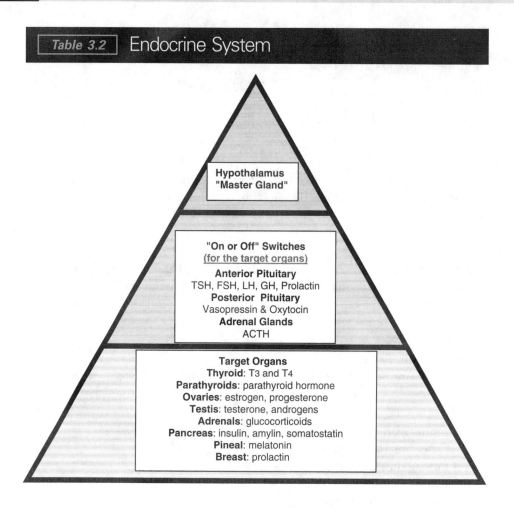

Hypothalamus
"Master Gland"

"On or Off" Switches
(for the target organs)
Anterior Pituitary
TSH, FSH, LH, GH, Prolactin
Posterior Pituitary
Vasopressin & Oxytocin
Adrenal Glands
ACTH

Target Organs
Thyroid: T3 and T4
Parathyroids: parathyroid hormone
Ovaries: estrogen, progesterone
Testis: testerone, androgens
Adrenals: glucocorticoids
Pancreas: insulin, amylin, somatostatin
Pineal: melatonin
Breast: prolactin

| Fast Facts | Disease Review |

TSH (thyroid stimulating hormone)

The best screening test for both hypothyroid and hyperthyroid disease.

- Used to monitor response to thyroid replacement therapy
- Used to monitor response to treatment for hyperthyroid disease

Hyperthyroid

Elevated free T4 and low TSH can detect majority of hyperthyroid cases. If positve results, order thyroid uptake scan. If nodules present, order ultrasound and refer to specialist.

GRAVES DISEASE

An autoimmune disorder causing hyperfunction and production of excess thyroid hormones (T3 and T4). It is the most common cause of hyperthyroidism in this country (60% to 80%). Higher incidence in women (8:1 ratio). These women are also at higher risk for other autoimmune diseases such as rheumatoid arthritis, pernicious anemia, lupus.

Classic Case

Middle-aged female loses a large amount of weight rapidly, becomes irritable, anxious and hyperactive. Insomnia with more frequent bowel movements (looser stools). Amenorrhea and heat intolerance. Enlarged thyroid (goiter) present.

Objective

Goiter: diffusely enlarged gland without nodules
Hands/fingers: fine tremors, sweaty palms
Cardiac: tachycardia
Eyes: exophthalmos in later sases

Labs

Suppressed TSH, increased free T4 (free T4 better measure than total T4).

Medications

Propylthiouracil (PTU): shrinks thyroid gland/decreases hormone production
Methimazole (Tapazole): shrinks thyroid gland/decreases hormone production

Adjunctive Treatment

Given before thyroid under control to ameliorate symptoms such as hyperstimulation (i.e., anxiety, tachycardia, palpitations), which is treated with beta-blocker propranolol (Inderal)

Radioactive Iodine

Permanent destruction of thyroid gland results in hypothyroidism for life. These patients need thyroid supplementation for life after thyroid is destroyed.

Pregnancy: Hyperthyroidism

PTU is preferred treatment. Give lowest effective dose possible.

Exam Tips

1) Radioactive iodine treatment results in hypothyroidism for life. Supplemented with thyroid hormone (i.e., Synthroid) for life.

2) PTU preferred for pregnant women.
3) Thyroid cancer risk factors (history neck irradiation in childhood or a painless nodule larger than 2.5 cm).
4) Chronic amenorrhea and hypermetabolism from hypothyroidism may result in osteoporosis. Supplement: calcium with vitamin D, Fosamax, weight-bearing exercises.

Thyroid Gland Tests

Thyroid gland ultrasounds: used to detect: goiter (generalized enlargement of gland), multinodular goiter, single nodule, and solid versus cystic masses
Thyroid cancer: single painless nodule >2.5 cm, history of neck irradiation in childhood
Thyroid scan: shows metabolic activity of thyroid gland
Cold spot: not metabolically active (more worrisome; rule out thyroid cancer)
Hot spot: metabolically active nodule and usually benign

DIABETES MELLITUS

A metabolic disorder affecting the body's metabolism of carbohydrates and fat.

Type 1 Diabetes

An autoimmune reaction stimulated by a viral infection. Massive destruction of beta cells in the islets of Langerhans (pancreas) causes abrupt cessation of insulin production. Results in ketoacidosis if uncorrected because of the breakdown of fatty stores that the body uses for fuel. If uncontrolled, ketosis will progress into coma or DKA (diabetic ketotic acidosis). Most patients are juveniles; occasionally adults (MODY or maturity onset diabetes of the young).

Type 2 Diabetes

Markedly decreased secretion with peripheral insulin resistance resulting in a chronic state of hyperglycemia and hyperinsulinemia. Results in microvascular (retinopathy, nephropathy) as well as macrovascular (acute MI, strokes, atherosclerosis or plaques on blood vessels) damage.

Target organs: the eyes, heart, vascular system, kidneys, and peripheral nerves, especially in the feet. Diabetes is the most common reason for chronic renal failure requiring dialysis and lower limb amputations in the United States.

Type 2 Diabetes Mellitus (85% to 90% of U.S. cases)

Stronger genetic component compared to type 1 diabetes. Usually presents at age 40 or older (may appear at younger ages)
Usually overweight or obese (BMI 30 or greater)
Hispanic, African American, Asian, or American Indian or positive family history

Metabolic syndrome (insulin resistance syndrome) present
  ■ Defined as obese patient with hypertension, hyperglycemia, and dyslipidemia

Diabetes Mellitus: Three Ways to Diagnose

Symptoms of diabetes (polyuria, polydipsia, polyphagia) plus random blood
  glucose >200 mg/dL
OR
Fasting blood glucose ≥ 126 mg/dL on two separate occasions
OR
2-hour blood glucose ≥ 200 mg/dL during an OGTT (oral glucose tolerance test)
  with a 75 g glucose load

Glycemic Parameters
Fasting blood glucose: less than 126 mg/dL
Postprandial (2 hours after large meal): less than 200 mg/dL

Impaired Glucose Tolerance
A fasting blood glucose between 110 mg/dL and 126 mg/dL. These patients are
considered at higher risk for type 2 diabetes. Another name for this condition is
prediabetes.

Labs

Hemoglobin A1c (HgbA1c): the average blood glucose levels over previous 3
months. No fasting required. Excess glucose attaches to the hemoglobin of the
red blood cells.
  Normal value for glycated Hgb or Hgb A1c: 4% to 6%.

1) Goal of treatment:
   ■ HgbA1c of 6% or less
2) Newly diagnosed diabetics: check HgbA1c every 3 months until blood glucose
   controlled.
3) Lipid profile at least once a year (or more if elevated).
4) Urinalysis once a year. If urinalysis is normal:
   ■ Check urine for microalbuminuria
   ■ If positive, order 24-hour urine for protein and creatinine
5) Other: electrolytes (potassium, magnesium, sodium), liver function panel,
   TSH.

Treatment Plan

Every visit: check BP, weight, blood sugar diary
Check feet at every visit (5.07 U monofilament tool)
    ■ Check for vibration sense, light and deep touch, numbness

Recommendations: Preventive Care

1) Flu shot every year.
2) Aspirin 81 mg per day.
3) Pneumovax vaccine age 60 (or earlier if in high-risk category).
4) Ophthalmologist: yearly dilated eye exam.
5) Podiatrist: once to twice a year especially with older diabetics.
6) BP: 130/80 mm Hg.

Diabetic Issues

Hypoglycemia

High risk: 50 mg/dL or less

Look for: sweaty palms, tiredness, dizziness, rapid pulse, strange behavior, confusion, and weakness. Final result is syncope if not treated with glucose. Be aware that for patients who are on beta blockers, the hypoglycemic response can be blunted or blocked.

Treatment: hard candy, 4 oz. orange juice, regular soft drink, glucose tabs/gel.

Type 1 diabetics—also can use glucagon injections

During Illness

1) Keep taking insulin or oral meds as scheduled unless FBG lower than normal.
2) Eat small amounts of food every 3 to 4 hours to keep FBG as normal as possible.
3) Check urine for ketones. If levels moderate to high—call healthcare giver.
4) Drink fluids. If dehydrated, call healthcare giver (cracked lips,etc.)
5) Contact healthcare giver if: blood glucose >300 mg/ldL, urine ketones moderate to high, feel sleepier than normal or cannot think clearly, unable to keep fluids down, diarrhea > 6 hrs.

Exercise

1) Increases glucose utilization and promotes weight loss. Some patients may have to reduce their usual dose of medicine or eat snacks before the activity and afterward.
2) If patient does not compensate for the increased glucose utilization from exercising such as reducing the dose of insulin or increasing caloric intake, there is a higher risk of hypoglycemic episodes.

   Example: if patient exercises in the afternoon, higher risk of hypoglycemia at night/bedtime if doesn't compensate by eating snacks or lowering insulin dose.

Snacks for Exercise

■ Simple carbohydrates (candy, juices) before or during exercise
■ Complex carbohydrates (granola bars) after exercise (avoids post exercise hypoglycemia)

3) Older diabetics: stress EKG. Rule out preexisting CHD before starting.

Diabetes Mellitus: Specific Eye Findings

- Microaneurysms due to neovascularization
- Neovascularization (growth of fragile small arterioles in retina rupture easily, causing bleeding and scarring on the retina)

Diabetic Foot Care

Patients with peripheral neuropathy should avoid excessive running or walking to minimize the risk of foot injury.

1) Never go barefoot.
2) Wear shoes that fit properly.
3) Check feet daily, especially the soles of the feet (use mirror).
4) Trim nails squarely (not rounded) to prevent ingrown toenails.
5) Report redness, skin breakdown, or trauma to health care giver immediately (main cause of lower leg amputations in the United States).

Antidiabetic Agents

Thiazolidinediones
Rosiglitazone (Avandia), pioglitazone (Actos)
Reduces peripheral tissue resistance and reduces hepatic glucagon production (gluconeogenesis). Take daily at breakfast with a meal.
Contraindication:
- History of moderate to severe CHF due to medication's effect of water retention and edema (aggravates or will precipitate heart failure)

Labs

1) Monitor LFTs (liver function studies). Check baseline, then periodically thereafter.
2) Discontinue if liver functions tests elevated >3 times the upper limit of normal AST and ALT, muscle soreness, or jaundiced.

Sulfonylureas
First generation: chlorpropamide (Diabenase) daily or BID
- Longer half-life with higher risk of hypoglycemia.
- Avoid in elderly or patients with history of hypoglycemic episodes.
Second generation: glyburide (Diabeta) daily to BID, glipizide (Glucotrol XL) daily
Stimulates the pancreas to secrete more insulin. Take at least 30 minutes before meals
Contraindication:
- Ketoacidosis

Adverse reactions: hypoglycemia, photosensitivity, GI symptoms, other

Biguanides

Metformin (Glucophage)

Decreases gluconeogenesis and decreases peripheral insulin resistance. Very rarely may cause hypoglycemia. Preferred for obese patients (can cause weight loss)

Contraindications:

■ Renal disease, acidosis, alcoholics, renal insufficiency, hypoxia

Increased risk lactic acidosis (pH < 7.25):

■ During hypoxia, hypoperfusion, renal insufficiency

IV contrast dye testing: hold metformin on day of procedure and 48 hours after. Check baseline creatinine and recheck after procedure. Serum creatinine must be normalized before drug can be resumed.

Acarbose (Precose)

Inhibits the enzyme alpha-glucosidase in the small intestine, which reduces carbohydrate absorption. Does not cause hypoglycemia

Side effects:

■ Commonly GI effects such as bloating, flatulence, abdominal cramping, and pain

■ Common reason for noncompliance. Start patient on a low dose and titrate up slowly

Repaglinide (Prandin)

A nonsulfonylurea drug. Rapid-acting with a very short half-life (<1 hour)

Indicated for type 2 diabetics with postprandial hyperglycemia

■ Defined as a blood sugar of >200 mg/dL 2 hours after a meal

Take before meals or up to 30 minutes after a meal. Because of its extremely short half-life, it is useful for treating the elderly and in patients with renal disease. Metabolized in liver

Exam Tips

1) Do not use any oral antidiabetic drugs on Type 1 diabetics.
2) Memorize the specific eye findings of diabetes versus hypertension.
3) Moderate to severe heart disease or heart failure is a contraindication because it causes water retention, which may precipitate CHF.
4) Mild type 2 diabetics do not need drug therapy if able to control blood glucose by diet and exercise alone.

Diabetes Mellitus: Management

1) Lifestyle changes are first-line treatment along with oral antidiabetics.
2) Weight loss improves metabolic control in type 2 diabetics.
3) Exercise increases cellular glucose uptake in the body.
4) Type 2 diabetics not well controlled on multiple oral agents; diet and lifestyle changes are good candidates for basal insulin therapy.

Types of Insulin
This is not an inclusive list. Only three types of insulin are listed.

Short-Acting Insulin (regular)
Onset: 30 minutes
Peak: 3 to 4 hours
Duration: 6 to 8 hours

Intermediate-Acting Insulin (NPH or Lente)
Onset: 1 to 2 hours
Peak: 6 to 12 hours
Duration: 18 to 24 hours

Lantus (insulin glargine-recombinant)
Considered a "basal insulin".
Onset: 1 hour
Duration: 24 hours with no pronounced peaks. Give once a day at the same time
Not indicated at present for children younger than 6 years of age

Diabetes: Possible Complications

Eyes: cataracts, diabetic retinopathy, blindness
Cardiovascular: hyperlipidemia, CAD, MI, hypertension
Kidneys: renal disease, renal failure
Feet: foot ulcers, skin infections, peripheral neuropathy, amputation
Gyne/GU: balanitis (candidal infection of the glans penis), candidal vaginitis

Diabetes: Other Findings

Dawn Phenomenon
This is a normal physiologic event. An elevation in the fasting blood glucose (FBG) occurs daily early in the morning. This is due to an increase in insulin resistance between 4:00 AM and 8:00 AM caused by the physiologic spike in growth hormone (anterior pituitary), glucagon (beta cells pancreas), epinephrine and cortisol (adrenals).

Somogyi Effect (rebound hyperglycemia)
Severe nocturnal hypoglycemia stimulates counterregulatory hormones such as glucagon to be released from the liver. The high levels of glucagon in the systemic circulation result in high fasting blood glucose by 7:00 a.m. The condition is due to overtreatment with the evening and/or bedtime insulin (dose is too high).

Diagnosis: check blood glucose very early in the morning (3 a.m.) for 1 to 2 weeks.
Treatment: snack before bedtime, or eliminate dinnertime NPH dose or lower the
    bedtime dose

Head, Eyes, Ears, Nose, and Throat (HEENT)

EYES

Herpes Keratitis

Acute onset of severe eye pain, photophobia, and blurred vision in one eye. Diagnosed by using fluorescein dye. A black lamp in a darkened room is used to search for fernlike lines in the corneal surface. In contrast, corneal abrasions appear more linear.

Infection permanently damages corneal epithelium, which may result in corneal blindness.

Acute Angle-Closure Glaucoma

Elderly patient with acute onset of severe eye pain accompanied by severe headache, tearing, photophobia, nausea, vomiting, and blurred vision. Examination reveals an oval-shaped pupil that is mid-dilated and appears cloudy. Ophthalmologic emergency.

EARS/NOSE/SINUS

Cholesteatoma

"Cauliflowerlike" growth accompanied by foul-smelling ear discharge. Hearing loss on affected ear. On exam, no tympanic membrane or ossicles are visible because of destruction by the tumor. History of chronic otitis media infections. The mass is not cancerous, but it can erode into the bones of the face and damage the facial nerve (CN7). Treated with antibiotics and surgical debridement. Refer to specialist (HEENT).

Battle Sign

Acute onset of a bruise behind the ear over the mastoid area after a recent history of trauma. Indicates a fracture of the basilar skull. Search for a clear golden serous discharge from the ear or nose (see below). Refer to ER (emergency room) for skull x-rays and antibiotics.

Clear Golden Fluid Discharge from the Nose/Ear

Indicative of a basilar skull fracture. CSF (cerebrospinal fluid) slowly leaks through the fracture. Testing the fluid with a urine dipstick will show that it is positive for glucose whereas plain mucus or mucupurulent drainage will be negative. Refer to ER.

Cavernous Sinus Thrombosis

A rare but life-threatening complication with a high mortality rate. Patient with history of a sinus or facial infection will manifest with a severe headache accompanied by a high fever. Rapid worsening of level of consciousness terminating in coma and death. Refer to ER.

PHARYNX

Peritonsillar Abscess

Severe sore throat and difficulty swallowing, odonophagia, trismus, and a "hot potato" voice. One-sided swelling of the peritonsillar area and soft palate. Affected area is markedly swollen and appears as a bulging red mass with the uvula displaced away from the mass. Accompanied by malaise, fever and chills. Refer to ER for incision and drainage (I&D).

Diphtheria

Sore throat, fever, and markedly swollen neck ("bull neck"). Low-grade fever, hoarseness and dysphagia. The posterior pharynx, tonsils, uvula, and soft palate are coated with a gray- to yellow-colored pseudomembrane that is hard to displace. Very contagious. Refer to ER.

Fast Facts Normal Findings

EYES

Fundi: the veins are larger than arteries
Cones: for color perception
Rods: for detecting light, depth perception, night vision
Macula and fovea: central vision
Cobblestoning: inner conjunctiva with mildly elevated lymphoid tissue resembling "cobblestones"

EARS

TMs (tympanic membrane): translucent off-white to gray color with the "cone of light" intact

Tympanogram: most objective measure for presence of fluid inside middle ear (results in a straight line vs. a peaked shape)

External portion of the ear has large amount of cartilage

Cartilage does not regenerate and injuries need referral to plastic surgeon

NOSE

Only the inferior nasal turbinates are usually visible in the primary care arena. The medial and superior turbinates are not visible without special instruments.

Lower 1/3 of the nose is cartilage. Cartilage tissue does not regenerate; if damaged, refer to plastic surgeon.

MOUTH

Look for leukoplakia on the surface and under the tongue. May be cancerous. Patients with a history of chewing tobacco are at high risk of oral cancer.

TONSILS

Butterfly-shaped glands with small porelike openings that may secrete white to yellow-colored exudate.

POSTERIOR PHARYNX

Look for postnasal drip (acute sinusitis, allergic rhinitis), redness

Posterior pharyngeal lymph nodes that are mildly enlarged distributed evenly on the back of the throat (allergies, allergic rhinitis)

Hard palate: look for any openings (cleft palate), ulcers, redness

Fast Facts | Benign Variants

Torus Palatinus

Painless bony protuberance midline on the hard palate (roof of the mouth) which may be asymmetrical. Skin should be normal. Does not interfere with normal function.

Fishtail or Split Uvula

Uvula is split into two sections ranging from partial to complete. May be a sign of an occult cleft palate (rare).

Nystagmus

A few beats of nystagmus on prolonged extreme lateral gaze that resolve when the eye moves back toward midline is normal. Vertical nystagmus is always abnormal.

Fast Facts | Abnormal Findings

ABNORMAL PHYSICAL EXAM FINDINGS

Papilledema

Optic disc swollen with blurred edges due to increased ICP (intracranial pressure) secondary to bleeding, brain tumor, abscess, pseudotumor cerebri.

Hypertensive Retinopathy

Copper and silver wire arterioles

Diabetic Retinopathy

Microvascularization and microaneurysms

Cataracts

Opacity of the corneas

Allergic Rhinitis

Blue-tinged or pale and swollen (boggy) nasal turbinates

Koplik's Spots

Small-sized red papules with blue-white centers inside the cheeks by the lower molars
Pathognomic for measles

Hairy Leukoplakia

Elongated papilla on the lateral aspects of the tongue
Rule out HPV (human papilloma virus) infection

Leukoplakia of the Oral Mucosa/Tongue

A bright white plaque caused by chronic irritation such as chewing tobacco (snuff) (rule out oral cancer) or on the inner cheeks (buccal mucosa)

Vocabulary

Buccal mucosa: mucosal lining inside the mouth
Palpebral conjunctiva: mucosal lining inside eyelids
Bulbar conjunctiva: mucosal lining covering the eyes
Soft palate: refers to the area where uvula, tonsils, anterior of throat are located
Hard palate: the "roof of the mouth"

Fast Facts EVALUATION AND TESTING

VISION

Distance Vision

The Snellen chart measures central distance central vision
Patient must stand 20 feet away from the chart

Near Vision

Ask patient to read small print

Peripheral Vision

The "visual fields of confrontation" exam
Look for blind spots (scotoma) and peripheral visual field defects

Color Blindness

Use the Ishihara chart.

Visual Test Results

1) Definition of a Snellen test result 20/60
   Top number (or numerator): the distance in feet at which the patient stands from the Snellen or picture eye chart (always 20 feet and never changes)
   Bottom Number (or denominator): the number of feet that the patient can see compared to a person with normal vision (20/20 or less). Number changes, dependent on patient's vision. In this example, the patient can see at 20 feet what a person with normal vision can see at 60 feet

2) Legal blindness: defined as a distance vision of 20/200 in the better eye with corrective lenses or a visual field less than 20 degrees (tunnel/vision).

HEARING TESTS

Weber Test

Place the tuning fork placed midline on the forehead
Normal finding: no lateralization. If lateralization (hears the sound in only one ear), abnormal finding

Rinne Test

Place tuning fork first on mastoid process, then front of the ear. Time each area.
Normal finding: air conduction last longer than bone conduction

---

Fast Facts **Disease Review**

EYES

Herpes Keratitis

Damage to corneal epithelium due to herpes virus infection secondary to shingles.

Classic Case
Complains of acute onset of eye pain, photophobia, and blurred vision of the affected eye. Look for a herpetic rash of the side of the temple and on the tip of the nose (rule out shingles of the trigeminal nerve or CN 5).

Objective
Use fluorescein dye strips with a black lamp in darkened room. Appears as fernlike lines. In contrast, abrasions appear more linear.

Treatment Plan
1) Refer to ophthalmologist stat (immediately) or to ER.
2) Treated with high-doses of Zovirax or Valtrex BID until resolved by ophthalmologist.
3) Avoid steroid ophthalmic drops (will worsen it).

Hordeolum (stye)

A painful acute bacterial infection of a hair follicle on the eyelid.

Classic Case

Complains of an itchy eyelid and an acute onset of a pustule on either upper or lower eyelid that eventually becomes painful.

Treatment Plan

1) Antibiotic drops or ointment (i.e., sulfa drops, gentamicin gtts, etc.).
2) Warm packs BID to TID until pustule drains.

Chalazion

A chronic inflammation of the meibonian gland (specialized sweat gland) of the eyelids.

Classic Case

Complains of a gradual onset of a small superficial nodule that is discrete and movable on the upper eyelid that feels like a bead. Painless. Can slowly enlarge over time. Benign.

Treatment Plan

1) If nodule enlarges or does not resolve in few weeks, biopsy to rule out squamous cell cancer. If large and affects vision, surgical removal an option.

Pinguecula

A yellow triangular thickening of the bulbar conjunctiva (skin covering eyeball). Located on the inner and outer margins of the cornea. Caused by UV (ultraviolet light) damage to collagen.

Pterygium

A yellow triangular (wedge-shaped) thickening of the conjunctiva that extends to the cornea on the nasal or temporal cornea. Due to UV-damaged collagen from chronic sun exposure. Usually asymptomatic. Can be red/inflamed at times.

Treatment Plan (both pinguecula and pterygium)

1) If inflamed, use weak steroid eye drops only during exacerbations.
2) Recommend use of good-quality sunglasses.
3) Removed surgically if encroaches cornea and affects vision.

Subconjunctival Hemorrhage

Blood that is trapped underneath the conjunctiva and sclera secondary to broken arterioles. Can be caused by coughing, sneezing, heavy lifting, vomitting, or can occur spontaneously. Resolves within 1 to 3 weeks (blood reabsorbed) like a bruise with color changes from red, green to yellow. Increased risk if on aspirin, anticoagulation, and hypertension.

Classic Case

Complains of sudden onset of bright red blood in one eye after an incident of severe coughing, sneezing, or straining. May also be due to trauma such as a fall. Denies visual loss and pain.

Treatment Plan

1) Watchful waiting and reassure patient. Follow up until resolution.

Primary Open-Angle Glaucoma

Gradual onset of increased intraocular pressure (IOP) due to blockage of the drainage of aqueous humor inside the eye. The retina (CN 2) undergoes ischemic changes and, if untreated, becomes permanently damaged. Most common type of glaucoma (60% to 70%).

Classic Case

Most commonly seen in elderly patients, especially those of African background or diabetics. Complains of gradual changes in peripheral vision (lost first) and then central vision. Results in permanent blindness if not treated.

Treatment Plan

1) Check IOP (intraocular pressure). Normal range IOP: 10 to 22 mm Hg.
2) Refer patient to ophthalmologist for annual exams.

Medications

Betimol (timolol): Beta-blocker eyedrops that lower IOP

Side effects and contraindications: same as oral form. Include bronchospasm, fatigue, depression, heart failure, bradycardia

Contraindicated: asthma, emphysema, COPD (chronic obstructive lung disease), second- to third-degree heart block, heart failure

Complication

1) Blindness due to ischemic damage to retina (CN I)

Primary Angle Closure Glaucoma

Sudden blockage of aqueous humor causes marked increased of the IOP causing ischemia and permanent damage to the optic nerve (CN 2).

Classic Case

An older patient complains of acute onset of a severe frontal headache or severe eye pain with blurred vision and tearing. Seeing halos around lights. May be accompanied by severe nausea and vomiting.

Objective

Eyes: fixed and mid-dilated cloudy pupil that looks more oval than round-shaped. Conjunctival injection with increased lacrimation.

Treatment Plan
Refer to ER.

Macular Degeneration

Gradual changes in the pigment of the macula (area of central vision) result in blindness. Cause is unknown. Leading cause of blindness in the elderly in this country. More common in the elderly and smokers. Two types: atrophic (dry form) and exudative (wet form).

Classic Case

Elderly smoker complains of gradual or sudden and painless central vision loss. During the early phase of visual loss, may not notice blurred and distorted central vision until a large area is involved. Peripheral vision is preserved.

Labs

Check central vision with Amsler Grid test (center of grid is distorted, blind spot or scotoma, or wavy lines).

Treatment Plan

Increase intake of antioxidants (vitamins C and E, beta carotene, zinc) and the herbs lutein and bilberry. Refer to ophthalmologist.

NOSE

Allergic Rhinitis

Inflammatory changes of the nasal mucosa due to allergy to certain allergens. Atopic family history. May have seasonal or daily symptoms.

Classic Case

Complains of constant nasal congestion with clear mucus discharge. Sometimes accompanied by nasal itch and frequent sneezing. Coughing from postnasal drip that worsens when supine.

Objective

Nose: blue tinge or pale boggy nasal turbinates. Mucus clear. Postnasal drip with clear to white-colored mucus.

Treatment Plan

Nasal steroid sprays daily (i.e., fluticasone/Flonase)
Cromolyn sodium (Intal) nasal spray QID (4 times a day)
Zyrtec 10 mg daily or PRN or combined with decongestants
Decongestants (i.e., pseudoephedrine or Sudafed) PRN

Complications
1) Acute sinusitis
2) Acute otitis media

Rhinitis Medicamentosa

Prolonged use of topical nasal decongestants (>3 days) causes rebound effects that result in severe and chronic nasal congestion if nasal decongestant use is discontinued abruptly.

Patients present with severe nasal congestion and clear watery mucous nasal discharge.

Epistaxis (nosebleeds)

Trauma and/or laceration to nasal passages results in bleeding. Posterior nasal bleeds can result in severe hemorrhage. Anterior nasal bleeds are milder. Patients on aspirin, cocaine abuse, severe hypertension, and anticoagulants (i.e., warfarin sodium or Coumadin) are at higher risk.

Classic Case

Complains of acute onset of nasal bleeding secondary to trauma. Bright red blood may drip externally through the nasal passages and/or the posterior pharynx. Profuse bleeding can result in vomiting of blood.

Treatment Plan

Bend head back and apply pressure over nasal bridge for several minutes. Nasal decongestants (i.e., Afrin) to shrink tissue. Nasal packing. Antibiotic prophylaxis for staph and strep as needed.

Complications

1) Posterior nasal bleeds may hemorrhage (refer to emergency room).

THROAT

Strep Throat

An acute infection of the pharynx caused by the beta streptococcus (gram positive) Group A bacteria. Rare sequelae are scarlet fever and rheumatic fever.

Classic Case

All ages affected, but most common in children. Acute onset of pharyngitis, pain on swallowing, and mildly enlarged submandibular nodes. Not associated with rhinitis, watery eyes, or congestion (coryza) from a viral infection. Submandibular nodes mildly enlarged.

Objective
Pharynx is dark pink to bright red
May have tonsillar exudate
Submandibular lymph nodes mildly enlarged
Sometimes, mild fever

Treatment Plan
Throat C&S (culture and sensitivity)
Penicillin QID × 10 days
Ibuprofen (Advil) or acetaminophen (Tylenol) for throat pain and fever
Symptomatic treatment: salt water gargles, throat lozenges
Repeat culture if high risk: history of MVP (mitral valve prolapse)

PCN Allergy

Z-Pack (azithromycin) × 5 days
Levaquin (levofloxacin) × 10 days (contraindicated if age < 18)

Complications
1) Scarlet fever: sandpaper texture to pink rash, acute pharyngitis findings.
2) Rheumatic fever: inflammatory reaction to strep infection that may affect the heart and the valves, joints, and the brain.
3) Peritonsillar abscess: displaced uvula, red bulging mass on anterior pharyngeal space on one side, dysphagia, fever. Refer to ER stat.

EARS

Acute Otitis Media (purulent otitis media)

An acute infection of the middle ear cavity with bacterial pathogens due to mucus that becomes trapped in the middle ear secondary to temporary eustachian tube dysfunction. The infection is usually unilateral, but may at times involve both ears.

Organisms
Streptococcus pneumoniae (gram positive). High rates of beta-lactam resistant strains
Haemophilus influenzae (gram negative)
Moraxella catarrhalis (gram negative)

Classic Case
Complains of ear pain, popping noises, muffled hearing. Recent history of a cold or flare-up of allergic rhinitis. Adult infections usually develop much more slowly than in children. Afebrile or low grade fever.

Objective

Tympanic membrane (TM): bulging or retraction with displaced light reflex (displaced landmarks)

Erythematous TM (may be due to coughing or crying in children)

Decreased mobility with flat line tracing on tympanogram (most objective finding)

Treatment Plan

Listed under "Acute Sinusitis." Treatment plans are combined for both acute otitis media and acute sinusitis because of the many similarities in the drugs used.

Acute Sinusitis (acute rhinosinusitis)

An infection of the sinuses by both gram-positive and gram-negative bacteria. The maxillary and frontal sinuses are most commonly affected.

Organisms

Streptococcus pneumoniae (gram positive). High rates of beta-lactam resistant strains.

Haemophilus influenzae (gram negative)

Moraxella catarrhalis (gram negative)

Classic Case

Complains of unilateral facial pressure that worsens when bending down along with pain in the upper molar teeth (maxillary sinusitis) or frontal headache (frontal sinusitis). Coughing is made worse when supine (i.e., during sleep). Self-treatment with over-the-counter cold and sinus remedies provides no relief of symptoms.

Objective

Posterior pharynx: purulent mucoid postnasal drip

Infected sinus: tender to palpation

Transillumination: positive ("glow" of light on infected sinus is duller compared with normal sinus)

Treatment Plan (both AOM and acute sinusitis)

Duration of treatment: 10 to 14 days

First-line

1) Amoxicillin is the gold standard for any age group.
2) High beta-lactam resistant strains: do not use amoxicillin.
3) Close follow-up infants and children. Evaluate again in 3 days. If not responding to amoxicillin, switch to second-line antibiotic.

Second-Line

Second-line antibiotic treatment criteria: history of antibiotic use in the past 6 months or no response to amoxicillin.

1) Amoxicillin/clavulanate (Augmentin) po BID.
2) Cefuroxime (Ceftin) po BID.
3) Trimethoprim sulfamethazole (Bactrim DS) po BID.
4) Cephalosporins
   - Second generation (cefprozil or Cefzil)
   - Third generation (ceftriaxone or Rocephin)

Penicillin-Allergic Patients
1) Azithromycin (Z-Pack).
2) Trimethoprim sulfamethazole (Bactrim DS) po BID.
3) Levofloxacin (Levaquin) if 18 years or older daily.

Pain
1) Naproxen sodium (Anaprox DS) po BID or ibuprofen (Advil) po QID as needed.
2) Acetaminophen (Tylenol) every 4 to 6 hours PRN.

Drainage
1) Oral decongestants such as pseudoephedrine (Sudafed).
2) Topical decongestants (i.e., Afrin): use only for 3 days maximum or will cause rebound.

Complications
1) Cholesteatoma: cauliflowerlike growth accompanied by foul-smelling ear discharge. No tympanic membrane or ossicles are visible (destroyed). History of chronic otitis media infections. Mass is not cancerous, but it can erode into the bones of the face and cause damage to the facial nerve (CN7).
2) Mastoiditis: red and swollen mastoid that is tender to palpation. Treat with antibiotics.
3) Preorbital or orbital cellulitis (more common in children).
   - Edema and redness periorbital area and diplopia
   - Abnormal EOM (extraorbital muscles) testing
   - Pain, fever, toxicity
4) Meningitis: stiff neck, headache, photophobia, fever.
5) Cavernous sinus thrombosis:
   - Life-threatening with high mortality; refer to ER
   - Complains of headache, abnormal neuro exam, confused, febrile, toxic

Otitis Externa (swimmer's ear)

Bacterial infection of the skin of the external ear canal (rarely fungal). More common during warm and humid weather (i.e., summer).

Organisms
Pseudomonas aeruginosa (gram negative)
Staphylococcus aureus (gram positive)

Classic Case

Complains of external ear pain, swelling, and green purulent discharge. History of recent activities that involve swimming or wetting ears.

Objective

Ear: pain with manipulation of the external ear or tragus. Purulent green discharge Erythematous and swollen ear canal that is very tender

Treatment Plan

Corticosporin ear drops QID × 7 days. Keep water out of ear during treatment.

Complications

1) Malignant otitis media:
   - Seen in diabetics, aggressive spread of infection to surrounding soft tissue/bone.
   - Hospitalize for high-dose antibiotics and surgical debridement.

Acute Mononucleosis (infectious mononucleosis)

Infection by the Epstein-Barr virus (EBV). Transmitted through oral contact. EBV virus lies latent in pharyngeal tissue. Can become reactivated and cause symptoms. Classic triad: fatigue, acute pharyngitis, lymphadenopathy.

Classic Case

Teenage patient presents with new onset of sore throat, enlarged cervical nodes, and fatigue. Sore throat and fatigue may last weeks to months. May have abdominal pain due to hepatomegaly and/or splenomegaly. History of intimate kissing.

Objective

Nodes: enlarged cervical nodes
Pharynx: erythematous. Tonsils red, sometimes with exudate (off-white)
Hepatomegaly and splenomegaly. Avoid vigorous palpation of the abdomen until resolves

Treatment Plan

Order abdominal ultrasound (sonogram), especially if patient is an athlete. Avoid all contact sports until resolution (repeat abdominal ultrasound). Symptomatic treatment.

Complications

1) Ruptured spleen.
2) Airway obstruction.
3) Encephalitis, coma.
4) Blood dyscrasias (atypical lymphocytes). Repeat CBC until lymphocytes normalized
5) Hepatitis, etc.

CHEILOSIS

Skin fissures and maceration at the corners of the mouth. Multiple etiologies such as oversalivation, iron-deficiency anemia, secondary bacterial infection, vitamin deficiencies.

Treatment Plan

Apply triple antibiotic ointment BID to TID until healed.
Remove or treat underlying cause.

HEENT EXAM TIPS

1) Ruptured spleen is a catastrophic event. Avoid contact sports (several weeks) until ultrasound documents resolution.
2) Betimol (timolol) has the same contraindications as oral beta-blockers.
3) Cholesteatoma, periorbital sinusitis complication.
4) Do not use amoxicillin if previous antibiotic past 6 months.
5) Penicillin-allergic patients, use macrolides, sulfas (also avoid cephalosporins).
6) Learn to recognize a description of eye findings such as pinguecula, pterygium, chalazion.
7) Weber or Rinne: testing the acoustic or the eighth cranial nerve.
8) Lateralization on the Weber exam is an abnormal finding.
9) Remember what 20/40 vision means: patient can see at 20 feet what a person with normal vision can see at 40 feet.

Cardiac System

Fast Facts Danger Signals

Acute Myocardial Infarction (MI)

Middle-aged or older male complains of midsternal chest pain that feels like heavy pressure on the chest. The pain is associated with numbness and/or tingling in the left jaw and the left arm. The patient is diaphoretic with cool clammy skin and a sensation of doom. There is a history of diabetes, hypertension, hyperlipidemia, smoking, and/or a positive family history.

Aortic Abdominal Aneurysm (AAA)

Usually asymptomatic. Elderly white male complains of pulsating-type sensation in abdomen and/or low back pain. With impending rupture, sudden onset of low back pain that steadily becomes sharp and excruciating. If rupture occurs, cardiovascular collapse causes death. Higher risk with hypertension, COPD, and smokers. May have undiagnosed Marfan syndrome.

Congestive Heart Failure (CHF)

Elderly patient complains of a gradual or acute onset of dyspnea, dry cough, and swollen feet and ankles. Sudden or gradual increased weight and crackles on the lung base along with an S3 heart sound are present. History of preexisting heart disease or previous episode of heart failure. Usually taking diuretics, lanoxin, and antihypertensive medications.

Bacterial Endocarditis

Patient presents with fever, chills, and malaise associated with skin findings found mostly on the fingers/hands and toes/feet. These are splinter hemorrhages on the nailbed (subungal hemorrhages), petechiae on the, palate, painful violet-colored nodes on the fingers or feet (Osler nodes), and tender red spots on the palms/soles (Janeway lesions).

A heart murmur may be present on cardiac exam.

Fast Facts **Normal Findings**

ANATOMY

Most of the left ventricular mass is located behind the right ventricle. The right ventricle sits anteriorly toward the chest. Most of the atria is located posteriorly facing the back. The lower border of the left ventricle is where the apical impulse is generated.

Apical impulse: at the 5th ICS (intercostal space) about 8 cm from the mid-sternal line.

Deoxygenated Blood

Enters the heart through the superior vena cava and inferior vena cava
Right atrium → tricuspid valve → right ventricle → pulmonic valve → pulmonary
    artery → lungs (pulmonary vein)

Oxygenated Blood

Exits the lungs through the pulmonary veins and enters the heart
Left atrium → mitral valve → left ventricle → aortic valve → aorta → general
    circulation

Systole and Diastole

The mnemonic to use is "Motivated Apples." These two words give you several clues. They will remind you of the names of the valves (which produce the sound) and the type of valve.

MOTIVATED
M (mitral valve)
T (tricuspid valve)
AV (atrioventricular valves)

APPLES
A (aortic valve)
P (pulmonic valve)
S (semilunar valves)

Normal Heart Sounds

S1 (systole)
- Closure of the mitral and tricuspid valves
- Atrioventricular or AV valves (3 leaflets)

S2 (diastole)
- Closure of the aortic and pulmonic valves
- Semilunar valves (2 leaflets)

S3 Heart Sound
- Pathognomic for CHF (congestive heart failure)
- Occurs during early diastole (ventricular gallop)
- Always considered abnormal if it occurs after the age of 40
      May be a normal variant in some children or young adults if there are no signs or symptoms of heart or valvular disease.

S4 Heart Sound
Caused by the increased resistance due to a stiff left ventricle. Usually indicates left ventricular hypertrophy. Considered as normal finding in some elderly (slight thickening of left ventricle).
- S4 occurs during late diastole (atrial gallop or "atrial kick").
- Best heard at the apex (mitral area) using the bell of the stethoscope
Summation gallop:
- All heart sounds are present (from S1 to S4) and sound like a galloping horse
- A pathologic finding

Stethoscope Skills

Bell of Stethoscope
- Low tones such as the extra heart sounds (S3 or S4)
- Mitral stenosis
Diaphragm of the stethoscope
- Mid- to high-pitched tones such as lung sounds
- Mitral regurgitation
- Aortic stenosis

Fast Facts | Benign Variants

Benign Split S2

Best heard over the pulmonic area (or second ICS left side of sternum). Due to splitting of the aortic and pulmonic components. A normal finding if it appears during inspiration and disappears at expiration.

Benign S4 in the Elderly

Some healthy elderly patients have an S4 (late diastole) heart sound. Also known as the "atrial kick" (the atria have to squeeze harder to overcome resistance of a stiff left ventricle). If there are no signs or symptoms of heart/valvular disease, it is considered a normal variant. Otherwise it is associated with LVH (left ventricular hypertrophy).

Exam Tips

1) S3 is a sign for CHF; S4 is a sign of LVH.
2) A split S2 is best heard at the pulmonic area.
3) Memorize the mnemonic "Motivated Apple" to help you remember the valves responsible for producing S1 and S2.
4) Grading murmurs: first time thrill palpated is at Grade IV.

Clinical Tips

1) S3 is pathognomic for CHF. Look for the sign if you suspect a patient has heart failure.

SOLVING QUESTIONS: HEART MURMURS

To solve a murmur question correctly, there are two pieces of information needed to solve it. These two are the timing (systole or diastole) and location of the murmur. All the murmurs seen on the test will fit into these two mnemonics.

Timing of Murmur

Systolic murmurs:

■ Use the MR. TRAS mnemonic

Diastolic murmurs:

■ Use the MS. PRAR mnemonic

Location of Murmurs

Auscultatory Areas

It is necessary to memorize the locations of the auscultatory areas. This will assist in solving questions about heart murmurs. There are only three sites to remember for the exam.

Mitral Area

- Fifth ICS (intercostal space) on the left side of sternum medial to the mid-clavicular line
- Apical murmur
- Apex of the heart

Pulmonic Area

- Second ICS on the left side of the sternum
- Left side of the upper sternum at the base (of the heart)

Aortic Area

- Second ICS to the right side of the sternum
- Right side of the upper sternum at the base (of the heart)

Mnemonic (discussed later)

Systole: MR. TRAS
Diastole: MS. PRAR

Shortcuts

1) Only one auscultatory area on the right side of the sternum: aortic area.
2) Aortic area is described as: the right side of the upper sternum or the base of the heart on the right side.
3) Aortic murmur (systole): aortic stenosis.
4) Aortic murmur (diastole): aortic regurgitation.
5) Mitral murmurs are described as the apex, apical area, or the fifth intercostal space on the left lower edge of the sternum by the midclavicular line. The word *mitral* will not be used because it is an obvious clue.
6) Mitral murmur (systole): mitral regurgitation.
7) Mitral murmur (diastole): mitral stenosis.
8) Systole: pansystolic, holosystolic, early or late systole, S1.
9) Diastole: early or late diastole, S2.

Mnemonics

MR. TRAS (use for all systolic murmurs)

These murmurs are also described as occurring during S1, or as holosystolic, pansystolic, early systolic, late systolic, or midsystolic murmurs.

MR (mitral regurgitation)
A pansystolic (or holosystolic) murmur:

- Heard best at the apex of the heart or the apical area

- Radiates to axilla
- Loud blowing and high-pitched murmur (use the diaphragm of the stethoscope)

TR (tricuspid regurgitation)
- Not on the test at present

AS (aortic stenosis)
A midsystolic ejection murmur:
- Best heard at the second ICS at the right side of the sternum
- Radiates to the neck
- A harsh and noisy murmur (use diaphragm of stethoscope)

Increased risk of sudden death. Patients with aortic stenosis should avoid physical overexertion. Monitored by serial cardiac sonograms with Doppler flow studies. Surgical valve replacement if worsens.

MS. PRAR
Diastole is also known as the S2 heart sound, early diastole, late diastole, or mid-diastole.
Diastolic murmurs are always indicative of heart disease (unlike systolic murmurs).

MS (mitral stenosis)
A low-pitched diastolic rumbling murmur:
- Heard best at the apex of the heart or the apical area
- Also called an "opening snap" (use bell of the stethoscope)

PR (pulmonic regurgitation)
- Not on the test at present

AR (aortic regurgitation)
A high-pitched diastolic murmur:
- Best heard at the second ICS at the right side of the sternum
- High-pitched blowing murmur (use diaphragm of the stethoscope)

Heart Murmurs: Grading System

Grade I
- Very soft murmur. Heard only under optimal conditions

Grade II
- Mild to moderately loud murmur

Grade III
- Loud murmur that is easily heard once the stethoscope is placed on the chest

Grade IV
- First time a thrill is felt. A louder murmur

Grade V
  ■ Very loud murmur heard with edge of stethoscope off chest
Grade VI
  ■ The murmur is so loud that it can be heard even with the stethoscope off the
    chest

Fast Facts Abnormal Findings

Pathologic Murmurs

1) All diastolic murmurs are abnormal.
2) Late systolic murmurs.
3) Loud murmurs, pansystolic or holosystolic murmurs.
4) Murmurs associated with a thrill.

Exam Tips

1) Memorize the auscultatory locations and mnemonics.
2) Systolic murmurs use MR. TRAS.
3) Diastolic murmurs use MS. PRAR.
4) All murmurs with "mitral" in their names are described as located:
   ■ On the apex of the heart or the apical area
   ■ Or the 5th ICS on the left side of the sternum medial to the midclavicular
     line.
5) There is only one auscultatory area on the right side of the sternum (aortic).
6) If you forget on which side of the sternum the aortic or pulmonic area lies (left?
   or right?):
   ■ The "r" in aortic is for the "right side"
   ■ The "l" in pulmonic is for the "left" side

Fast Facts Disease Review

PULSUS PARADOXUS

Also known as a paradoxical pulse. Measured by using the BP cuff and a stethoscope.

During inspiration: systolic pressure normally decreases slightly due to a
slight increase of the pressure inside the chest cavity (positive pressure)

Certain pulmonary and cardiac conditions cause an exaggerated decrease of
the systolic pressure of >10 mm Hg

Pulmonary cause:
   ■ Asthma, emphysema (increased positive pressure)

Cardiac cause:
- ■ Tamponade, pericarditis, cardiac effusion (decreases movement of left ventricle)

ATRIAL FIBRILLATION (AF)

Any condition or substance that irritates or overstimulates the heart can cause atrial fibrillation. For example: hyperthyroidism, cocaine, caffeine or alcohol, heart failure.

May be asymptomatic. Rate of stroke is 10 times higher in older patients.

Classic Case

Older patient complains of sudden onset of heart palpitations that may be associated with feeling weak or dizzy. May be accompanied by chest pain or syncope.

Treatment Plan

Diagnostic test is the 12-lead EKG
INR (internationalized normal ratio) is used to monitor response to anticoagulation

Medications

Anticoagulants decreases risk of thrombosis and emboli. For acute episodes of embolization, patient is hospitalized and started on heparin IV. Before discharge, switched to warfarin sodium (Coumadin) 2–10 mg/day.

Complications

1) Death from thromboembolic event (i.e., stroke, pulmonary embolism)

Anticoagulation Guidelines

Atrial Fibrillation
INR (international normalized ratio): 2.0 to 3.0 times normal

Synthetic Valves
INR: 2.5 to 3.5 times normal

HYPERTENSION

Majority of patients have essential hypertension (90–95% of cases). A multifactorial disorder that results from genetic, renal (renin/angiotensin), sympathetic nervous system, and environmental factors.

Blood pressure (BP): peripheral vascular resistance (PVR) × CO (cardiac output)
Any change in the PVR or CO results in a change in BP (increase/decrease).

Examples:

Na+ (sodium):
- Water retention increases vascular volume (increased CO)

Angiotensin I to angiotensin II:
- Increased vasoconstriction (increased PVR)

Sympathetic system stimulation:
- Epinephrine secretion causes tachycardia and vasoconstriction (increased PVR)

Vasodilation (beta blockers):
- Decreased resistance (decreased PVR)

Severe hemorrhage:
- Less blood volume (decreased CO)

Correct Blood Pressure Measurement

1) Avoid smoking or caffeine intake 30 minutes before measurement.
2) Patient should be seated on a chair with back and arm supported.
3) Begin BP measurement after 5 minutes of rest (mercury sphygmomanometer preferred over digital machines).
4) Two or more readings separated by 2 minutes should be averaged per visit.
5) Higher number determines BP stage (BP 140/100 is stage II instead of stage I).

Secondary Hypertension (HTN)

Most common causes are renal conditions (i.e., renal artery stenosis, renal failure).
Rule out secondary cause if the following:
- If onset of hypertension is younger than age 35 years
- Severe hypertension or abrupt onset
- Refractory to treatment

Physical Exam Findings

Eyes
- Silver and/or copper wire arterioles
- AV nicking (arteriovenous junction nicking)
- Flame-shaped hemorrhages, papilledema

Heart
- S3 (heart failure)
- S4 (left ventricular hypertrophy)
- Carotid bruits (narrowing due to plaque)
- Peripheral edema (CHF or kidney disease)
- Decreased or absent peripheral pulses (PVD)

Table 3.3 — Hypertension Diagnosis and Management: JNC 7 Treatment Guidelines

Stage	Systole/Diastole	Treatment Recommendations
Normal	<120 mm Hg <80 mm Hg	Healthy lifestyle. Exercise
Prehypertension	120 to 139 mm Hg 80 to 89 mm Hg	Lifestyle changes. Lose weight. Exercise
Stage I	140 to 159 mm Hg 90 to 99 mm Hg	*Thiazide diuretics preferred for most cases* If indicated or compelling condition: ACE inhibitors, ARBs, Beta-blockers, CCB or combination drug
Stage II	>160 mm Hg >100 mm Hg	Two-drug combination for most patients. Thiazide diuretic plus ACE inhibitor, ARB, beta-blocker, calcium channel blocker, or a combination drug
Compelling Indications	Diabetes Kidney disease Heart failure Recurrent stroke prevention	ACEI, ARB, thiazide diuretic, beta-blocker, CCB ACEI, ARB Thiazide diuretic, beta blocker, ACEI, ARB, etc Thiazide diuretic, ACEI
	Dietary intake	Magnesium, potassium, calcium

Note. ACEI: ACE inhibitor, ARB: ACE receptor blocker, CCB: Calcium channel blocker. Adapted from Joint National Committee on Prevention, Detection, Evaluation, and Treatment of High Blood Pressure (JNC 7), 2003. Cardiac Risk Equivalents (JNC 7): Conditions determined to markedly increase the risk of heart disease or hypertension. Goal BP for these patients is 130/80. Cardiac risk equivalents: Diabetics, chronic renal disease, microalbuminuria.

Renal Artery Stenosis

▪ Epigastric or upper abdominal quadrant bruit

Pheochromocytoma

▪ Labile increased BP, sudden onset anxiety
▪ Paroxysms of sweating
▪ Severe headaches, palpitations

Hyperthyroidism

▪ Weight loss, tachycardia, fine tremor, moist skin, anxiety
▪ Atrial fibrillation

Kidneys
- Bruit (renal artery stenosis)
- Cystic renal masses (polycystic kidney)
- Increased creatinine (renal insufficiency, renal failure)

Sleep Apnea
- Increases blood pressure
- Marked hypoxic episodes during sleep

Exam Tips

1) Eye findings: learn to distinguish the findings in hypertension (copper and silver wire arterioles, AV nicking) from those in diabetes (neovascularization, microaneurysms.

Current Treatment Guidelines

Joint National Committee for the Assessment, Evaluation and Treatment of High Blood Pressure in Adults, 7th Report (2003).

Stage I (BP 140–139 or 90–99 mm Hg)
- Thiazide-type diuretics preferred for most patients

Stage 2 (systolic $\geq$ 160 or diastolic $\geq$ 100 mm Hg)
- Two-drug therapy for most patients
- Thiazide-type diuretic and another drug class antihypertensive agent
- If other disease(s) with compelling indications, prescribe drug

Diabetics and CAD (coronary artery disease)
- Goal is BP < 130/80 mm Hg

Compelling Indications

Diabetes Mellitus (DM)
Unless contraindicated, all diabetics should be on angiotensin reuptake inhibitors or angiotensive receptor blockers because of their renal protective properties.

Angiotensin reuptake (ACE) inhibitors:
- Captopril (Capoten)

Angiotensin receptor blockers (ARBs):
- Losartan (Cozaar)

Beta-blockers:
- Propranolol (Inderal LA)

Calcium channel blockers (CCBs):
- Nifedipine (Norvasc)

Systolic Hypertension in the Elderly
- Diuretics preferred or long-acting dihydropyridine CCBs (i.e., Norvasc)

Heart Failure
- ACE inhibitors or ARBs
- Diuretics
- Beta-blockers

Post Myocardial Infarction (MI)
- Beta blockers, ACE inhibitors, aldosterone antagonists

Target Organs
Rule out target organ damage.
Brain: strokes
Eyes: retinopathy, bleeding, blindness
Heart: left ventricular hypertrophy, heart disease, acute MI, congestive heart failure (CHF)
Kidneys: proteinuria, renal failure

Lifestyle Recommendations
This is the first-line therapy for both hypertension and diabetes.
1) Lose weight.
2) Stop smoking.
3) Reduce stress level.
4) Reduce dietary sodium:
    - Less than 2.4 grams per day
5) Maintain adequate intake of potassium, calcium, and magnesium.
6) Limit alcohol intake:
    - 1 ounce (30 mL) or less per day men
    - 0.5 ounce or less per day women
7) Eat fatty cold-water fish (salmon, anchovy):
    - 3 times a week
8) Exercise moderately:
    - 30 to 45 minutes most days of the week

OBESITY

BMI Calculation (body mass index): weight (in kilograms) $\times$ (height in meters)^2

Exam Tips

1) Remember BMI calculation factors (weight $\times$ height)
2) Do not confuse BMI formula with the PEF (peak expiratory flow)
3) PEF is height, age, gender (mnemonic is "HAG")
    - Weight is not a factor used for the PEF formula

Table 3.4	Basal Metabolic Index (BMI)
	BMI
Underweight	<18.5
Normal weight	18.5 to 24.9
Overweight	25 to 29.9
Obese	30 to 39.9
Grossly obese	>40.0

Dietary Sources of Recommended Minerals

Calcium (low-fat dairy)

Potassium (most fruits and vegetables)

Magnesium (dried beans, whole grains, nuts)

Avoid high sodium intake

- Cold cuts, ready-made foods, any pickled foods (cucumbers, eggs, pork parts)

Omega 3 oils

- Salmon, anchovies (sardines), flaxseed oil

Labs

Kidneys: creatinine, urinalysis

Endocrine: thyroid profile, fasting blood glucose

Electrolyte: potassium (K^+), Sodium (Na^+), calcium (Ca^{2+})

Heart: cholesterol, HDL, LDL, triglycerides (complete lipid panel)

Anemia: complete blood count

Baseline EKG and chest x-ray (to rule out cardiomegaly)

Medications

Beta-Blockers

Avoid abrupt discontinuation after chronic use. May precipitate severe rebound hypertension. Wean slowly.

Action: decreases vasomotor activity, cardiac output, inhibits renin and norepinephrine release

Blocks beta receptors on the heart and the peripheral vasculature. Two types of beta blocker receptors: B1 (cardiac effects) and B2 (lungs and peripheral vasculature)

Contraindications
- Second- to third-degree heart block (okay to use with first-degree block)
- Asthma, COPD, or chronic lung disease
- Sinus bradycardia

Other Uses

Migraine headache: for prophylaxis only (not for acute attacks)

Glaucoma: to reduce intraocular pressure or IOP (i.e., Betimol Ophthalmic Drops)

Resting tachycardia, angina, post MI

Hyperthyroidism and pheochromocytoma: to control symptoms until primary disease treated

Beta blockers: ends with "-olol":
- Metoprolol (Lopressor) 100 mg QD to BID
- Propranolol (Inderal LA) 40 mg BID (only long-acting form used for HTN)

Propranolol (plain Inderal): shorter half-life (not for HTN treatment)

Calcium Channel Blockers (CCBs)

Blocks calcium channels in the arterioles, resulting in systemic vasodilation, which results in decreasing PVR. Depresses heart muscle and the AV node (decreases cardiac output).

Side Effects
- Headaches (vasodilation)
- Ankle edema (from vasodilation; considered benign)
- Heart block or bradycardia (depresses cardiac muscle and AV node)

Contraindications
- Second- and third-degree AV block
- Bradycardia
- Congestive heart failure

Examples

Dihydropyridines ("-pine" ending):

Nifedipine (Procardia XL), amlodipine (Norvasc)

Nondihydropyridine: Verapamil (Calan), diltiazem (Cardizem CD)

Ace Inhibitors and Angiotensin Receptor Blockers

Blocks conversion of angiotensin I to II (more potent vasoconstrictor)

Diabetes Mellitus: drug of choice (protects kidneys) for diabetics

Pregnancy Category C
- Fetal kidney malformations and fetal hypotension

Side Effects
Dry hacking cough (up to 10% with ACEs; less with ARBs)
Hyperkalemia, angioedema (rare but may be life-threatening)

Contraindications
Renal disease or renal artery stenosis
    ■ Precipitates acute renal failure if given ACE or ARB
Hyperkalemia (this is also a side effect for ACE and ARBs, will have additive effect)

Examples
ACE inhibitors: Captopril (Capoten), enalapril (Vasotec), lisinopril (Zestril)
Angiotensin receptor blockers (ARBs): Losartan (Cozaar)

Alpha-1 Blockers
Also known as alpha-1 inhibitors or agonists (instead of blockers). Block alpha receptors in peripheral arteries, resulting in profound vasodilation (large number of alpha-1 receptors in arterioles). Used to treat males with benign prostatic hyperplasia (BPH) and hypertension.

Side Effect
■ Dizziness, postural hypotension

Start at very low doses and titrate up slowly until good BP control. Given at bedtime because of common side effect of postural hypotension.

Example
Terazosin (Hytrin)

Exam Tips

1) ACE inhibitors: the drug of choice for diabetics, causes a dry cough (10%).
2) Avoid combining ACE inhibitors with potassium-sparing diuretics (i.e., triamterene, spironolactone) because of increased risk for hyperkalemia.
3) Renal artery stenosis: ACE inhibitors precipitate acute renal failure.
4) Alpha blockers are not first-line drugs for hypertension except if patient has preexisting BPH.

Clinical Tips

1) High cholesterol is not considered a risk factor for heart disease over the age of 75.
2) Over age 75: screening depends on life expectancy and functional status.
3) Start niacin at low dose and gradually titrate up to avoid unpleasant side effects of flushing and headache. Advise to take with food and warn patient about side effects. Side effects usually fade by 2 weeks. Can be taken with ibuprofen 30 minutes before to minimize them.

CONGESTIVE HEART FAILURE (CHF)

Left Ventricular Failure

Crackles, cough, decreased breath sounds, dullness to percussion
Paroxysmal nocturnal dyspnea, orthopnea

Right Ventricular Failure

JVD (jugular venous distention), enlarged liver, enlarged spleen
Anorexia, nausea, abdominal pain, lower extremity edema

Summary

Here is an easy way to remember whether a sign or symptom is from the left or right side of the heart: Both *left* and *lung* start with the letter L. Therefore, any question asking you to identify a sign/symptom is made easier. Left is for *lung* and right is the GI tract (by default).

DEEP VEIN THROMBOSIS (DVT)

Thrombi develop inside the deep venous system of the legs or pelvis secondary to stasis, trauma to vessel walls, inflammation, or increased coagulation.

Etiology of DVT (divided into three categories)

1) Venous stasis: prolonged travel/inactivity, bedrest, CHF.
2) Inherited coagulation disorders: Factor C deficiency, Leiden, and so forth.
3) Increased coagulation due to external factors: OC use, pregnancy, bone fractures especially of the long bones, trauma, recent surgery, malignancy.

Classic Case

An adult or elderly patient complains of gradual onset of swelling on a lower extremity after a history of travel (>3 hours) or prolonged sitting. The patient complains of a painful lower extremity that is red and warm.

Treatment Plan

Homan's Sign: lower leg pain on dorsiflexion of the foot
CBC, platelets, clotting time (PT/PTT, INR)
Contrast venography (gold standard)
B-mode ultrasound with Doppler flow study, MRI (magnetic resonance imaging)
Hospital admission, heparin IV; then warfarin po (Coumadin) for 3 to 6 months (first episode) or longer. For recurrent DVT or elderly, antithrombotic treatment may last a lifetime

Complications

1) Pulmonary emboli
2) Stroke and other embolic episodes

Exam Tips

1) A case of DVT will have a positive Homan's sign (in the exam). In real-life practice, most cases of DVT are asymptomatic.
2) Choose *low-tech* procedures (i.e., ankle and brachial BP) over invasive or expensive tests unless the low-tech procedure has already been done.

SUPERFICIAL THROMBOPHLEBITIS

Inflammation of a superficial vein due to local trauma. Higher risk if indwelling catheters, intravenous drugs (i.e., potassium), secondary bacterial infection (*Staphylococcus aureus*).

Classic Case

Adult patient complains of an acute onset of a painful and warm vein on an extremity. The patient is afebrile with normal vital signs.

Objective

Indurated cordlike vein that is warm and tender to touch with a surrounding area of erythema.

Treatment Plan

NSAIDs (nonsteroidal anti-inflammatory drugs) such as ibuprofen or naproxen sodium (Anaprox DS) BID. Warm compresses. Elevate limb. If septic cause, admit to hospital.

PERIPHERAL VASCULAR DISEASE (OCCLUSIVE ARTERIAL DISEASE)

Gradual narrowing and/or occlusion of medium to large arteries in the lower extremities. Blood flow to the extremities gradually decreases over time resulting in permanent ischemic damage (sometimes gangrene). Higher risk with hypertension, smoking, diabetes, and hyperlipidemia.

Classic Case

Older patient who has a history of smoking and hyperlipidemia complains of worsening pain on ambulation (intermittent claudication) that is instantly relieved by rest. Over time, the symptoms worsen until the patient's walking distance is greatly limited.

Objective

Skin: atrophic changes (shiny and hyperpigmented ankles that are hairless and cool to touch

CV (cardiovascular): decreased to absent dorsal pedal pulse (may include popliteal and posterior tibial pulse), increased capillary refill time, and bruits over partially blocked arteries

Treatment Plan

Initial method (low tech): ankle and brachial BP before and after exercise

Diagnostic tests: Doppler ultrasound flow study, angiography

Smoking cessation (smoking causes vasoconstriction) and daily ambulation exercises

Pentoxifylline (Trental) if indicated. Percutaneous angioplasty or surgery for severe cases

Complications

1) Gangrene of foot and/or lower limb with amputation

RAYNAUD'S PHENOMENON

Reversible vasospasm of the peripheral arterioles on the fingers and toes. Cause is unknown. Associated with an increased risk of autoimmune disorders (i.e., thyroid disorder, pernicious anemia, rheumatoid arthritis). Most patients are females (60 to 90%) with a gender ratio 8:1.

Classic Case

An adult to middle-aged woman complains of episodes of color changes on her fingertips. The colors range from blue, white, and red and is accompanied by numbness and tingling. Attacks last for several hours. Hands and feet become numb with very cold temperatures.

Treatment Plan

1) Avoid touching cold objects, cold weather.

2) Smoking cessation. Nifedipine (Norvasc), captopril (Capoten).
3) Do not use any vasoconstricting drugs (i.e., Imitrex, ergots), beta-blockers, and so forth.

Complications

1) Small ulcers in the fingertips and toes,

Exam Tip

1) Think of the colors of the American flag as a reminder of this disorder.

BACTERIAL ENDOCARDITIS

Bacterial infection of the endocardial surface of the heart. Presentation ranges from full-blown disease to subacute endocarditis. Bacterial pathogens are gram positives (i.e., viridans strep, staph aureus, etc.). Also known as infective endocarditis.

Higher Risk

Poor dental hygiene
Prosthetic valvular implants
Mitral valve prolapse
IV drug users

Classic Case

Adult middle-aged male presents with fever, chills, and malaise that are associated with skin findings (mostly on the fingers/hands and toes/feet).

Objective

Nails: splinter hemorrhages on the nailbed (subungal hemorrhages)
Mouth: petechiae on the palate
Fingers and toes: painful violet-colored nodes on the fingers or feet (Osler nodes)
Palms/soles: tender red spots on the skin (Janeway lesions)
A heart murmur may be present on cardiac exam

Treatment Plan

Blood cultures × 3 (first 24 hours) with C&S
Transesophageal ultrasound, echocardiogram

CBC with differential: leukocytosis
Sedimentation rate: elevated
RF (rheumatoid factor): positive

Treatment Plan

IV antibiotic with penicillin, gentamicin, vancomycin, and so forth.

Complications

1) Valvular destruction.
2) Abscess (myocardium).
3) Emboli, and so forth.

Endocarditis Prophylaxis

High-Risk Patients
Mitral valve prolapse with thickened redundant leaflets
Prosthetic heart valves (bioprosthetic and homografts)
Hypertrophic cardiomyopathy and so forth

High-Risk Procedures
Dental (i.e., cleaning, root canals)
Certain types of respiratory or throat surgery (i.e., tonsillectomy, bronchoscopy)
Certain GU procedures (i.e., prostatectomy, vaginal hysterectomy), terminations

Standard Regimen
Adults: amoxicillin 2 g po 1 hour before procedure
Younger than age 18: amoxicillin 50 mg/kg 1 hour before procedure

Penicillin Allergy
One hour before procedure: clindamycin 600 mg or clarithromycin (Biaxin) 500 mg or cephalexin (Keflex) 2 g.

*Adapted from American Heart Association Guidelines, 1997.

MITRAL VALVE PROLAPSE

Normal sinus rhythm associated with an S2 "click" followed by a systolic murmur. More common in tall and thin adult females. Higher risk of thromboemboli and bacterial endocarditis. If thickened redundant leaflets, needs endocarditis prophylaxis. Diagnosed by cardiac ultrasound.

Classic Case

Adult female patient complains of fatigue, palpitations, lightheadedness that is aggravated by heavy exertion. May be asymptomatic.

CARDIAC ARRHYTHMIAS

Paroxysmal Atrial Tachycardia

Tachycardia with peaked QRS complex and p waves present. May be terminated with carotid massage, calcium-channel or beta blockers. Heart rate ranges from 100 to 250 beats/minute. Cause: digitalis toxicity, hyperthyroid, and so forth. An uncommon arrhythmia.

Classic Case

Patient complains of palpitations, lightheadedness, dyspnea, and so on.

Atrial Fibrillation

An irregularly irregular rhythm with no p waves seen on the EKG. Heart rate ranges from 80 to 180 beats/minute. Common arrhythmia.

Cause: heart disease, hyperthyroid, excess alcohol or stimulants, and so forth.

Classic Case

Patient may be asymptomatic or may complain of palpitations, dyspnea, angina, and so forth.

Exam Tips

1) No EKG strips are included in the exam.
2) Atrial fibrillation and paroxysmal atrial tachycardia (PAT) are usually in the exams.
3) PAT and AF have many causes, such as alcohol intoxication, hyperthyroid, stimulants such as theophylline, decongestants, cocaine, heart disease.

HYPERLIPIDEMIA

Screening Guidelines

1) Complete lipid profile (fasting) every 5 years starting at age 20.
2) Over age 40 years, screen every 2 to 3 years.
3) Preexisting hyperlipidemia, screen annually or more frequently.

Total Cholesterol

Normal: <199 mg/dL
Borderline: between 200 and 239 mg/dL
High: >240 mg/dL

HDL (high-density lipoprotein)

HDL: >40 mg/dL

- If <40 mg/dL, associated with Increased risk of CAD even if normal LDL or cholesterol

LDL (low-density lipoprotein)

LDL: <130 mg/dL for low-risk patients with fewer than 2 risk factors

Triglycerides

Normal: <150 mg/dL

High risk of acute pancreatitis: >500 mg/dL

If a patient with high cholesterol also has high triglycerides, must treat hyper-triglyceremia first before LDL or total cholesterol.

Coronary Risk Equivalent

High risk: defined as a coronary heart disease risk of >20% (chances of an MI over next 10 years is 20%). These patients are treated the same as if they had preexisting heart disease. Diabetes is a coronary risk equivalent. Therefore, their goal is an LDL <100 mg/dL.

*Adapted from the Third Report of the Expert Panel on Detection, Evaluation and Treatment of High Blood Cholesterol in Adults (2001).

Exam Tips

You must memorize some values. These are (not inclusive):

1) Borderline cholesterol, high cholesterol, HDL, LDL goal for CHD or DM.
2) Low HDL (<40 mg/dL) is a risk factor of CHD even though total cholesterol, triglyceride and LDL are normal.

Risk Factors: Heart Disease

1) Hypertension
2) Family history of premature heart disease (women with MI before age <65 years or men with MI age <55 years)
3) Diabetes mellitus (considered a CHD risk equivalent even if patient has no history of preexisting heart disease)
4) Dyslipidemia
5) Low HDL cholesterol: <40mg/dL
6) Age (men older than 45 or women older than 55)
7) Cigarette smoker
8) Obesity (BMI $\geq$30 kg/m^2)
9) Microalbuminuria

*Adapted from JNC 7 (May 2003)

Treatment Plan: Hyperlipidemia

1) Lifestyle changes such as weight loss, exercise most days of the week, better diet low in saturated fat, smoking cessation.
2) Encourage use of soluble fiber in diet (i.e., psyllium, fruit, vegetables) to enhance lowering of LDL (lowers LDL by blocking absorption in GI tract up to 10%).
3) If no changes in lipids after a trial of 6 months of lifestyle changes, consider antilipidemic drugs if >2 risk factors.

Treatment Goal

1) Decrease LDL first except if patient has very high triglyceride levels (high risk of acute pancreatitis).
2) High triglyceride levels >500 mg/dL must be treated first before treating high LDL level.

American Heart Association: Therapeutic Lifestyle Changes Diet

Cholesterol: less than 200 mg per day

Total fat: 25 to 35%

Saturated fat: less than 7%

Monounsaturated fat: up to 20%

Polyunsaturated fat: up to 10%

Carbs: 50% to 60% should be from complex carbohydrate foods (i.e., whole grains, fruits and vegetables)

Protein: 15% (soy can replace some animal products)

Medications

Patient Education

1) Do not drink alcohol while on these drugs because it increases hepatotoxicity. Avoid prescribing to alcoholics.
2) Advise patient to report symptoms of hepatitis or rhabdomyolysis. Stop taking drug if suspect reaction.
3) Rhabdomyolysis: muscle pain and aches that persist and are not associated with muscular exertion.
   Labs: order CPK and LFTs (will be elevated)
4) Acute hepatitis: anorexia, nausea, dark colored urine, jaundice, fatigue
   Labs: order LFTs (elevated ALT (SGPT) and AST (SGOT)

HMG CoA Reductase Inhibitors (statins)

Pravastatin (Pravachol), lovastatin (Mevacor), simvastatin (Zocor), others

Best agent for decreasing LDL. Some statins also elevate HDL (i.e., Zocor)

Increased risk of hepatitis or rhabdomyolysis (rare) if on combination therapy with fibrates or nicotinic acid

Side effects: hepatic toxicity, rhabdomyolysis (breakdown of skeletal muscle = acute renal failure)

Nicotinic Acid

Niacin (over the counter) daily to TID, Niaspan (slow-release niacin) daily

Very good agent for lowering triglycerides and elevating HDL level

Combining this drug with statins, fibrates, or alcohol increases risk of hepatotoxicity

Side effects: flushing, itching, tingling, hepatotoxicity; GI effects such as abdominal pain

Fibrates

Gemfibrozil (Lopid), fenofibrate (Tricor)

Great for reducing triglycerides and elevating HDL

Combining this drug with statins, niacin, or alcohol increases risk of hepatotoxicity

Side effects: hepatic and renal effects

Bile Acid Sequestrants

Cholestyramine (Questran Light), colestipol (Colestid), colesevelam (WelChol)

Work locally in the small intestines to interfere with the absorption of fats

May be used in combination with other medications (statins, fibrates, niacin) without increasing risk for hepatotoxicity. An alternative drug for patients who cannot tolerate statins, fibrates, and niacin. Not as effective as other agents. No hepatotoxicity

Interferes with absorption: fat-soluble vitamins (take MVI tabs daily), tetracycline, digoxin, others

Side effects: bloating, flatulence, abdominal pain. Start at low doses and titrate up slowly

PULMONARY SYSTEM

Fast Facts | Danger Signals

Pulmonary Emboli (PE)

Older adult complains of sudden onset of dyspnea and coughing. Cough may be productive of pink-tinged frothy sputum. Other symptoms are tachycardia, pallor, and feelings of impending doom. Any condition that increases risk of blood clots will increase risk of PE. These patients have a history of atrial fibrillation, estrogens, surgery, pregnancy, long bone fractures, and prolonged inactivity.

Impending Respiratory Failure (asthmatic patient)

Asthmatic patient presents with tachypnea (>25/min) tachycardia or brady cardia, cyanosis, and anxiety. The patient appears exhausted, fatigued and diaphoretic and uses accessory muscles to help with breathing. Physical exam reveals cyanosis and "quiet" lungs with no wheezing or breath sounds audible.

Treatment

Adrenaline injection stat. Call 911. Oxygen at 4–5 L/min., albuterol nebulizer treatments, parenteral steroids and antihistamines (diphenhydramine and cimetidine).

After treatment, a good sign is if breath sounds and wheezing are present (a sign that bronchi are becoming more open). Usually discharge with oral steroids for several days (i.e., Medrol Dose Pack).

Fast Facts | Normal Findings

Normal Findings

Lower lobes: vesicular breath sounds (soft and low)
Upper lobes: bronchial breath sounds (louder)

Egophony

Normal: will hear "eee" clearly instead of "bah"
Abnormal: will hear "bah" sound
Normal: the "eee" sound is louder over the large bronchi because larger airways are better at transmitting sounds. The lower lobes have a softer sounding "eee"

Tactile Fremitus

Instruct patient to say "99" or "1,2,3." Use finger pads to palpate lungs and feel for vibrations.

Normal: stronger vibrations palpable on the upper lobes and softer vibrations on lower lobes.

Abnormal: the findings are reversed. May palpate stronger vibrations on one lower lobe (i.e., consolidation). Asymmetrical findings are always abnormal.

Percussion

Normal: resonance
Tympany or hyperresonance: COPD, emphysema (overinflation)
Dull tone: bacterial pneumonia with lobar consolidation, pleural effusion (fluid or tumor)
Use middle finger or index finger as the pleximeter finger on one hand. The finger on the other hand is the hammer. The liver sounds dull. The stomach area may be tympanic

Whispered Pectoriloquy

Normal: voice louder and easy to understand in the upper lobes. The voice is muffled and harder to understand on the lower lobes

Abnormal: clear voice sounds in the lower lobes or muffled sounds on the upper lobes

Instruct patient to whisper "one, two, three." Compare both lungs

---

Fast Facts Disease Review

CHRONIC OBSTRUCTIVE PULMONARY DISEASE (COPD)

COPD is a term that includes both emphysema and chronic bronchitis. Most patients have a mixture of both; one or the other may predominate. The disease is characterized by the loss of elastic recoil of the lungs and alveolar damage that takes decades. The most common risk factor is chronic cigarette smoking and older age. Currently, COPD affects 14 to 16 million Americans and is projected to increase as the baby boomer generation gets older.

Chronic Bronchitis

Defined as coughing with excessive mucus production for at least three or more months for a minimum of two or more consecutive years.

Emphysema

Permanent alveolar damage and loss of elastic recoil results in chronic hyperinflation of the lungs. Expiratory respiratory phase is markedly prolonged.

Risk Factors
■ Chronic smoking (etiology in up to 90% of cases of COPD), older age (>40)
■ Occupational exposure (coal dust, grain dust)
■ Alpha-1 trypsin deficiency: rare condition. Patients have severe lung damage at earlier ages. Alpha-1 trypsin protects lungs from oxidative and environmental damage

Classic Case

Elderly male with a history of many years of cigarette smoking complains of gradually worsening dyspnea over several years that is starting to limit physical activity. The patient complains of getting easily short of breath upon physical exertion. Accompanied by a chronic cough that is productive of large amounts of white to light yellow sputum.

Objective

Emphysema component: increased AP (anterior-posterior) diameter or barrel chest, decreased breath and heart sounds, hypoxia especially at night in sleep, weight loss

Percussion: hyperresonance

Tactile fremitus and egophony: decreased
Chest x-ray: flattened diaphragms with hyperinflation
Chronic bronchitis component: productive cough, wheezing and coarse crackles
Acute exacerbations: fever, purulent sputum, increased symptoms of wheezing and dyspnea
Treatment: Bactrim DS, Augmentin, Ceftin, Floxin BID × 10 days, Medrol Dose Pack PRN

Treatment: COPD

1) Ipratropium (Atrovent) QID (anticholinergic)
2) Add albuterol (short-acting B2 agonist) inhaler or atrovent/albuterol mix (Combivent)
3) Add long-acting theophylline (Theo-Dur) (serum levels 8 to 12 mcg/mL)
4) Start oxygen therapy by nasal cannula at 2 to 3 L/minute
5) Consider prednisone (10 to 14 days) for exacerbations (up to 10% benefit)

Start oxygen therapy earlier. Usually started at bedtime (oxygen desaturation worsens in the night). It is the only therapy for COPD shown in studies to prolong life.

Exam Tips

1) Ipratropium (Atrovent) is an anticholinergic.
2) The only treatment known to prolong life in COPD patients is supplemental oxygen therapy.

BACTERIAL PNEUMONIA

Bacterial lung infection results in inflammatory changes and damage to the lungs. The bacteria causing the most deaths in outpatients is the pneumococcus (gram positive).

Organisms

Streptococcus pneumoniae or *Pneumococcus* (gram positive)
Haemophilus influenzae: more common in smokers (gram negative)
Mycoplasma or *Chlamydia pneumoniae* (atypical bacteria), others

Classic Case

Middle-aged to elderly adult complains of a sudden onset of fever, chills, and a productive cough. The phlegm is a green to rusty color. The patient complains of pleuritic chest pain with coughing and appears tired and ill.

Objective

Auscultation: crackles and decreased breath sounds (affected lobe)
Tactile fremitus: increased
Abnormal whispered pectoriloquy (whispered words louder)
Percussion: Dullness over affected lobe

Labs

Sputum for gram stain and culture, chest x-ray (gold standard), complete blood count (CBC)

CBC: leukocytosis (>10.5) with a possible "shift to the left" (increased band forms). Seen more in serious bacterial infections

Chest x-ray:

- Lobar consolidation or diffuse patchy infiltrates
- If smoker or high risk, repeat chest x-ray post-treatment (8 to 10 weeks) because it may be a presenting sign of lung cancer (due to mass blocking bronchioles)

American Thoracic Society (ATS) Guidelines for Outpatient Community-Acquired Pneumonia (CAP)*

Below Age 60 With No Comorbidity (i.e., asthma, diabetes, heart disease)

1) Macrolides are preferred
   - Clarithromycin (Biaxin) BID × 10 days
   - Azithromycin (Z-Pack) daily × 5 days
   - Erythromycin QID × 10 days

Ages 60 Years or older and Younger Patients With Comorbidity

1) Second generation cephalosporin or IM Ceftriaxone preferred
   - Cefuroxime axetil (Ceftin) BID × 10 to 14 days
   - Amoxicillin clavulanate (Augmentin) BID × 10 to 14 days
2) Consider adding a macrolide or doxycycline if high suspicion of atypical bacterial infection
3) OR antipneumococcal quinolone as ONE drug therapy
   - Levaquin 500 mg QD × 7 to 14 days

Pneumococcal Vaccine (Pneumovax)

Healthy patients:
- Single dose usually sufficient at age 65 years (lifetime)
- 60% to 70% effectiveness

Underlying disease:
- 50% effective

---

* Adapted from the American Thoracic Society CAP Guidelines (2001).

Severely immunocompromised:

■ Only 10% effective

Recommended for:
1) Persons aged 65 years or older
   ■ Nursing home residents
2) Preexisting heart and lung disease
   ■ Asthma, congenital heart disease, emphysema, others
3) Impaired immunity
   ■ Alcoholics/cirrhosis of the liver
   ■ Splenectomy or asplenia
   ■ HIV infection
   ■ Chronic renal failure
4) Blood disorders
   ■ Sickle cell anemia
   ■ Hodgkin's lymphoma, multiple myeloma

High-Risk Patients
Repeat vaccine in 5 to 7 years (boosts antibodies):

■ HIV infection
■ Asplenia, chronic renal failure
■ Blood cancers: lymphoma, Hodgkin's disease, leukemia
■ Organ transplant patients (immunosuppressive therapy)

ATYPICAL PNEUMONIA

An infection of the lungs by atypical bacteria. More common in children and young adults. Seasonal outbreaks. Also known as "walking pneumonia."

Organisms

Mycoplasma pneumoniae (atypical bacteria)
Chlamydia pneumoniae (atypical bacteria)
Legionella pneumoniae (atypical bacteria): found in areas with moisture such as air conditioners (more severe with higher mortality)

Classic Case

A teenage to young adult complains of several weeks of fatigue and severe coughing that is mostly nonproductive. Gradual onset of symptoms. Illness started with a sore throat, clear rhinitis, and low-grade fever. Complains of malaise. Continues to go to work/school despite symptoms. May have co-workers with same symptoms.

Objective

Auscultation: wheezing and diffused crackles/rales
Nose: clear mucus
Throat: red with no pus
Chest x-ray: diffuse interstitial infiltrates

Medications

1) Macrolides:
   - Azithromycin (Z-Pack) × 5 days
   - Clarithromycin (Biaxin) 500 mg BID × 10 days
   - Erythromycin stearate 500 mg QID × 10 days
2) Antitussives (dextromethorphan, Tessalon perles) as needed (PRN).
3) Increase fluids and rest.

Poor Prognosis: Pneumonia

1) Elderly: age 60 years or older.
2) Multiple lobar involvement.
3) Leukopenia.
4) Alcoholics (aspiration pneumonia).

ACUTE BRONCHITIS

Acute viral or bacterial infection of the bronchi causes inflammatory changes that result in increased reactivity of the upper airways. Mainly manifested with dry cough that may last from 4 to 6 weeks.

Classic Case

Young adult complains of frequent episodes of severe cough that is nonproductive or productive of a small amount of phlegm. May complain of mild wheezing. Cough keeps patient awake at night. Patient complains of chest pain from severe coughing.

Objective

Lungs: ranges from clear to severe wheezing. Normal or prolonged expiration
Percussion: resonant
Chest x-ray: normal
Afebrile to low-grade fever

Treatment Plan

1) Treatment is symptomatic. Increase fluids and rest. Stop smoking (if smoker).
2) Dextromethorphan (Robitussin), Tessalon perles (antitussives) PRN for cough.

Table 3.5	Common Lung Infections

Disease	Signs and Symptoms
Acute Bacterial Pneumonia (Community-acquired or CAP) *Strep. pneumoniae* (G. Pos.) *Mycoplasma pneum.* (G. Neg.)	Acute onset. High fever and chills. Productive cough & large amount of green to rusty-colored sputum. Chest pain w/cough. Crackles; decreased breath sounds. CBC: leukocytosis; elevated neutrophils. Band forms may be seen. CXR: lobar consolidation
Atypical Pneumonia Macrolide antibiotics *Mycoplasma pneumoniae*	Gradual onset. Low grade fever. Headache, Sore throat. Cough. Wheezing. Sometimes, rash. CXR: interstitial to patchy infiltrates
Viral Pneumonia Influenza, RSV (respiratory synctial virus) Prophylactic antibiotics Common: secondary infection with bacteria	Fever. Cough. Pleurisy. Shortness of breath. Scanty sputum production. Myalgias. Breath sounds: decreased breath sounds. Rales. CXR: patchy to interstitial infiltrates
Acute Bronchitis Symptomatic treatment only. *No* antibiotics. Antitussives, mucolytics (guaifenesin)	Starts with coldlike symptoms: sore throat, runny nose. Progresse to paroxysms of dry and severe cough. Can last up to 4 to 6 weeks.
Allergic Rhinitis Antihistamines, nasal steroid sprays, decongestants (oral) Antihistamine nasal spray (Astelin)	Nasal stuffiness. Itchy nose. Clear mucus. Sneezing. Tearing. Itchy eyes. Postnasal drip cough worse when supine.

Note. Adapted from the ATS (American Thoracic Society) CAP Guidelines (2001).

3) Guaifenesin (expectorant/mucolytic) PRN.
4) Albuterol inhaler (Ventolin) QID or nebulized treatment for wheezing.

Complications

1) Exacerbation of asthma (increased risk of status asthmaticus).

Classic Findings: Respiratory Infections

Bacterial pneumonia:
- Sudden onset, toxic, fever
- Cough productive of green to rusty-colored sputum

Atypical pneumonia:
- Gradual onset, low-grade fever
- Always tired but continues working
- Cough

Acute bronchitis:
- Frequent paroxysms of dry cough in a young adult
- Usually afebrile

Exam Tips

1) Recognize a classic case of bacterial pneumonia compared to atypical pneumonia.
2) Preferred treatment for atypical pneumonia is macrolides (azithromycin, erythromycin).
3) Do not pick antibiotics as a treatment option for acute bronchitis.

Clinical Tips

1) Pneumovax vaccine is underutilized. Offer vaccine to high-risk patients and repeat dose in 5 to 7 years if immunocompromised.
2) Emphasize importance of adequate fluid intake (thins out mucus).

COMMON COLD (VIRAL UPPER RESPIRATORY INFECTION)

A mild viral upper respiratory infection caused by up to 200 different types of viruses (i.e., rhinovirus and adenovirus). Self-limiting infection (range of 4 to 10 days). Most contagious from day 2 to day 3. More common in crowded areas and in small children.

Transmission is by respiratory droplets and fomites. The common cold occurs throughout the year, but most cases occur in the winter months.

Classic Case

Patient complains of an acute onset of sneezing accompanied by nasal itchiness that progresses to a sore throat. Nasal congestion, runny eyes, and clear mucoid rhinitis (coryza) follows shortly, along with a low-grade fever and malaise.

Objective

Nasal turbinates: swollen with clear mucus
Anterior pharynx: reddened
Cervical nodes: smooth, mobile, and small or "shotty" nodes (0.5 cm size or less) in the submandibular and anterior cervical chain
Lungs: clear

Treatment Plan

Symptomatic treatment. Increase fluids and rest
Oral decongestants (i.e., pseudoephedrine/Sudafed) PRN
Antitussives (i.e., dextromethorphan/Robitussin) PRN
Antihistamines (i.e., diphenhydramine/Benadryl) PRN
Frequent handwashing

Complications

1) Acute sinusitis.
2) Acute otitis media.

TUBERCULOSIS (TB)

A lung infection caused by mycobacterium tuberculosis bacteria. Transmission is through respiratory droplets. Most common site of infection is the lungs (85%). Other sites include the kidneys, brain, lymph nodes, adrenals, and bone. TB infection is controlled by an intact immune system. Macrophages sequester the bacteria in the lymph nodes (mediastinum) in the form of granulomas.

The majority of cases (90%) of active disease in the United States are reactivated infections. Reactivation occurs when the immune system is compromised or is less active (child below age 3 years and elderly).

Miliary Tuberculosis

Also known as *disseminated TB disease*. Infects multiple organ systems. More common in younger children (below the age of 5) and the elderly. Chest x-ray will show classic "milia seed" pattern.

Classic Case

Immunocompromised adult patient complains of fevers, anorexia, fatigue, and night sweats along with a mild nonproductive cough (early phase). Aggressive infections (later sign) will have productive cough with blood-stained sputum (hemoptysis) along with weight loss (late sign).

Labs

Screening: PPD (purified protein derivative) subdermally (Mantoux test)
Tine test is not acceptable test for screening
Sputum culture and AFB (acid fast bacilli) stain (takes from 3 to 6 weeks)

Treatment Plan

1) Active disease: use three drugs initially because of higher rates of resistant strains against INH (isoniazid) and rifampin. Narrow down number of medications only after C&S results. Treat a minimum of 6 months until culture negative.
2) HIV: treat for at least 12 months and culture negative.
3) Ethambutal (causes optic neuritis). Avoid in patients with abnormal vision (i.e., blindness, retinal vein occlusion, and so forth).

DOT (direct observed treatment)

Highly recommended for pediatric and noncompliant patients

How: patient is observed by a nurse when he or she takes the medications. Mouth, cheek, and area under the tongue checked to make sure the pill was swallowed adequately

Recent PPD Converters

Recent converters: defined as person with history of negative PPD results who then converts to a positive (becomes infected)

At higher risk of active TB disease (up to 10%) in the first 1 to 2 years after seroconversion.

Prophylaxis:
- Offer if under age 35 with no history liver disease or alcohol abuse
- Prophylaxis not recommended if older than age 35; higher risk of drug hepatitis

INH 300 mg daily × 6 months. If HIV positive, treat for at least 12 months

Also give pyridoxine (vitamin B6) if on INH. Order baseline liver function tests (LFTs)

Before Prophylaxis

Chest x-ray must be negative with no signs/symptoms of active TB disease.

History of BCG (bacille Calmette-Guerin) Vaccination

Affects PPD testing adversely with higher risk of false positive results. Commonly given to patients from areas where TB is endemic (Asia, Africa, Latin America).

Anergy Testing

Used for patients suspected of being immunocompromised to rule out false-negative result (immune system too weak to respond even if positive for TB disease).

Procedure

1) The PPD is administered on the volar aspect of the left lower arm (as usual) and the "control" antigen is given on the right lower arm. "Control" agents used are tetanus, candida, or mumps antigens.
2) Do not mix the two. Use tuberculin syringe to administer each agent.

3) If control side is negative, unable to do PPD (invalid result). Consider other methods for detecting infection (i.e., bronchoscopy).

Booster Phenomenon

Two-step testing:
- Recommended for elderly
- Reduces incidence of false-negative PPDs

Elderly patient's immune system "forgets" how to react to the PPD antigens

When given a second dose of PPD in 7 to 10 days, helps decrease false negatives

Explanation

1) A person is negative after many years of no PPD testing.
2) When redone again (first time), there is no reaction (false negative).
3) If PPD repeated in 7 to 10 days, it will be positive (if TB infection present). Otherwise, if still a negative, more likely to be a true negative result.

PPD Testing Results (Mantoux)

Look for an induration (feels harder). The red color is not as important. If a PPD result is a bright red color but is not indurated (skin feels soft), it is a negative result.

≥5 mm

- HIV (+)
- Positive chest x-ray findings or close contact with a person with active TB
- Any child with TB symptoms (especially before the age of 5)

≥10 mm:

- Immunocompromised (i.e., chemo, bone marrow transplant, renal failure, diabetes, others)
- Intravenous (IV) drug user, health care worker, prisoner, homeless
- Comes from a high-prevalence country (Asia, Latin America, Africa, India)

Exam Tips

1) A PPD result may be listed as 9.5 mm. It is a negative (by definition) unless the patient has the signs/symptoms and/or chest x-ray findings suggestive of TB.
2) Memorize the criteria for the 10-mm results
3) Small children exposed to active TB have a high chance of coming down with the disease.

ASTHMA

Chronic inflammation of the bronchial tree results in increased airway responsiveness to stimuli (internal or external). Reversible airway obstruction. Genetic predisposition with positive family history of allergies, eczema, and allergic rhinitis. Exacerbations can be life-threatening (status asthmaticus).

Classic Case

Young to middle-aged patient complains of worsening symptoms after a recent bout of a viral upper respiratory infection. Complains of shortness of breath, wheezing, and chest tightness that is sometimes accompanied by a dry cough in the early morning (i.e., 3:00 a.m.). The patient reports increasing the frequency of albuterol inhaler usage to self-treat symptoms.

Trigger Factors for Asthma

Viral URIs, airborne allergens
Food allergies: sulfites, red and yellow dye, seafood
Cold air or cold weather and fumes from chemicals or smoke
Emotional stress and exercise (exercise-induced asthma)
GERD (reflux of acidic gastric contents irritates airways)
ASA or NSAIDs

Objective

Wheezing with prolonged expiratory phase. As asthma worsens, the wheezing occurs during both inspiration and expiration.

Exacerbations

Nebulizer treatments using albuterol/saline solution. May repeat in 15 minutes if poor relief of symptoms. If unable to reverse attack, call 911. Epinephrine stat.
   Discharge home with Medrol Dose Pack or prednisone tabs 40 mg per day ×
4 days (no weaning necessary if 4 days or less).

Maintenance Medications

Inhaled corticosteroid BID
Depending on severity of asthma, can add leukotriene inhibitors (Singulair), mast
   cell stabilizers (great for kids), long-acting B2 agonist mixture (salmeterol
   combined with corticosteroid), and/or sustained-release theophylline
Respiratory distress: tachypnea, using accessory muscles (intercostals, abdominal) to breathe, diaphoresis, fatigue

Exam Tips

1) First-line treatment for severe asthmatic exacerbation or respiratory distress is an adrenaline injection.
2) Severe respiratory distress: tachypnea, disappearance of or lack of wheezing, accessory muscle use, diaphoresis, and exhaustion.

Treatment Algorithm: Asthma*

Step 1: Mild Intermittent
▦ Albuterol (Ventolin) metered dose inhaler as needed

Step 2: Mild Persistent Asthma
▦ Albuterol (Ventolin) metered dose inhaler

PLUS
▦ Low dose steroid metered dose inhaler
▦ And/or cromolyn/nedocromil (Intal inhaler)
Consider sustained release theophylline (5 to 5 mcg/mL).

Step 3: Moderate Persistent Asthma
▦ Albuterol metered dose inhaler
PLUS
▦ Low to medium-dose steroid metered dose inhaler mixed with salmeterol (i.e., Advair)
OR
▦ Leukotriene inhibitors (i.e., Singulair), theophylline

Exercise-induced Asthma
Premedicate 20 minutes before the activity with 2 puffs of an inhaled steroid or mast cell stabilizer.

Asthma Medications

"Rescue" Medicine
These drugs are used to relieve wheezing as needed (PRN).
1) Short-acting B2 agonists MDI (metered dose inhalers) or by nebulizer
   ▦ Albuterol (Ventolin) or pirbuterol (Alupent) 2 inhalations every 4 to 6 hours PRN
   ▦ Levalbuterol (Xopenex) nebulizer solution
2) Quick onset (15 to 30 minutes) and last about 4 to 6 hours.
   ▦ Used to relieve symptoms (wheezing) but does not treat underlying inflammation

---

* Expert Panel Report II: Guidelines for the Diagnosis and Management of Asthma, Feb. 1997.

Maintenance Medications

1) These drugs are anti-inflammatories. They must be taken daily to be effective.
   - Steroids: triamcinolone (Azmacort) BID, etc.
   - Mast cell stabilizers: cromolyn sodium (Intal) QID
   - Leukotriene inhibitors: zafirlukast (Singulair)
2) The only exception is this is the long-acting B2 agonist formoterol (Foradil) BID.
3) Long-acting B2 agonists are *not* rescue drugs. Although taken daily, they are used to relieve bronchospasm. Slow onset of action (3 hours); use daily to maintain a blood level.

Theophylline (Theo-24)

Drug class: methylxanthine or xanthine
Now used as third-line drug for asthma because of risk of toxicity and multiple drug interactions such as the following:
   - Macrolides, quinolones
   - Cimetidine
   - Anticonvulsants such as phenytoin, carbamazepine (Tegretol)
   - Check blood levels: normal is 12 to 15 mg/dL

Asthma Treatment: In a Nutshell...

1) Every patient should be on a short-acting B2 agonist (albuterol) PRN.
2) For children: mast cell stabilizers (Intal, Tilade) work well (give 4-week trial).
3) Inhaled corticosteroids. Dose depends on class of asthma.

Leukotriene inhibitors, long-acting B2 agonist mixture (salmeterol combined with corticosteroid), and sustained-release theophylline are added depending on severity of asthma and the response.

Exam Tips

1) Do not confuse asthma "rescue" drugs with "maintenance" or "control" drugs.

Clinical Tips

1) Chronic use of high-dose inhaled steroids can cause osteoporosis, mild growth retardation in children, glaucoma, cataracts, immune suppression, HPA suppression, other effects.
2) Consider supplementing with calcium with vitamin D 1500 mg tabs QD for menopausal women and other high-risk patients (i.e., on long-term steroids).
3) Bone density testing, annual eye exams if long-term steroids (cataracts and glaucoma)
4) Monitor growth in children.

Peak Expiratory Flow (PEF)

Mnemonic: HAG
PEF is based on height (H), age (A), and gender (G), or HAG

Peak Expiratory Flow Rate: PEFR or PEF
Used by asthmatics to measure effectiveness of treatment, worsening symptoms and exacerbations. Correlates well with the FEV_1 (forced expiratory volume at 1 second).

Spirometer Parameters
Green Zone: 80% to 100% of expected volume
- Maintain or reduce medications

Yellow Zone: 50% to 80% of expected volume
- Maintenance therapy needs to be increased or patient is having an acute exacerbation

Red Zone: below 50% of expected

If after treatment, patient's PER still below 50% expected, call 911. If in respiratory distress, give epinephrine injection. Call 911.

Pulmonary Function Tests (PFTs)
Measures severity of obstructive or restrictive pulmonary dysfunction.

1) Obstructive dysfunction (reduction in airflow rates)
   - Asthma, COPD (chronic bronchitis and emphysema), bronchiectasis, others
2) Restrictive dysfunction (reduction of lung volume due to decreased lung compliance)
   - Pulmonary fibrosis, pleural disease, diaphragm obstruction, others

Exam Tips

1) Do not confuse the formula for the PEF with the BMI.
   PEF formula is based on: height, age and gender (or sex)
   BMI formula is based on height and weight

HEMATOLOGY

Fast Facts Danger Signals

Vitamin B12 Deficiency

Gradual onset of peripheral neuropathy starting in the hands and/or feet (or both) that slowly ascends. Other signs and symptoms of anemia seen (i.e., fatigue, pallor, glossitis). Peripheral smear reveals a macrocytic or megaloblastic anemia and multisegmented neutrophils.

Hodgkin's Lymphoma

Night sweats, fevers, and pain with ingestion of alcoholic drinks. Generalized itching not associated with hives. Painless and enlarged lymph nodes. Anorexia and weight loss. Higher incidence from teen and older adults (>50 years), males, and White people.

A cancer of the beta lymphocytes.

Acute Leukemia

Fever, fatigue, and weight loss. Bleeding gums, nosebleeds (epistaxis), pallor, easy bruising, petechiae, and so forth. Bone pain. A cancer of the hematopoietic progenitor cells.

Acute Hemorrhage

Sudden and rapid drop in the hemoglobin (<6 g/dL) and hematocrit values. Signs and symptoms of shock such as pallor, clammy skin, tachycardia, and hypotension are present.

Neutropenia

Frequent infections (especially bacterial). Fever, sore throat, oral thrush, and so forth.

Defined as an absolute neutrophil count of less than $1,500/mm^3$.

Thrombocytopenia

Easy bruising, bleeding gums, spontaneous nosebleeds, hematuria, and so forth. Normal Platelet count: $100,000/mm^3$. Platelet count $<20,000/mm^3$ increases risk of spontaneous bleeding.

Fast Facts | Laboratory Testing

Laboratory Norms

1) Hemoglobin
   Males: 13.0 to 18.0 g/dL
   Females: 12.0 to 16.0 g/dL
2) Hematocrit
   The proportion of red blood cells (RBCs) in 1 mL of plasma.
   Males: 37% to 49%
   Females: 36% to 46%

3) MCV (mean corpuscular volume)

A measure of the average size of the red blood cells in a sample of blood. Decreased in microcytic anemias. Elevated in macrocytic anemias

Normal: MCV 80 to 100 fL

4) MCHC (mean corpuscular Hgb concentration)

A measure of the average color of the red blood cells in a sample of blood. Decreased in iron-deficiency anemia and thalassemia. Normal in macrocytic anemias

Normal: 31.0 to 37.0 g/dL

5) MCH (mean corpuscular hemoglobin)

Indirect measure of the color of RBCs. Decreased values means pale or hypochromic RBCs. Decreased in iron-deficiency anemia and thalassemia. Normal with the macrocytic anemias

Normal: 25.0 to 35.0 pg/cell

6) TIBC (total iron binding capacity)

A measure of available transferrin that is left unbound (to iron). Transferrin is used to transport iron in the body. Elevated in iron-deficiency anemia. Normal in thalassemia, B12, and folate-deficiency anemia

Normal: 250 to 410 mcg/dL

7) Serum ferritin

The storage form of iron. Produced in the intestines. Stored in body tissue such as the spleen, liver, and bone marrow. Correlates with iron storage status in a healthy adult

Markedly decreased in iron-deficiency anemia but normal to high in thalassemia trait

Normal: 20 to 400 ng/mL

8) Serum iron

Decreased in iron-deficiency anemia. Normal to high in thalassemia and the macrocytic anemias. Not as sensitive as ferritin. Affected by recent blood transfusions. Avoid iron supplements 24 hours before testing

Normal: 50 to 175 mcg/dL

9) RDW (red cell distribution width)

A measure of the variability of the size of red blood cells in a given sample. Elevated in iron-deficiency anemia

10) Reticulocytes (also called stabs)

Immature red blood cells that still have their nuclei. After 24 hours in circulation, reticulocytes lose their nuclei and mature in a red blood cell (no nuclei). The bone marrow normally will release small amounts to replace damaged red blood cells. RBCs survive 120 days before being broken down by the spleen into iron and globulin (recycled) and bilirubin.

Normal: 0.5% to 2.5% (of total red cell count)

11) Reticulocytosis (>2.5%)

An elevation of reticulocytes is seen when the bone marrow is stimulated by supplementation of iron, folate, or B12 (after deficiency) and after acute bleeding episodes. Chronic bleeding does not cause elevation of the reticulocytes

If there is no reticulocytosis after an acute bleeding episode or after appropriate supplementation, considered abnormal. Rule out bone marrow failure

12) Serum folate and B12

Low values if deficiency exists. Deficiency will cause a macrocytic anemia

Normal folate level: 3.1 to 17.5 ng/mL

Normal B12 level: >250 pg/mL

White Blood Cells and Platelets

White cell differential: percentage of each type of leukocyte in a sample. The differential for each type of white blood cell should add up to 100%

Normal White Blood Cell count: 4.5 to 10.5 × 10^3 (4,500 to 10,5000/10 mm³)

- Neutrophils or segs (segmented neutrophils): 45% to 75%
- Band forms or stabs (immature neutrophils): 0% to 5%
- Lymphocytes: 16% to 46%
- Monocytes: 4% to 11%
- Eosinophils: 0% to 8%
- Basophils: 0% to 3%

Fast Facts Hemoglobin

Hemoglobin (high altitude): adaptation to oxygen-thin air (hypoxic conditions) in higher elevations by certain ethnic groups (Andean) is done by the bone marrow producing higher levels of hemoglobin in the circulation.

Heavy smokers and COPD: may have secondary polycythemia (versus polycythemia vera) with elevated levels of hemoglobin/hematocrit as a response by the body to chronic hypoxia.

Fast Facts Disease Review

ANEMIAS

Anemia is simply defined as a decrease in the hemoglobin/hematocrit value below the norm for the patient's age and gender.

Iron-Deficiency Anemia

Microcytic and hypochromic anemia (small and pale RBCs) cause by deficiency in iron.

The most common type of anemia in the world for all races, ages, and gender.

Table 3.6	Laboratory Findings: Anemia	
Type of Anemia	**Diagnostic Tests**	**Red Blood Cell Changes**
Iron Deficiency	**Ferritin/serum iron** ↓ TIBC ↑ RDW ↑ (red cell distribution width)	MCV < 80 (microcytic) MCHC ↓ (hypochromic) Poikilocytosis (variable shapes) Anisocytosis (variable sizes)
Thalassemia Minor	**Hemoglobin electrophoresis**	MCV < 80 (microcytic) MCHC ↓ (hypochromic)
Pernicious Anemia	**Antiparietal antibodies** ↑	MCV > 100 (macrocytic) Megaloblastic RBCs Normal color (normochromic)
Folate Deficiency	**Folate level** ↓	MCV > 100 (macrocytic) Megaloblastic RBCs Normal color (normochromic)
B12 Deficiency	**B12 level** ↓ Hypersegmented Neutrophils	MCV > 100 (macrocytic) Megaloblastic RBCs Normal color (normochromic)
Normocytic Anemia	**MCV between 80 and 100** History of chronic inflammatory disease such as rheumatoid arthritis (RA)	MCV between 80 and 100 (normal-sized RBCs)
Sickle Cell Anemia	**Hemoglobin electrophoresis** Hemoglobin S seen	Sickle-shaped RBCs with shortened lifespan 10 to 20 days (norm is 120 days) Target cells. Hemolytic anemia

Note. Bolded lab tests are diagnostic or the "gold standard" for the exams.

Classic Case

Pallor of the conjunctiva and nailbeds. Complains of daily fatigue and a sore red tongue (glossitis). Cravings for nonfood items such as ice or dirt (pica). Severe anemia will have spoon-shaped nails (koilonychia), dyspnea, and tachycardia.

Etiology

Most common cause is chronic bleeding. In reproductive-aged females (heavy periods) and in males/menopausal females (GI blood loss—rule out cancer). Chronic gastritis (NSAIDs), post gastrectomy, increased physiologic requirements such as in pregnancy.

Infants: rule out chronic intake of cow's milk before 12 months of age (causes GI bleeding)

Labs

Decreased:

- Hemoglobin and hematocrit
- MCV<80 fL
- MCHC (pale color)
- Ferritin and iron

Increased

- TIBC (total iron binding capacity)
- Ferritin level

Abnormal peripheral smear: anisocytosis (variations in size) and poikilocytosis (variations in shape).

Treatment Plan

Identify cause of anemia and correct if possible.

Ferrous sulfate 325 mg po BID (twice daily) to TID (three times a day) × 3 to 6 months

Treat iron-deficiency anemia for 3 to 6 months to restore ferritin

Common side effects to iron: constipation, dark stools, stomach upset

Thalassemia Minor or Trait

A genetic disorder of the bone marrow where it manufactures small, pale red blood cells, which results in a mild hypochromic microcytic anemia. The bone marrow produces abnormal hemoglobin (defective alpha or beta globin chains) along with reduction in hemoglobin synthesis. Affects ethnic groups: Mediterranean (Italians, Greeks) or Asian.

Classic Case

Discovered incidentally because of abnormal CBC results, which reveal microcytic and hypochromic red blood cells. Total red blood cell count may be mildly elevated. Ethnic background is either Mediterranean or Asian. Patient asymptomatic.

Treatment Plan

"Gold standard" diagnostic test: hemoglobin electrophoresis

Hemoglobin electrophoresis

- In beta thalassemia abnormal (elevated Hgb. A2, Hgb F)
- In iron-deficiency anemia, it is normal

Blood smear: microcytosis, anisocytosis, poikilocytosis

Serum ferritin and iron level normal (not a "deficiency" anemia)

Educate of the possibility of having a child with the disease if partner also with trait (1 in 4 [25%] chance of having a child with the actual disease).

Exam Tips

1) Learn to differentiate thalassemia from iron-deficiency anemia.

Macrocytic/Megaloblastic Anemias

Vitamin B12 Deficiency Anemia

Caused by a deficiency in vitamin B12, which is necessary for the health of the neurons and the brain.

Total body supply of B12 lasts 3 to 4 years. Chronic deficiency results in peripheral neuropathy, which is progressive and can result in dementia if not corrected. Neurologic damage may not be reversible. Highest incidence in older women. Most common cause of vitamin B12 deficiency is pernicious anemia (most common cause of B12 anemia).

Differential diagnosis: folate-deficiency anemia

Pernicious Anemia

An autoimmune disorder caused by the destruction of parietal cells in the fundus (anti-parietal antibodies) resulting in cessation of intrinsic factor production. Intrinsic factor is necessary in order to absorb vitamin B12 from the small intestine

Other causes: gastrectomy, strict vegans and small bowel disease

Vitamin B12 sources: all foods of animal origin (meat, poultry, eggs, milk, cheese)

Classic Case

Older to elderly female complains of gradual onset of paresthesias on her feet and/or hands that is slowly getting more severe.

Neuropathic symptoms may include any of the following:

- Tingling/numbness of hands and feet
- Neuropathy starts in peripheral nerves and migrate centrally
- Difficulty walking (gross motor)
- Difficulty in performing fine motor skills (hands)

Objective

Decreased reflexes in affected extremity, weak hand grip, decreased sensation, and so forth

Inflamed tongue or glossitis (not a specific finding since it is found in other disorders)

Treatment Plan

Check for both B12 level and folate level (both levels must always be checked together)

Positive: anti-parietal antibody (to rule out pernicious anemia), 24-hour urine for methylmalonic acid (MMA), Schilling test

Peripheral blood smear: macro-ovalocytes, hypersegmented neutrophils
Decreased B12 level (less than 100 pg/L)

Medications
Lifetime supplementation of B12 (100-mcg injections, oral or nasal B12 spray).

Exam Tips
Pernicious Anemia (PA) results in:
1) B12-deficiency anemia.
2) Macrocytic/megaloblastic anemia.
3) Neurologic symptoms.

Clinical Notes
1) Missing a diagnosis of B12 deficiency can result in irreversible neurological damage.
2) Any patient complaining of neuropathy should have B12 levels checked.

Folic Acid Deficiency Anemia

Deficiency in folate results in red blood cell changes (macrocytosis), which manifests as macrocytic anemia. Total body supply of folate lasts 2 to 3 months
Most common cause: inadequate dietary intake.
Higher risk: alcoholics, elderly, overcooking vegetables
Increased physiologic need in pregnancy, chronic illness
Drugs interfering with folate absorption: phenytoin, trimethoprim-sulfa, methotrexate, others

Classic Case
An alcoholic older male complains of tiredness, fatigue, and a reddened and sore tongue (glossitis). Pallor. No neurological complaints.

Treatment Plan
CBC: decreased hemoglobin and hematocrit, increased MCV
Peripheral smear: macro-ovalocytes, hypersegmented neutrophils
Below-normal folate level
Food sources: leafy green vegetables (kale, collard greens), grains, beans, liver

Medications
1) Correct primary cause. Improve diet. Stop overcooking vegetables.
2) Folic acid 1 to 5 mg per day

Exam Tips
1) Pernicious anemia results in B12 deficiency.
2) Pernicious anemia is a macrocytic anemia.
3) Learn food groups for both folate and B12.
4) Red blood cell size is described in many ways such as:

MCV < 80: microcytic and hypochromic RBCs, small and pale RBCs

MCV > 100: macrocytes or macro-ovalocytes, larger than normal RBCs, or RBCs with enlarged cytoplasms

5) Ethnic background may not be mentioned in a thalassemia problem, or it may be a distractor. Be careful.

6) Only B12-deficiency anemia has neurologic symptoms (tingling, numbness).

7) Summary: microcytic anemias

Iron-deficiency anemia versus thalassemia trait:

Ferritin level
- Low in iron deficiency
- Normal to high in thalassemia

Serum iron
- Decreased in iron deficiency
- Normal to high in thalassemia

TIBC
- Elevated in iron deficiency
- Normal or borderline thalassemia

MCHC or color
- Decreased in iron deficiency
- Normal in thalassemia

Hgb. electrophoresis
- Normal iron deficiency
- Abnormal thalassemia

Ethnic background
- Ethnicity or age does not matter in iron-deficiency anemia
- Iron-deficiency anemia is the most common anemia overall in any age group or gender
- Thalassemia is seen in Mediterranean background (i.e., Greeks, Italians, etc.) and Asians (i.e., Chinese)

Anemia Exam Tips

1) Some questions on iron-deficiency anemia may mention a patient's descent (i.e., Italian descent).

2) As mentioned before, ethnic background does not matter with this anemia. The MCV, ferritin level, TIBC are what matters.

GASTROINTESTINAL SYSTEM

| Fast Facts | Danger Signals

Acute Appendicitis

Patient who is a teen or adult complains of an acute onset of periumbilical pain that is steadily getting worse. Over a time period of 12 to 24 hours, the pain starts to localize at McBurney's point. The patient has no appetite (anorexia).

When the appendix ruptures, clinical signs of acute abdomen present such as involuntary guarding, rebound, and a boardlike abdomen. The psoas and obturator signs are positive.

Colon Cancer

Very gradual (years) with vague GI symptoms. Tumor may bleed intermittently and patient may have iron-deficiency anemia. Changes in bowel habits, changes in stool or bloody stool. Heme-positive stool, dark tarry stool, mass on abdominal palpation. Older patient (>50 years of age) especially if history of multiple polyps or Crohn's disease.

Zollinger-Ellison syndrome

A gastrinoma located on the pancreas or the stomach; secretes gastrin, which stimulates high levels of acid production in the stomach. The end result is the development of multiple and severe ulcers in the stomach and duodenum. Complains of epigastric to midabdominal pain. Stools may be a tarry color. Screening by serum fasting gastrin level.

Crohn's Disease

Right lower quadrant intermittent abdominal pain. Lower abdominal pain 1 hour after eating. Diarrhea with mucus. Fever, malaise, and mild weight loss. Abnormal liquid stools. Patients with Crohn's disease at higher risk for colon cancer.

Fast Facts Normal Findings

Route of food or drink from the mouth:

Esophagus → stomach (hydrochloric acid, intrinsic factor) → duodenum (bile, amylase, lipase) → jejunum → ileum→ colon → cecum → rectum→ anus

Abdominal Contents

Right upper quadrant: liver, gallbladder, ascending colon, kidney (right), pancreas (small portion). Right kidney is lower than the left because of displacement by the liver.
Left upper quadrant: stomach, pancreas, descending colon and kidney (left)
Right lower quadrant: appendix, ileum, cecum, ovary (right)
Left lower quadrant: sigmoid colon, ovary (left)
Suprapubic area: bladder, uterus, rectum

Fast Facts Benign Variants

Appendix can be located in any quadrant of the abdomen.

Fast Facts | Abdominal Maneuvers

Acute Abdomen or Peritonitis

Psoas/Ilipsoas (supine position)

Used for acute appendicitis or any suspected retroperitoneal area acute process (i.e., ruptured ectopic pregnancy). Flex hip 90 degrees, ask patient to push against resistance (examiner's hand) and to straighten the leg.

Obturator Sign (supine position)

Used for acute appendicitis or any suspected retroperitoneal area acute process (i.e., ruptured ectopic pregnancy). Rotate right hip through full range of motion. Positive sign if pain with the movement or flexion of the hip.

Rovsing's Sign (supine position)

Deep palpation of the left lower quadrant of the abdomen results in referred pain to the right lower quadrant.

McBurney's Point

Area located between the superior iliac crest and umbilicus in the right lower quadrant. Tenderness or pain is a sign of a possible acute appendicitis.

Markle Test (Heel Jar)

Instruct patient to raise heels, then drop them suddenly. An alternative is to ask the patient to jump in place. Positive if pain elicited or if patient refuses to perform because of pain.

Involuntary Guarding

With abdominal palpation, the abdominal muscles reflexively become tense or boardlike.

Rebound Tenderness

Patient complains that the abdominal pain is worse when the palpating hand is released compared to the pain felt during deep palpation.

Fast Facts | Disease Review

IRRITABLE BOWEL SYNDROME (IBS)

A chronic functional disorder of the colon (normal colonic tissue) marked by exacerbations and remissions. Spontaneous remissions. Commonly exacerbated by excess stress.

Classic Case

A young adult to middle-aged female complains of intermittent episodes of moderate to severe cramping pain in the lower abdomen, especially on the left lower quadrant. Bloating with flatulence. Relief obtained after defecation. Stools range from diarrhea to constipation or both types with increased frequency of bowel movements.

Objective

Abdominal exam: tenderness in lower quadrants during an exacerbation. Otherwise the exam is normal
Rectal exam: normal with no blood or pus
Heme-negative stools

Treatment Plan

1) Increase dietary fiber. Supplement fiber with Metamucil (psyllium).
2) Antispasmodics (i.e., Bentyl) as needed. Decrease life stress.
3) Rule out: amoebic, parasitic, or bacterial infections, inflammatory disease of the GI tract, and so forth. Stool for ova and parasites (especially diarrheal stools) with culture.

GASTRIC ULCER AND DUODENAL ULCER DISEASE

Gastric ulcers have higher risk for malignancy (up to 10%) compared to duodenal ulcers, which are mostly benign. Duodenal ulcers are five times more prevalent than gastric ulcers (seen more in elderly).

Etiology

Helicobacter pylori or *H. pylori* (gram negative bacteria)
Chronic NSAIDs, which disrupt prostaglandin production. Results in reduction of GI blood flow with reduction of protective mucus layer.

Classic Case

Middle-aged to older adult complains of epigastric pain, burning/gnawing pain, or ache (80%). Pain relieved by food and/or antacids (50%) with reoccurrence from 2 to 4 hours after a meal. Self-medicating with over-the-counter antacids. May be taking NSAIDs or aspirin.

Objective

Abdominal exam: normal or mildly tender epigastric area during flare-ups
Hemoccult can be positive if actively bleeding

Treatment Plan

"Gold standard": biopsy of gastric and/or duodenal tissue (by upper endoscopy)
Urea breath test: not as sensitive as a biopsy; positive with active infection
Titers: *H. pylori* IgM and IgG levels
Fasting gastrin levels to rule out Zollinger-Ellison syndrome as needed

H. pylori Negative Ulcers (antibiotics not recommended)

Do not use any antibiotics, because there is no infection. Treat symptoms. Lifestyle
   changes.
First-line: H2 blockers
   ▪ Ranitidine (Zantac) × 4 to 6 weeks
If no relief or poor result, switch to a proton pump inhibitor (PPI)
   ▪ Omeprazole (Prilosec) daily × 4 to 6 weeks

H. pylori Positive Ulcers

Two types of regimens:
1) Omeprazole (Prilosec) QD plus:
   Clarithromycin (Biaxin) BID plus
   Amoxicillin 1 g BID
   Add an H2 antagonist or PPI × 4 to 6 weeks after
2) Triple therapy:
   Bismuth subsalicylate tab 600 mg QID plus
   Metronidazole tab 250 mg QID plus
   Tetracycline 500-mg caps QID × 2 weeks
   Plus: ranitidine 150 mg daily × 4 to 6 weeks after

Exam Tips

1) Distinguish whether question about *H. pylori* negative ulcers or *H. pylori* positive ulcers.
2) Both treatment regimens have appeared on the exams before.

Clinical Notes

1) Today, most clinicians start with PPIs rather than H2 antagonist. But in the test, follow the foregoing rules.

GASTROESOPHAGEAL REFLUX DISEASE (GERD)

Acidic gastric contents regurgitate from the stomach into the esophagus. Chronic GERD causes damage to squamous epithelium of the esophagus and may result in Barrett's esophagus (a precancer), which increases risk of squamous cell cancer.

Classic Case

Middle-aged to older adult complains of chronic heartburn of many years duration. Symptoms associated with large and/or fatty meals and are worsened when supine. Long-term history of self-medication with OTC antacids. May be on chronic NSAIDs, aspirin, or alcohol.

Objective

Acidic or sour odor to breath
Reflux of sour acidic stomach contents especially with overeating
Thinning tooth enamel due to increased hydrochloric acid
Sore red throat (not associated with a cold)
Chronic coughing

Labs

Gold standard: esophageal motility studies.

Treatment Plan

Lifestyle changes include: avoid large or high-fat meals especially 3 to 4 hours before bedtime, lose weight, avoid mints (relaxes gastric sphincter), avoid caffeine, alcohol, ASA, and NSAIDs.

Medications

H2 blockers (ranitidine) × 4 to 6 weeks. If no relief, start on proton pump inhibitor (PPI) such as omeprazole (Prilosec) × 4 to 6 weeks.

Complications

Barrett's esophagus (a precancer for esophageal cancer).

Exam Tips

1) Barrett's esophagus is a precancer.

Clinical Tip

1) Any patient with at least a decade or more history of chronic heartburn should be referred to a gastroenterologist for an endoscopy to rule out Barrett's esophagus.

DIVERTICULITIS

Diverticula are small pouchlike herniations on the external surface of the colon secondary to a chronic lack of dietary fiber. Diverticulitis is infected diverticula. Higher incidence in Western societies.

Classic Case

Elderly patient presents with acute onset of fever with left lower quadrant abdominal pain with anorexia, nausea, and/or vomiting.

Constipation or diarrhea
Hematochezia (bloody stool) if hemorrhaging

Objective

If signs of an acute abdomen are present (i.e., rebound, boardlike), refer to ER
If diverticula not inflamed, normal abdominal exam

Labs

Sigmoidoscopy. Barium enema (can see diverticula the best) but not during acute exacerbation.

Treatment Plan

1) Chronic therapy: high-fiber diet with fiber supplementation such as psyllium (Metamucil) or methylcellulose (Citrucel).
2) Outpatient treatment for very mild cases only. If no response in 72 hours or worsens, refer to ER.

Medications

Trimethoprim/sulfamethazole BID or Cipro BID plus metronidazole 500 mg q 6 hours × 7 to 10 days. Close follow-up. Moderate to severe cases: hospitalize.

ACUTE PANCREATITIS

Acute inflammation of the pancreas secondary to many factors such as elevated triglyceride levels, cholecystitis, cholelithiasis, alcohol abuse, infections
Elevated triglycerides (>800 mg/dL) at very high risk of acute pancreatitis

Classic Case

Adult to older patient complains of an acute onset of guarding and tenderness over the epigastric area or the upper abdomen. The classic finding is of epigastric abdominal pain that radiates to the midback and anorexia. May be accompanied by fever, tachycardia and signs and symptoms of shock. Refer patient to ER.

Objective

Cullen's sign: bluish discoloration around umbilicus (hemorrhagic pancreatitis)
Gray Turner's sign: bluish discoloration on the flank area (hemorrhagic pancreatitis)
Hypoactive bowel sounds (ileus), jaundice, guarding, and boardlike upper abdomen if peritonitis

Labs

Elevated pancreatic enzymes such as serum amylase, lipase, and trypsin
Elevated AST, ALT, GGT, bilirubin, leukocytosis, and so forth

Complications

1) Death.
2) Acute hepatic injury.
3) Diabetes, others.

VIRAL HEPATITIS

Fast Facts | Laboratory Tests

HEPATITIS A, B, AND C

Hepatitis A

No chronic or carrier state exists
Transmission: fecal and oral route from contaminated food
Self-limiting infection. Treatment is symptomatic. Vaccine available (Havrix) and recommended for travelers to areas where hepatitis A is endemic

IgG Anti-HAV (Hepatitis A antibody IgG type) Positive
▪ Antibodies present (immune)
▪ No virus present and not infectious

How: history of hepatitis. An infection or vaccination with hepatitis A vaccine (Havrix).

IgM Anti-HAV (Hepatitis A antibody IgM type) Positive
- Acute infection
- Hepatitis A virus still present (infectious). No immunity yet

Hepatitis B

Transmission; sexual (semen, vaginal secretions, and saliva), blood, blood products, organs.

HBsAg (Hepatitis B surface antigen)
- Screening test for hepatitis B
- If positive, patient has a current infection and infectious

May be due to either an acute infection or chronic hepatitis B infection.

Anti-HBs (Hepatitis B surface antibody) positive means:
- Antibodies present and immune against hepatitis B virus
- Not infectious

May be due to either a past infection or vaccination with hepatitis B vaccine.

HbeAg (Hepatitis B "e" antigen")
- Indicates active viral replication. Infectious
- Persistence indicates chronic hepatitis B

Chronic Hepatitis Infection: Two Types
- Chronic infection with mildly elevated LFTs
- Chronic and active infection with elevated LFTs (active viral replication). Patient is at higher risk of cirrhosis, liver failure, and liver cancer

Hepatitis C

Transmission: intravenous drug use (50%), blood or blood products, sexual intercourse. In 40% of cases, the mode is unknown

High-risk groups: IV drug users, hemophiliacs, or anyone with history frequent transfusions

Highest risk for chronic hepatitis infection and cirrhosis (30%). Cirrhosis markedly increases the risk for liver cancer or liver failure. Refer to GI for management

Treatment: alpha interferon injections and ribavirin. Liver biopsy to stage disease

Anti-HCV (antibody Hepatitis C virus)
- Screening test for hepatitis C
- Up to 85% of cases become carriers

Unlike hepatitis A and B, a positive anti-HCV (antibody) does not always mean that the patient has recovered from the infection and has developed immunity. It may instead indicate current infection.

    If this test is positive:

- Order HCV RNA or HCV PCR (polymerase chain reaction)
- If positive, indicates current infection

LIVER FUNCTION TESTS (LFTs)

1) Serum aspartate aminotransferase (AST)
   Also known as serum glutamic oxaloacetic transaminase (SGOT). Normal: 0 to 45 mg/dL
   - Present in the liver, heart muscle, skeletal muscle, kidney, and lung
   - Not specific for liver injury because it is also elevated in other conditions (i.e., acute MI)
2) Serum alanine aminotransferase (ALT)
   Also known as serum glutamic pyruvic transaminase (SGPT). Normal: 0 to 40 mg/dL
   This enzyme is found mainly in the liver. A positive finding indicates liver inflammation
   - More specific for hepatic inflammation than AST
3) AST/ALT ratio (or SGOT/SGPT ratio)
   - A ratio of 2.0 or higher may be indicative of alcohol abuse
4) GGT (serum gamma glutamyl transferase)
   Sensitive indicator of alcohol abuse. May be a "lone" elevation
   - Elevated in liver disease and acute pancreatitis
5) Alkaline phosphatase
   An enzyme derived from bone, liver, gallbladder, kidneys, GI tract, and placenta
   Normally elevated during growth spurts (i.e., teenagers)
   - Higher levels seen during growth spurts in children and teens
   - Also may be elevated with healing fractures, osteomalacia, malignancy, others

Exam Tips

1) PCR tests are not antibody tests. They are testing for presence of viral RNA. A positive result means that the virus is present.
2) Hepatitis C has highest risk of cirrhosis and liver cancer.
3) A lone elevation in the GGT is a sensitive indicator of possible alcoholism.
4) The alkaline phosphatase is normally elevated during the teen years.

Fast Facts | Disease Review

ACUTE HEPATITIS

An acute liver inflammation with multiple causes. Examples include viral infection, hepatotoxic drugs (i.e., statins), excessive alcohol intake, toxins.

Classic Case

Sexually active adult complains of a new onset of fatigue, nausea, and dark-colored urine for several days. New sexual partner (less than 3 months).

Objective

Skin and sclera have a yellow tinge (jaundiced or icteric)
Liver: tenderness over the liver from percussion and deep palpation

Labs

ALT and AST: elevated up to 10× normal during the acute phase of the illness
Other liver function tests may be elevated such as the serum bilirubin and GGT

Treatment Plan

Remove and treat the cause (if possible). Avoid hepatotoxic agents such as alcoholic drinks, acetaminophen, and statins (i.e., pravastatin or Pravachol). Treatment is supportive.

Fast Facts | Case Studies for Viral Hepatitis

Patient A

HBsAg: negative
Anti-HBs: positive
HBeAg: negative

Results are indicative of either:
▪ History of old hepatitis B infection that has resolved
▪ Or history of vaccination against hepatitis B

Patient B

HBsAg: positive
HBeAg: positive

anti-HBs: negative
anti-HAV: positive
anti-HCV: negative

Results are indicative of

- Hepatitis B infection
- History of previous hepatitis A infection and immune

This patient is an infectious carrier of the Hepatitis B virus. If the HBeAg is positive, it means that the patient is a carrier (either lowly or highly contagious).

Exam Tips

1) There will be a serology question (as just shown). You will have to figure out what type of viral hepatitis the patient has (A, B, or C?). It is usually a patient with Hep. B.

RENAL SYSTEM

Fast Facts Danger Signals

Acute Pyelonephritis

Patient presents with acute onset of high fevers, chills, dysuria, frequency, and flank pain. The flank pain is described as a deep ache. May have history of recent bladder infection.

Acute onset of high fevers, chills, dysuria and frequency. Complains of unilateral flank pain or a deep ache that is associated with nausea and/or vomiting. May have recent history of urinary tract infection (UTI).

Recurrent Urinary Tract Infections (child)

Child complains of painful urination, frequency, and is taking longer than normal to void (if toilet trained). May have hematuria. A sign of renal or urologic abnormality. Refer.

Acute Renal Failure

Peripheral edema, weight gain (water retention) and oliguria. May be anorexic and lethargic.

Rapid decrease in renal function. Elevated urinary and serum creatinine.

Fast Facts | Normal Findings

Kidneys

The kidneys are located in the retroperitoneal area. The lower half of the right kidney falls below the rib cage. It is lower than the left kidney due to displacement by the liver.

The basic functional unit of the kidneys are the nephrons which contain the glomeruli.

Function

Kidneys are the body's regulators of electrolytes, fluids, and bicarbonate (affects blood pH). It also produces the hormone erythropoietin which stimulates bone marrow into producing more red blood cells. Water is reabsorbed back to the body by the action of antidiuretic hormone and aldosterone. Kidneys excrete water soluble waste as urine. The average daily urine output is 1500 mL.

Fast Facts | Laboratory Testing

Serum Creatinine

Male 0.7 - 1.3 mg/dL
Female 0.6 - 1.1 mg/dL

Serum creatinine is an indirect measure of renal function. Creatinine is the end product of creatine metabolism which comes mostly from muscle. Creatinine clearance is fairly constant and is not affected by fluid status or dietary intake of meat.

Creatinine clearance is doubled for every 50% reduction of the GFR (glomerular filtration rate). Elevated values are seen during acute or chronic renal failure, nephrotoxic drugs, etc.

Urinalysis

Epithelial cells
  - Large amounts in a urine sample indicate contamination

Leukocytes
Normal WBC in urine: $\leq$ 10 WBCs/mcL qL
  - Presence of leukocytes in urine (pyuria) is abnormal in males and indicates infection

The urinalysis is a more sensitive test for infection in males compared to females.

Urine for culture and sensitivity
  - $\geq 10^5$ CFU/mL of bacteria (CFU or "colony forming units") indicates infection
  - Lower values indicative of bacteuria

Red blood cells
  - Seen in kidney stones and some lower UTIs
Protein
  - Indicates kidney damage
  - May be present in acute pyelonephritis. May also see casts.
  - Urine dipsticks only pick up albumin, not microalbumin (Bence-Jones proteins).
Nitrites
  - Indicative of infection
  - Due to breakdown of nitrates to nitrates by certain bacteria.

Fast Facts | Disease Review

URINARY TRACT INFECTIONS (UTIs)

Infection of the lower urinary tract predominantly due to gram-negative bacteria such as *Escherichia coli* (*E. coli*) (85%). Others are *Staphylococcus saprophyticus* (4%) and *Klebsiella* (3%). UTIs in children younger than age 3 are more likely to progress to pyelonephritis.

Risk Factors

Failure to void after sex or increased sexual intercourse (i.e., honeymoon bladder)
Diaphragm and spermicide use
Diabetes mellitus
Pregnancy
History of a recent UTI

Other risk factors: renal calculi, ureteral strictures, tumors.

Classic Case

A sexually active female complains of new onset of dysuria, frequency, frequent urge to urinate, and nocturia. May also complain of suprapubic discomfort.

Treatment Plan

Urinalysis: leukocyte positive (WBCs $\geq 10/\text{mcL}$), positive nitrites, red blood cells.
Urine for C&S (culture and sensitivity)

Medications

Treat $\times$ 3 days if uncomplicated UTI. Treat $\times$ 7 days for complicated UTIs.
Trimethoprim/sulfoxazole (Bactrim, Septra) BID, amoxicillin (Amoxil) TID

Nitrofurantoin (Macrodantin) BID
Ciprofloxacin (Cipro) or ofloxacin (Floxin) BID (age 18 years of older)

Complications

Acute pyelonephritis.

Urinary Tract Infections: Uncomplicated vs. Complicated

Uncomplicated UTIs

Healthy females aged 18 years or older can have the "3-day" treatment regimen. These patients do not need urine C&S before or after treatment. Studies show that women reporting UTI symptoms have 90% sensitivity in identifying their infection.

Complicated UTIs

Must treat these patients for a minimum of 7 days or longer.

Diabetics
Pregnant women
Children
Elderly
HIV patients or anyone who is immunocompromised
History of one kidney only (or only one functioning kidney)

Labs

Urinalysis and urine C&S before and after treatment to document resolution.

Urinary Tract Infections: Special Categories

Elderly

Do not treat asymptomatic bacteriuria in elders with chronic indwelling Foley catheters.

Males

UTIs are never "normal" in males. Rule out ureteral stricture, infected kidney stones, anatomic abnormality, acute prostatitis, STDs, and so forth. Must be evaluated further. Refer to urologist.

RECURRENT CYSTITIS

Three or more per year for females. Never normal in males.
Rule out urologic abnormality: infected stones, reflux, fistulas, ureteral stenosis, and so forth
Consider prophylactic antibiotics for 6 to 12 months after ruling out pathology

Medications

Trimethoprim sulfa (40 mg/200 mg) 1/2 tab at HS
Nitrofurantoin (Furadantin) 100-mg tablet at HS
Postcoital UTIs: one tab (Bactrim DS) after sex

ACUTE PYELONEPHRITIS

Acute bacterial infection of the kidney(s) most commonly due to gram-negative bacteria. Bacteria gain entry through the urethra and ascend the urinary tract into the kidney.

Most common pathogens are gram-negative bacteria such as *E. coli*, *Proteus*, and *Klebsiella* (gram-negative anaerobe).

Classic Case

Patient presents with acute onset of high fever, chills, and one-sided flank pain. Complains of dysuria, frequency, and urgency. Anorexia with nausea and/or vomiting. May appear toxic.

Physical Exam

CVA tenderness on one kidney (sometimes both)
Urine dipstick: leukocytes, blood, casts, protein
Urine C&S: presence of 10^5 CFU (colony-forming units)/mL
CBC: leukocytosis, neutrophilia (>75%)
Bands or stags (immature neutrophils) may be seen on the CBC (shift to the left)

Treatment Plan

1) Treat outpatient if not toxic (adults) with close follow-up.
2) Ciprofloxacin (Cipro) or ofloxacin (Floxin) BID × 14 days (do not use if < 18 years).
3) Trimethoprim/sulfoxazole (Bactrim, Septra) BID × 14 days.
4) Close follow-up: 12–24 hours.
5) Coexisting condition that compromises immune system or toxic: refer or hospitalize.

Children and pregnant women: must hospitalize for IV antibiotics.

Exam Tips

1) Right kidney sits lower than the left kidney because of displacement by the liver.
2) Large numbers of epithelial cells in the urine mean contamination.

3) Memorize the normal WBC count (10.5) and the neutrophil (or segs).
4) Neutrophils make up from 50% to 75% of all the WBCs in a sample.
5) If band forms (immature WBCs) are seen, it is indicative of a serious bacterial infection.
6) The serum creatinine is preferred to BUN when checking renal function.

Clinical Tips

1) Do not use fluoroquinolones or quinolones in pregnant women, children, or any patient below the age of 18 years (interferes with cartilage development).

MEN'S HEALTH

Fast Facts Danger Signals

Testicular Cancer

Teenage to young adult males complains of nodule, sensation of heaviness or aching, one larger testicle, and/or tenderness in one testicle. Testicular cancer can present as a new onset of a hydrocele (from tumor pressing on vessels). Usually painless and asymptomatic until metastasis. More common in White males ages 15 to 30 years. Rare in African Americans.

Prostate Cancer

Older to elderly male complains of a new onset of low back pain, rectal area/perineal pain or discomfort accompanied by obstructive voiding symptoms such as weaker stream and nocturia. May be asymptomatic. More common in Black men, positive family history of prostate cancer, age > 50 years.

Priapism

Continuous penile erection of at least 4 hours or longer unrelated to sexual desire or stimulation. May have recently taken drugs for erectile dysfunction (ED), either oral or intracavernous form, and/or have a history of sickle cell anemia or other blood clotting disorder, spinal cord injury (especially quadriplegia), medications (i.e., antipsychotics), and illicit drugs such as cocaine. A medical emergency.

Fast Facts Normal Findings

Spermatogenesis

1) Sperm production starts at puberty and continues for the entire lifetime of the male.

2) Sperm are produced in seminiferous tubules of the testes.
3) Sperm production takes 64 days (about 3 months).
4) Ideal temperature (sperm production) is from 1 to 2 degrees lower than core body temperature.

Prostate Gland

1) Heart-shaped gland that grows throughout the life cycle of the male.
2) Produces PSA (prostate specific antigen) and prostatic fluid.
3) Prostatic fluid (alkaline pH) helps the sperm survive in the vagina (acidic pH).
4) Up to 50% of 50-year-old males have BPH (benign prostatic hypertrophy).

Testes

1) Oval-shaped gland that feels rubbery and has a smooth surface.
2) he left testicle usually hangs lower than the right.

Epididymis

1) Sits like a cap on the upper pole of the testes.
2) Located on top and the sides of each testicle in a posterior lay.

Cremasteric Reflex

The testicle is elevated toward the body in response to stroking the ipsilateral inner thigh (or the thigh on the same side as the testicle).

Transillumination: Scrotum

Useful for evaluating testicular swelling, mass, or bleeding.

Direct a beam of light behind the scrotum
Serous fluid inside scrotum = brighter red glow (i.e., hydrocele)
Blood or mass = dull glow to no glow (i.e., cancerous tumor)

| Fast Facts | Disease Review

TESTICULAR CANCER

Most common tumor in males ages 15 to 30 years. Most likely a White male (rare in Black males).

Classic Case

Teenage to young adult males complains of nodule, sensation of heaviness or aching, one larger testicle, tenderness in one testicle. May present as a new onset of a hydrocele (from tumor pressing on vessels). Usually painless and asymptomatic until metastasis.

Objective

Affected testicle feels "heavier" and more solid
May palpate a hard fixed nodule (most common site is the lower pole of the testes)
- 20% will have concomitant hydrocele

Labs

Ultrasound of the testicle reveals solid mass
Gold standard of diagnosis: testicular biopsy
Refer to urologist. Surgical removal (orchiectomy).

PROSTATE CANCER

Most common cancer in older males (but lung cancer causes the highest mortality).

Objective

Hard fixed nodule or indurated area on the prostate gland on an older male. Painless
Indurated area or nodule on digital rectal exam (DRE)
Elevated PSA > 4.0 ng
Diagnostic test: biopsy. Screening test: PSA level with DRE

Treatment Plan

1) Most cancers not aggressive and slow-growing. Watchful waiting by urologist.
2) Serial PSA (every 4 to 6 months) and sonograms.
3) Surgery: high risk of impotence.
4) Drug therapy with antiandrogens (Proscar), hormone blockers (i.e., Lupron), others.

BLUE DOT SIGN

Torsion of a testicular appendage. Signs and symptoms may mimic testicular torsion.

Testicular appendage: pedunculated, polyplike; attached to the surface of a testicle.

Classic Case

Adult male complains of acute sudden onset of localized pain in one testicle with indurated and tender blue-colored mass (Blue Dot sign) underneath scrotal skin. No voiding or obstructive symptoms.

Objective

It does not cause the entire testicle to swell (compared to testicular torsion). Testicle itself is not involved. *Not* testicular torsion. Not a true surgical emergency, but it needs to be removed surgically.

BENIGN PROSTATIC HYPERTROPHY (BPH)

Also known as benign prostatic hyperplasia. Seen in 50% of males older than age 50 (up to 80% of males older than 70 years of age). Rarely seen in males younger than age 40 years.

Classic Case

Older male complains of urinary obstructive symptoms such as dribbling, decreased force of stream, postvoid dribbling, urinary retention and frequency. Nocturia very common.

Objective

PSA (prostate specific antigen) is mildly elevated (norm ranges from 0 to 4 ng/mL)
Enlarged prostate that is symmetrical in texture and size (rubbery texture)

Treatment Plan

Gold standard test: transurethral prostate biopsy.

Medications

1) Alpha-adrenergic antagonist: terazosin (Hytrin).
2) Anti-androgen: finasteride (Proscar).
3) Herbal: Saw palmetto (does not work for everybody).

Exam Tips

1) Proscar is a category X drug. Teratogenic. Should not be touched with bare hands if reproductive-aged female.

CHRONIC PROSTATIS

Gradual onset of symptoms such as frequency, burning, dribbling and nocturia. May be asymptomatic. More common in older males. Caused mostly by *E. coli*,

Pseudomonas, Klebsiella, Proteus mirabilis (gram negatives). If STDs, rule out *Neisseria gonorrheae* (gram negative) and *Chlamydia trachomatis* (atypical bacteria).

Classic Case

Older male with history of same signs and symptoms for weeks to months. Gradual onset. May complain of suprapubic discomfort or perineal discomfort. If prostate enlarged, will complain of nocturia and weaker stream, and dribbling.

Objective

Prostate may feel normal or "boggy" to palpation. Not tender.

Treatment Plan

Urine and prostatic fluid cultures. Uses three tubes: first, urethra; second, bladder; third, prostate (obtained after prostatic massage). Send for culture and STD testing.

Medications

Ofloxacin (Floxin) or Bactrim DS po BID × 12 weeks (3 months).

Exam Tips

1) Learn to distinguish between chronic prostatitis and acute prostatitis.
2) Chronic: gradual onset; prostate can feel normal (older males).
3) Acute: sudden onset; prostate swollen and very tender (younger males).
4) Proscar is a Category X drug.
5) "Blue dot" sign is not considered a true emergent condition (compared to testicular torsion) on the exam.

ACUTE BACTERIAL EPIDIDYMITIS

Bacteria ascends up the urethra (urethritis) and reaches epididymis, causing an infection
Sexually active males < 35 years old
   ■ More likely to be infected with an STD (chlamydia, GC)
Older males > 35 years old
   ■ Usually due to gram-negative *E. coli*

Classic Case

Adult to older male complains of systemic symptoms such as fever, chills, and anorexia accompanied by unilateral testicular pain. Markedly tender and indurated epididymitis.

Urethral discharge especially if gonorrheal (green color). Color and amount depend on organism. Also complains of voiding symptoms such as dysuria and frequency.

Positive Prehn's sign: relief of pain with scrotal elevation

Labs

CBC: leukocytosis with shift to the left
UA: leukocytes (pyuria), blood (hematuria), nitrites

Medications

1) If high-risk, treat for gonorrhea and/or chlamydia × 21 days. Treat sex partner.
2) Ofloxacin (Floxin) or ciprofloxacin (Cipro) BID × 21 days.
3) Bactrim DS BID for × 21 days.
4) Stool softeners (i.e., docusate sodium or Colace).
5) Analgesics or NSAIDS for pain and fever (i.e., Tylenol, ibuprofen, naproxen).
6) Bedrest if severe or hospitalize for IV antibiotics.
7) Scrotal elevation and scrotal ice packs.

ACUTE PROSTATIS

Acute infection of the prostate. Infection ascends urinary tract. May be secondary to untreated urethritis, cystitis or epididymitis
Sexually active males <35 years old: usually due to STDs.
Older males more likely due to gram-negative bacteria such as *E. coli*

Classic Case

Adult to older male complains of acute onset of fever, chills, and malaise accompanied by suprapubic or perineal pain/discomfort. Pain on defecation especially if constipated. Also complains of frequency and dysuria.

Objective

Gently examine prostate. Do not vigorously massage; can result in bacteremia. Prostate is extremely tender and warm to touch.

Labs

Urine before and post prostatic massage for C&S
Urine or Gen-Probe test for gonorrhea and chlamydia

Medications

1) Ofloxacin (Floxin), ciprofloxacin (Cipro) or Bactrim DS BID × 21 days.
2) Treat sex partner.

ERECTILE DYSFUNCTION (ED)

Inability to produce an erection firm enough to perform sexual intercourse. Vascular insufficiency, neuropathy (diabetics), medications (SSRIs, beta-blockers), smoking, alcohol, hypogonadism. May be psychic causation or mixture of both.

Organic Cause

Inability to have an erection under any circumstances. Due to neurovascular or vascular damage.

Psychic Cause

Early morning erections or can achieve a firm erection with masturbation.

Medications

Sildenafil citrate (Viagra) 25/50/100 mg; take one dose 1/2 to 1 hour before sex
Use only one dose every 24 hours
Other forms of treatment: intracavernous injections (Caverject)

Contraindications for Viagra

Concomitant nitrates. Recent post-MI, post-CVA, major surgery or any condition where exertion is contraindicated.

OTHER CONDITIONS

Peyronie's Disease

Crooked penile erection (may be painful). Palpable hard plaques beneath skin of penile shaft. Surgical correction an option if vaginal penetration problematic.

Balanitis

Candidal infection of the glans penis; more common in uncircumcised men.

Phimosis

Foreskin cannot be pushed back from the glans penis because of edema; usually seen in neonates.

Varicocele

Varicose veins in scrotal sac (feels like "bag of worms"). New-onset varicocele can signal testicular tumor (20%).

WOMEN'S HEALTH

Fast Facts | Danger Signals

Dominant Breast Mass/Breast Cancer

Middle-aged to older female with a dominant mass on one breast that feels hard and is irregular in shape. The mass is attached to sorrounding breast tissue or is immobile. One of the most common locations are the upper outer quadrants of the breast (the Tail of Spence). Skin changes may be seen, such as the "peau de orange" (localized area of skin that resembles an orange peel), dimpling, and retraction. Mass is painless or may be accompanied by serous or blood discharge. The nipple may be displaced or become fixed.

Paget's Disease of the Breast (ductal carcinoma in situ)

Older female reports a history of a chronic scaly red-colored rash resembling eczema on the nipple (or nipple and areola) that does not heal which slowly enlarges over time. The skin lesion slowly evolves to include crusting, ulceration, and/or bleeding. Some women complain of itching. Nipple discharge and/or a lump may be present.

Ectopic Pregnancy

Sexually active female who has not had a period (or had period but light to scant bleeding) in 6 to 7 weeks complains of lower abdominal/pelvic pain or cramping (intermittent, persistent, or acute).If ruptured, pelvic pain worsens and can be referred to the right shoulder. Pain worsens when supine or with jarring. If bleeding is profound, patient may be in shock. Past medical history of pelvic inflammatory disease (PID), tubal ligation, older age, and so forth. This is the leading cause of death for women in the United States during the first trimester of pregnancy.

Ovarian Cancer

Older women with complaints of vague symptoms such as low back pain, pelvic pain, abdominal bloating, and/or constipation. If metastases, symptoms depends on area affected. Symptoms may be bone pain, abdominal pain, headache, blurred vision, others.

Fast Facts   Normal Findings

Menarche

- Irregular the first year or two after menarche (not ovulating monthly yet)

Breasts (specialized sweat glands)

- Pubertal changes starts at Tanner stage II (breast buds)
- Areola/nipples develop first before other breast tissue (Tanner stage II)

Cervix

- Younger girls (before puberty) higher number of glandular cells on the surface
- Cells undergo metaplastic changes (transformation zone) during puberty
- Most cancers are located in the transformation zone area

Ovaries

- Female infants are born with 3 million eggs
- Eggs are stored as follicles in the ovaries

MENSTRUAL CYCLE

This example is based on a perfect 28-day menstrual cycle.

Follicular Phase (days 1 to 14)

FSH stimulates the ovaries into making new follicles (or the "eggs"). As follicles mature, produces estrogen until the end of the cycle Estrogen stimulates the growth of the endometrial lining.

Estrogen is the predominant hormone the first 2 weeks of the menstrual cycle.

Midcycle (day 14): Ovulation

LH is secreted by the anterior pituitary gland which induces ovulation.

Luteal Phase (days 14 to 28)

Progesterone is the predominant hormone. Stabilizes endometrial lining.

After ovulation, corpus lutea is left over. It produces progesterone until the end of the cycle

Menstruation

If not pregnant, both estrogen and progesterone fall drastically inducing menses. The low hormone levels stimulate the anterior pituitary and the cycle starts again.

MENOPAUSE

Defined as amenorrhea (no blood or spotting) for 12 consecutive months. Due to physiologic ovarian failure.
- Mean age 51 years (range 45 to 55 years)
- FSH >30 to 35 mIU/mL (follicle stimulating hormone)

Perimenopause

Classic signs/symptoms are hot flashes, night sweats, mood changes, insomnia. As ovaries gradually fail, periods become very irregular and eventually get lighter and disappear.

Fast Facts | Menopausal Body Changes

Ovaries

After several years of menopause, the ovaries are atrophied and a smaller size. Therefore, a palpable ovary is considered abnormal. Rule out ovarian cancer. Order an intravaginal/pelvic ultrasound. The CEA 125 is elevated later in ovarian cancer.

Labia and Vagina

Both become atrophic and thinner with less rugae. The vaginal canal becomes dry.

Dyspareunia (painful intercourse) is common. It is treated by lubricants, oral, or topical estrogens.

Urethra and Bladder

These organs atrophy increasing the risk of urinary incontinence and cystoceles. Cystoceles (prolapsed bladder) are treated by the use of a pessary or by surgery.

Urinary incontinence is treated medically with anticholinergic/antispasmodics (i.e., oxybutynin or Oxytrol), Kegel exercises, pads, fluid limitation, and/or surgical repair.

Hormone Replacement Therapy (HRT) or Estrogen Replacement Therapy (no uterus)

Increased risk of acute MI, thromboembolism, endometrial cancer, and breast cancer.

Recommendations

1) Use hormones at the lowest possible dose for the shortest amount of time and only for symptomatic women with moderate to severe symptoms who do not respond to other types of treatment (including alternative medications).
2) Evaluate hormone replacement annually.
3) Keep menstrual calendar for any episodes of breakthrough bleeding.
   ▪ Endometrial biopsy for breakthrough bleeding to rule out uterine cancer.

Fast Facts | Laboratory Procedures

Pap Smears

Screening test only. Diagnostic test is the cervical biopsy (done during a colposcopy)

High false-negative rate of 15% to 40%

Satisfactory specimen only if both squamous epithelial cells and endocervical cells present
   ▪ If endocervical cells are missing, repeat Pap (incomplete)

Endometrial cells
   ▪ If present, refer for endometrial biopsy

ASCUS (atypical squamous cells of undetermined significance)
   ▪ Check for HPV strain. Oncogenic types must be referred to gynecologist

AGCUS (atypical glandular cells of undetermined significance)
   ▪ Refer for endometrial biopsy

KOH (potassium hydroxide) Slide

Useful for helping with diagnosis of fungal infections (hair, nails, skin). KOH works by causing lysis of the squamous cells, which makes it easier to see hyphae and spores.

KOH is also used for the "whiff test" for bacterial vaginosis. A strong fishlike odor is released after one to two drops are added to the slide.

Tzanck Smear

Used as an adjunct for evaluating herpetic infections (oral, genital, skin). A positive smear will show large abnormal nuclei on the squamous epithelial cells.

Gram Stain

Useful for diagnosing gonorrhea in the clinical area. Under high power, the white blood cells are examined for gram-negative bacteria (*Neisseria gonorrheae*) after the specimen has been stained.

Fast Facts | Oral Contraceptives

Absolute Contraindications

1) History of thrombophlebitis or thromboembolic disorders (i.e., DVT)
2) CVA or CAD (coronary artery disease)
3) Migraine with focal aura (i.e., basilar migraines)
4) Known/suspected cancer of the reproductive system: breast, endometrium, ovary
5) Known or suspected estrogen dependent neoplasia
6) Undiagnosed genital bleeding
7) Cholestatic jaundice of pregnancy
8) Acute or chronic liver disease with abnormal LFTs
   - If acute infection of the liver (i.e., mononucleosis) with elevated LFTs, estrogen is contraindicated.
   - When LFTs are back to normal, can go back on birth control pills
9) Hepatic adenomas or carcinomas
10) Known or suspected pregnancy
11) Hypersensitivity
12) Smoking over age of 35 years
    - Relative contraindication since women younger than age 35 who smoke can have the pill if no other contraindications exist

Mnemonic "My CUPLETS"

My —Migraines with focal aura
C   CAD or CVA
U   Undiagnosed genital bleeding
P   Pregnant or suspect pregnancy
L   Liver tumor or active liver disease
E   Estrogen-dependent tumor
T   Thrombus or emboli
S   Smoking age 35 or older

Relative Contraindications

1) Migraine headaches
   - Migraines with focal neurological findings (basilar migraines mimic TIAs) are an absolute contraindication due to increased risk of stroke
2) Smoking below age of 35 years
3) Hypertension (uncontrolled by drugs)
4) Fracture or cast on lower extremities
5) Severe depression

Exam Tips

1) Problems on absolute versus relative contraindications of birth control pills are designed with answer options that list a true contraindication with a relative contraindication. For example, a question asking for a relative contraindication may have an answer choice such as "history of a blood clot that resolved" (absolute) and "migraine headache" (relative).
2) Any smoking at age 35 and older is an absolute contraindication.

Advantages of the Pill (after >5 years of use)

Ovarian cancer (decreased by 40%)
Endometrial cancer (decreased by 50%)
Lower risk of PID and pregnancy (due to thickened cervical mucous plug)

Decreased Incidence
Dysmenorrhea and cramps (decrease in prostaglandins)
Iron-deficiency anemia (less blood loss from lighter periods)
Acne and hirsutism (lower levels of androgenic hormones)
Ovarian cysts (due to suppression of ovulation)
Fibrocystic breasts (due to decreased progesterone)

New Prescriptions

There are two methods of starting the first pill pack. Rule out pregnancy first. All patients must use condoms in the first 2 weeks of the menstrual cycle during the first pill pack.

1) "Sunday Start": take first pill on the first Sunday during the menstrual period.
2) "Day One Start": take the 1st pill during the first day of the menstrual period.

Patient needs follow-up visit in 2 to 3 months to check BP and for side effects, questions, and so on.

Oral Contraceptive Pill Problems

Breakthrough Bleeding (BTB) and Spotting

Term used for menstrual bleeding that occurs out of usual cycle. Oral contraceptive pills contain hormones (estrogen/progesterone) the first 3 weeks of the pill cycle, the 4th week is hormone-free (when the period occurs).

1) If bleeding occurs in the first 2 weeks of the cycle
   - Increase estrogen (or decrease progesterone)
2) If bleeding occurs in the last 2 weeks of the cycle
   - Increase progesterone (or decrease estrogen)

   NSAIDs can also help decrease bleeding.

Missing Consecutive Days of Oral Contraceptive Pills

Missed 1 Day
Take two pills the next day and continue with same pill pack ("doubling up").

Missed 2 Consecutive Days
Take two pills the next 2 days to catch up and finish the birth control pill pack and use condoms until next pill cycle.

Drug Interactions of Oral Contraceptives

1) Anticonvulsants: phenobarbital, phenytoin.
2) Antifungals: griseofulvin (Fulvicin).
3) Certain antibiotics: ampicillin, tetracyclines, rifampin.

Pill Danger Signs

Thromboembolic events can happen in any organ of the body
These signs indicate a possible thromboembolic event. Advise patient to report these or to call 911 if symptoms of severe abdominal or chest pains, headaches, visual changes, severe leg pains, and so forth

Fast Facts | Other Contraceptives

Emergency Contraception ("Morning After Pill")

Rule out preexisting pregnancy first. Effective up to 72 hours after unprotected sex. Most effective if taken first 24 hours.

1) Progesterone only (i.e., Plan B - levonorgestrel 0.75 mg tabs). Effective up to 89%.
2) Estrogen/progesterone birth control pills (i.e., Ovral) high doses. Effective up to 75%.

Dosing: take first dose as soon as possible (no later than 72 hours after). Take the second dose in 12 hours. Birth control pills cause more vomiting. If vomits within 1 hour, repeat dose.

Advise patient that if she does not have a period in next 3 weeks, she should return to rule out pregnancy.

IUD (intrauterine device)

Copper-bearing IUDs (i.e., TCu 380A): 0.8%. Approved for 5- to 10-year use. Second most commonly used method of contraception in the world (female sterilization is the first).

Contraindications
- Recent infection of the reproductive tract (i.e., cervicitis, PID)
- Suspected or with STD or pregnant
- Uterine or cervical abnormality (i.e., bicornate uterus)
- Undiagnosed vaginal bleeding

Increased Risk
Endometrial and pelvic infections (first few months after insertion only)
Perforation of the uterus
Heavy or prolonged menstrual periods

Education
1) Check for missing or shortened string after each menstrual period. If the patient or clinician does not feel the string, order a pelvic ultrasound.

Depo-Provera (depot medroxyprogesterone)

0.03% failure rate
Each dose by injection lasts 3 months. Check for pregnancy before starting dose.
Start in first 5 days of cycle (day 1 to 5) because females are less likely to ovulate at this times

Risks of Long-Term Use (>5 years)
Increased risk for osteoporosis and weight gain. Be careful with women with anorexia nervosa because greatly increases risk of osteoporosis and fractures (may already have osteopenia). Recommend calcium with vitamin D and weight-bearing exercises.

All women on Depo-Provera for at least 1 year (or longer) have amenorrhea because of severe uterine atrophy from lack of estrogen.

Clinical Tips

Do not recommend to women who want to become pregnant in 12 to 18 months. Causes delayed return of fertility. It takes up to 1 year for most women to start ovulating; rarely it can take up to 2 years for some women to be fertile again.

Diaphragm with Contraceptive Gel (20% failure rate)

Latex dome-shaped device. Must be used with spermicidal gel. Will need additional spermicidal gel/foam inside vagina before every act of intercourse

Must use spermicide outside of the diaphragm and do not remove diaphragm until 6 to 8 after last ejection. Can leave diaphragm inside the vagina up to 24 hours

Increased risk:

■ UTIs and toxic shock syndrome (TSS) rare

Male Condoms (14% failure rate)
Female Condoms (20% failure rate)

Do not use with any oil-based lubricants, creams, etc.

Exam Tips

1) Menopausal female body changes (i.e., ovaries).
2) Contraindications to IUD, oral contraceptives.
3) Distinguish between relative and absolute contraindications.
4) Missing 2 consecutive days of the pill (take two pills next 2 days to finish cycle and use condoms until next cycle starts).
5) On the ANCC exam, questions will ask for the best birth control method for a case scenario. Remember the contraindications or adverse effects of the pill, IUD, diaphragms.

| Fast Facts | Benign Variants

Supernumerary Nipples

Nipples form a V-shaped line on both sides of the chest down the abdomen. Sides are symmetrically distributed.

| Fast Facts | Disease Review

FIBROCYSTIC BREAST

Monthly hormonal cycle induces breast tissue to become engorged and painful. Symptoms occur 2 weeks before the onset of menses (luteal phase) and resolve after menses start.

Classic Case

Adult female complains of tender, bloated, and lumpy breasts 1 to 2 weeks before her menstrual cycle for many years. Relief of symptoms occurs after onset of menses. Denies dominant mass, skin changes, nipple discharge, or enlarged nodes.

Objective

Multiple mobile and rubbery cystic masses on both breasts
Both breasts have symmetrical findings

Treatment Plan

Stop caffeine intake. Vitamin E and evening primrose capsules daily
Wear bras with good support
Refer: dominant mass, skin changes, fixed mass

POLYCYSTIC OVARY SYNDROME (PCOS)

Hormonal abnormality marked by anovulation, infertility, and excessive androgen production that increases risk for heart disease, breast, and uterine cancer.

Classic Case

Obese teen or young adult complains of excessive facial and body hair (hirsutism 70%), bad acne, and amenorrhea or infrequent periods (oligomenorrhea). Dark thick hair (terminal hair) is seen on the face and beard areas.

Treatment Plan

Pelvic/intravaginal US: enlarged ovaries with multiple follicular cyst ovaries
Serum testosterone and androstenedione are elevated. FSH levels normal or low

Medications

1) Low-dose OCs to suppress ovaries
2) Medroxyprogesterone 10 mg for first 10 days of each month to induce menses
3) Spironolactone to decrease and control hirsutism
4) Metformin (Glucophage) to induce ovulation if desires pregnancy
5) Weight reduction

Complications

Increased risk for:
1) Coronary heart disease (CHD).
2) Type 2 diabetes mellitus.
3) Breast cancer and endometrial cancer.

CANDIDA VAGINITIS

Overgrowth of *Candida albicans* yeast in the vulva/vagina. It results in a large amount of inflammation with symptoms of pruritis, swelling, and redness. The male penis can also be infected (balanitis). Diabetics, HIV, on antibiotics (i.e., amoxicillin) are at higher risk.

Classic Case

Adult female presents with complaints of white cheeselike vaginal discharge accompanied by pruritis, burning, redness, and irritation. A large amount of thick white discharge ("curdlike") is also seen.

Treatment Plan

Microscopy or wet mount is the preferred diagnostic test
Pseudohyphae, spores, and a large number of WBCs

Medications

Miconazole (Monistat), clotrimazole (Gyne-Lotrimin) are OTC (over-the-counter)
    Prescription: Diflucan 100-mg tab × 1 dose, terconazole (Terazol) vaginal cream/suppository

Exam Tips

1) Several questions on different types of vaginitis are on the exam.

BACTERIAL VAGINOSIS (BV)

Caused by anaerobic bacterial overgrowth due to unknown reasons or secondary to terminations and PID. Not an STD, therefore sexual partner does not need treatment.
    Pregnant women are at higher risk for intrauterine infections and premature labor.

Classic Case

Sexually active female complains of embarrassing, unpleasant, and fishlike vaginal odor that is worse after intercourse (no condom). Vaginal discharge is copious with thin and milklike consistency. Coats the vaginal walls, color is off-white to gray. There is no vulvar or vaginal redness or irritation.

Treatment Plan

Wet Smear Microscopy
Clue cells and very few WBCs. May see *Mobiluncus* bacteria
Clue cells: squamous epithelial cells with large amount of bacteria coating the surface that obliterates the edges of the cell

Whiff Test
Apply one drop of KOH (potassium hydroxide) to a cotton swab that is soaked with vaginal discharge.
Positive: a strong "fishy" odor is released.

Vaginal pH
Alkaline vaginal pH > 4.5. Normal vaginal pH is between 4.0 to 4.5 (acidic)

Medications

1) Metronidazole (Flagyl) BID × 7days or vaginal gel at HS (bedtime) × 5 days.
2) Watch for disulfuram (Antabuse) effect if combined with alcohol (severe nausea, HA, etc).
3) Clindamycin (Cleocin) cream at HS × 7 days.
4) Oil-based creams can weaken condoms.
5) Sex partners: treatment not recommended by the CDC because not an STD.
6) Abstain from sexual intercourse until treatment is done.

TRICHOMONAS VAGINITIS (TRICHOMONIASIS)

Unicellular protozoan parasite with flagella that infects genitourinary tissue (both males and females). Infection causes inflammation (pruritis, burning, and irritation) of vagina/urethra.

Classic Case

Adult female complains of very pruritic, reddened vulvovaginal area. Copious green and bubbly vaginal discharge. May have dysuria. Sex partner may have same symptoms.

Objective

"Strawberry cervix" from small points of bleeding on cervical surface.

Treatment Plan

Microscopy wet smear (use low power): mobile unicellular organisms with flagella (flagellates) and a large amount of WBCs.

Medications

Metronidazole (Flagyl) 2 g po × 1 dose or 500 mg BID × 7 days
Treat sexual partner because an STD. Test both for other STDs

ATROPHIC VAGINITIS

Chronic lack of estrogen in estrogen-dependent tissue of the urogenital tract results in atrophic changes in the genital tracts of menopausal women.

Classic Case

Menopausal female complains of vaginal dryness, itching, and pain with sexual intercourse (dyspareunia). Complains of a great deal of discomfort with speculum exams (i.e., Pap smears).

Objective

Atrophic labia with decreased rugae, dry, pale pink color to vagina.

Treatment Plan

Topical estrogens (i.e., Premarin Cream). Prolonged vaginal estrogens (if intact uterus) need progesterone supplementation to prevent endometrial hyperplasia.

OSTEOPOROSIS

A gradual loss of bone density secondary to estrogen deficiency and other metabolic disorders. Most common in menopausal females. Other risk groups include:
- Patients on chronic steroids (severe asthma, autoimmune disorders, etc.)
- Androgen deficiency, hypogonadism

Bone Density Test Scores

Osteoporosis: T scores of –2.5 or fewer standard deviations
Osteopenia: T scores between –1.5 and –2.4 standard deviations

Treatment Plan

1) Weight-bearing exercises several times a week
   - Swimming is not considered a weight-bearing exercise (good for severe arthritis)
2) Calcium with vitamin D 1200 mg (on hormones) or 1500 mg per day

Table 3.7	Vaginal Infections

Type	Signs/Sx	Labs
Bacterial Vaginosis Anaerobes	"Fishlike" vaginal odor Profuse milklike discharge Not itchy/vulva not red	Clue cells Whiff test: positive pH > 4.5 alkaline Few WBCs
Trichomonas Vaginitis	"Strawberry cervix" Bubbly discharge Vulvovagina red/irritated	Mobile protozoa with flagella Numerous WBCs
Candidal Vaginitis	Cheesy or curdlike white discharge Vulvovagina red/irritated	Pseudohyphae Spores Numerous WBCs
Atrophic Vaginitis	Scant to no discharge Less rugae, vaginal color pale. Dyspareunia (painful intercourse) complains of burning during intercourse	Atrophic changes on Pap test, FSH Can diagnose without labs; based on history

3) Bisphosphonates
   Fosamax (Alendronate) 5 to 10 mg/day or 70 mg weekly
   - Rebuilds bone and stops existing bone loss
   - Take upon awakening in a.m. with full glass water on empty stomach
   - Will cause severe esophagitis or esophageal perforation if lodged in the esophagus
   Contraindications: inability to sit upright, esophageal motility disorders, history of PUD or GI
4) SERM class (selective estrogen receptor modulator)
   Evista: Category X drug (synthetic estrogen)
   - Does not stimulate endometrium or breast tissue
   - Not for use in premenopausal women (aggravates hot flashes), history venous thrombosis
5) Other hormones
   Miacalcin (calcitonin salmon, derived from salmon)
   - Stops bone loss but does not rebuild bone
   - Good choice for relief of bone pain from vertebral fractures

Exam Tips

1) Bone Density Score for osteoporosis: T score $\geq$ −2.5 standard deviation.

SEXUALLY TRANSMITTED DISEASES (STDs) or Sexually Transmitted Infections (STIs)

Fast Facts | Danger Signals

Human Immunodeficiency Virus

High risk factors such as homosexual males (or men who have sex with men, MSM), injection drug use, female partners of high-risk males, infants of infected mothers, others. Early signs include hairy leukoplakia of the tongue, shingles in a healthy adult, lymphadenopathy, and so forth.

Disseminated Gonococcal Disease (disseminated gonorrhea)

Sexually active adult from high-risk population (e.g., homeless) complains of petechial skin rashes of hands/soles, swollen, red, and tender joints in one large joint (migratory asymmetrical arthritis) such as the knee. Accompanied by signs of STD (i.e., cervicitis, urethritis). If pharyngitis, will have severe sore throat with green purulent throat exudate that does not respond to usual antibiotics used for strep throat.

Syphilis

Painless chancres in the genitals or mouth that resolve in 2 weeks (first stage). More common in homosexual males and low socioeconomic status.

Organism: *Treponema pallidum* (spirochete).

Fast Facts | Normal Findings

Female normal findings covered under women's health section
Male normal findings covered under GU section

Fast Facts | Disease Review

STD Screening Recommended by the CDC

All sexually active adolescents and females ages 20 to 24 years.

Risk Factors

Sexually active single adult with history of multiple sexual partners, especially if new sexual partner (defined as 3 months or less). Inconsistent condom use.

CHLAMYDIA TRACHOMATIS

Obligate intracellular bacteria that infects squamous epithelial cells of the urinary/genital tracts. Chlamydia does not infect pharynx and rectum. Most common bacterial STD in United States. Majority of infections are asymptomatic.

Possible Sites of Infection

Both genders: urethritis
Females: cervicitis, endometritis, salpingitis (fallopian tubes), PID
Males: epididymitis, prostatitis

Uncomplicated Infections

Chlamydia (cervicitis, urethritis, sex partners)
1) Azithromycin 1 g po single dose.
2) Or doxycycline 100 mg BID × 7 days.
   - Side effect: abdominal pain, nausea, photosensitivity (avoid sun or use sunscreen)
3) Or cefixime (Suprax) 400 mg, or Cipro 500 mg or Floxin 400 mg × one dose.
   CDC prefers DOT (directly observed treatment) × one dose (i.e., azithromycin, ciprofloxacin)
   No test of cure is necessary for azithromycin or doxycycline

Pregnant Women
1) Erythromycin base QID × 7 days. Test of cure 3 weeks after completion of treatment because treatment is not as effective as azithromycin or doxycycline.

NEISSERIA GONORRHEA (GC)

A gram-negative bacterium that infects the urinary and genital tracts, rectum, and pharynx. Unlike chlamydia, GC can become systemic or disseminated if left untreated.

High rates of coinfection with chlamydia. If positive for GC, must cotreat for both even if negative chlamydial tests.

Possible Sites of Infection

Urethritis (dysuria, frequency)
Proctitis (rectal pain, tenesmus, purulent rectal discharge/stool)
Pharyngitis (severe sore throat unresponsive to typical antibiotics, purulent discharge on the posterior pharynx)

Cervicitis (mucopurulent cervical discharge, mild bleeding after intercourse)
Endometritis (heavy menstrual bleeding)
Salpingitis (fallopian tubes) and PID (pelvic or lower abdominal pain, adnexal pain, dyspareunia or painful intercourse)
Epididymitis and prostatitis (discussed in the men's health section)

Classic Case

Sexually active teenage to young adult female complains of purulent vaginal discharge, pelvic pain, dyspareunia, and pain on jarring pelvis (i.e., heel drop test). History of new male partner (less than 3 months) or multiple sexual partners. Inconsistent condom use.

Bimanual Exam Findings

Cervical motion tenderness (CMT), lower abdominal tenderness/one-sided adnexal pain
Mucopurulent cervical discharge (may pool in the posterior fornix of vagina)

Treatment Plan

Uncomplicated Infections
Cervicitis, urethritis, pharyngitis:

1) Ceftriaxone 125 mg IM × 1 dose plus co-treat for chlamydia.
2) Ciprofloxacin (Cipro) 400 mg po × one dose.
3) Must cotreat for chlamydia.

Complicated Infections
Acute epididymitis, acute prostatitis, acute proctitis, PID:

1) Ceftriaxone (Rocephin) 250 mg IM × one dose.
2) Must cotreat for chlamydia.

Risk Factors for PID

1) IUD: the first few months after insertion.
2) History of PID: 25% reoccurrence.
3) Multiple partners.
4) Age 24 or younger.

Oral contraceptives reduce the risk of PID (because of thickened mucous plug).

Labs

Reproductive-aged females: rule out pregnancy first

Gen Probe (use only on urethra and cervix)

- Do not use on the pharynx and rectum

Urine tests for chlamydia and gonorrhea

Gen-Probe preferred. Mandatory chlamydial cultures with sexual assault (any age)

Gonorrhea (anaerobic cultures) such as the Thayer-Martin or chocolate agar

- For pharyngeal and rectal areas but can be used for other sites if indicated

Cultures must be taken for all sexually abused children and sexual assault

Gram stain

- Useful for gonorrhea only. Look for gram-negative diplococci in clusters

Other STD testing: HIV, syphilis, hepatitis B, herpes type 2

Partners should be tested and treated. No sex until both complete treatment.

UNUSUAL COMPLICATIONS

Fitz-Hugh-Curtis Syndrome (Perihepatitis)

Chlamydial and/or gonococcal infection of the liver capsule (not the liver itself) resulting in extensive scarring between the liver capsule and abdominal contents (i.e., colon). Scars look like "violin strings" (seen on laparoscopy). A complication of disseminated GC and/or PID.

Classic Case

Sexually active female with symptoms of PID complains of RUQ (right upper quadrant) abdominal pain and tenderness on palpation. The liver function tests are normal.

Treated as a complicated gonorrheal/chlamydial infection (14-day treatment).

Jarisch-Herxheimer Reaction

The sudden massive destruction of spirochetes after a penicillin G injection causes an immune-mediated reaction that usually resolves spontaneously. Treatment is supportive.

Classic Case

Adult patient complains of severe chills, fever, myalgia, and tachycardia after being treated for syphilis. BP may be high, then falls. Care is supportive.

Reiter's Syndrome

An immune-mediated reaction secondary to infection with certain bacteria (i.e., chlamydia) that spontaneously resolves. More common in males. Treatment is supportive (i.e., NSAIDs).

Classic Case

A male with current history of chlamydia genital infection (i.e., urethritis) complains of dry red and swollen joints that come and go (migratory arthritis in large joints such as knee) and ulcers on the skin of the glans penis.

Mnemonic: "I can't see, pee, or climb up a tree."

Exam Tips

1) Older and well-known drugs such as doxycycline and ceftriaxone more likely to appear as treatment options.
2) If GC positive, always cotreat for chlamydia even if the chlamydial test result is negative.
3) Inverse not true. If chlamydia, do not prophylax against GC unless indicated.
4) Reiter's syndrome (learn signs/symptoms).
5) Erythromycin used for pregnant patients who have chlamydia. Test of cure after treatment.

Clinical Tips

1) Test of cure testing not necessary for azithromycin or doxycycline treatment.
2) PID is a clinical diagnosis. Do not treat a test, treat the patient.
3) Chlamydia is a hard organism to culture or to test for. Base decision to treat on patient risk factors and clinical signs or symptoms.
4) Fitz-Hugh-Curtis is frequently seen on the test.

SYPHILIS

Treponema pallidum (spirochete) infection. Becomes systemic if untreated.

Classic Case

Signs and symptoms dependent on stage of infection.

Primary
- Painless chancre (heals in 6 to 9 weeks if not treated)

Secondary (>2 years)
- Condyloma lata (infectious white papules in moist areas that look like white warts)
- Maculopapular rash on palms and soles that is not pruritic

Latent stage
- Asymptomatic

Tertiary (3 to 10 years)
- Neurosyphilis, gumma (soft tissue tumors), aneurysms, valvular damage, and so forth

Labs

Screening test: RPR or VDRL

Diagnostic test: darkfield exam, FTA-ABS (fluorescent antibody absorption antibody test)

Monitoring treatment response: RPR or VDRL titers (ratio of the decrease in titers used)

Treatment Plan

1) Procaine penicillin G IM (dose depends on stage of disease).
2) Doxycycline BID × 28 days (primary and secondary stages only).
3) Treat sex partner(s).
4) Recheck RPR or VDRL to monitor treatment response (look for at least a fourfold decrease in the pretreatment and posttreatment titers).

Exam Tips

1) Do not confuse *Condyloma acuminata* (genital warts) with *Condyloma lata*.
2) Screening test is RPR or VDRL.

Clinical Tips

1) Use the same serology and lab throughout treatment. If RPR used, continue with it.
2) The most common criterion clinicians use to diagnose PID is cervical motion tenderness.

HIV INFECTION (Human Immunodeficiency Virus)

Screening: ELISA test (enzyme-linked immunosorbent assay)
- Detects antibodies, not viral RNA
- Sensitivity/specificity > 99% (too sensitive with higher rates of false positives)
- If positive twice, lab will check Western blot automatically

Confirmatory test: Western blot
- Antibody test with high specificity for HIV

Window period
- 6 weeks to 6 months (<1% up to 36 months)

Diagnostic Tests (viral RNA test)

PCR (polymerase chain reaction)
- Detects viral RNA (actual viral presence)

Table 3.8	Sexually Transmitted Diseases: Treatment Guidelines

Organism	Uncomplicated Infections	Complicated Infections
Chlamydia trachomatis Pregnancy Erythromycin 500 mg QID × 7 days or Amoxicillin 500 mg TID × 7 days Note: Doxycycline, Cipro, Floxin are Category D: avoid in pregnancy	**Doxycycline 100 mg BID × 7 days Or azithromycin 1 gm × 1 dose** Mucopurulent cervicitis Urethritis Treat sexual partners	**Doxycycline 100 mg BID × 14 days** Pelvic inflammatory disease (PID) Salpingitis, tubo-ovarian abscess **Males** Epididymitis, prostatitis
Neisseria gonorrheae **Plus Chlamydia Tx** **Pregnancy** Treat GC drugs plus chlamydia pregnancy treatment Note: Doxycycline, Cipro, Floxin are Category D: avoid in pregnancy	**Ceftriaxone 125 mg IM × 1 dose plus Doxycycline 100 mg BID × 7 days** Mucopurulent cervicitis Urethritis Pharyngitis Proctitis Treat sexual partners	**Ceftriaxone 250 mg IM × one dose Plus doxycycline 100 mg BID × 14 days** PID, Salpingitis, Tubo-ovarian abscess **Males** Epididymitis, epididymo-orchitis Prostatitis **Disseminated GC** Above plus asymmetric arthritis and rash. (Treatment at www.cdc.gov)
Syphilis *Treponema pallidum* Pregnancy Same treatment, may repeat tx after 1 week if during 3rd trimester	**Benzathine penicillin G 2.4 mU IM × one dose** Early cases, primary, secondary or latent cases <1 year Treat sexual partners. *Retreat if clinical signs recur or sustained 4-fold titers*	**Benzathine penicillin G 2.4 mU IM weekly × 3 weeks** More than 1 year's duration (latent, indeterminate, cardiovascular, late benign) Maculopapular rash includes palms/soles *Follow-up all cases mandatory! (Any stage of disease)*

Note. Adapted from Centers for Disease Control, Sexually Transmitted Disease Treatment Guidelines (2006).

Viral load
- Number of RNA copies in 1 mL plasma. Test measures actively replicating HIV virus; progression of disease and response to antiretroviral treatment

P24 antigen
- Indicates active HIV replication

Risk Factors

Sex (especially men who have sex with men)
Drug use, blood products from 1975 to 1985
History of other STDs, multiple partners, homeless, and so forth

Vaccines

1) Annual flu shot.
2) Hepatitis B × 3.
3) Hepatitis A (anal to oral contact).
4) Td every 10 years.

Prophylaxis for PCP (*Pneumocystis carinii* pneumonia)

If the CD4 lymphocyte count is <200 cells/mcL, prophylaxis for PCP
PCP drugs: TMP-SMX (Bactrim), dapsone or pentamidine by nebulizer

HIV Education

1) Do not handle cat litter (toxoplasmosis).
2) Bird stool contains histoplasmosis spores.
3) Turtles and other amphibians may be infected with salmonella.
4) Do not eat uncooked meat.
5) Safe sex, get partner tested.

Exam Tips

1) PCP prophylaxis when CD4 < 200.
2) Bactrim DS used first; if allergic to sulfa, use pentamidine.
3) Screening test is the ELISA test (tests for antibodies only).
4) Confirmatory test is Western blot.
5) Example of a diagnostic test is PCR (viral RNA), viral load.
6) HIV infected pregnant women: start AZT in the second trimester.
7) Hairy leukoplakia of tongue: rule out HIV infection.

HIV Infection: Pregnant Women

No treatment: 5% to 25% of infants become infected
Breast feeding: transmission rate of 12% to 14%
Newborns: start treatment with zidovudine (AZT) within first 48 hours
Zidovudine

  ▪ Drug of choice for treating pregnant women
  ▪ Reduces rate of perinatal transmission by 60%
Start zidovudine during second trimester of pregnancy until delivery

CONDYLOMA ACUMINATA (Genital Warts)

Human papilloma virus (HPV) has 70 subtypes (only a few are oncogenic)
Genital sites: cervix, vagina, external genitals, urethra, anus
Other sites that can be infected are the larynx, nasal mucosa, oral mucosa, con-
   junctivae

HIV-Positive Women

Higher risk for aggressive HPV disease. Need to have Paps every 3 to 6 months to
monitor. Higher incidence of cervical cancer.

Pap Smears

1) Cervical cancer screening test is the Pap smear (false-negative rates of up to
   18%).
2) Koilocytotic changes (large cell nuclei): may signify human papilloma virus
   (HPV) infection, test for an infection and refer for a colposcopy.
3) If ASCUS (atypical squamous cells of unknown significance), test for HPV and
   refer to gynecologist.

Colposcope

A specialized microscope for evaluating and treating cervix. It is used to visualize
the cervix and to obtain cervical tissue biopsies. A biopsy is the gold standard for
diagnosing cervical cancer.

Acetowhitening

Areas of white-colored skin (HPV infected skin) on the cervical surface that appear
only after acetic acid (distilled vinegar) is swabbed on the cervix. This procedure
is done before starting a colposcopic examination and biopsy. HPV-infected skin
becomes a bright-white color from the acetic acid exposure.

Medications

1) Podofilox (Condylox): self-administered by the patient for external warts only.
   Podophyllin contraindicated in pregnancy.
2) Cryo, bichloroacetic or trichloroacetic acid (caustic acids) done in office.

HERPES SIMPLEX: HSV1 and HSV 2

HSV 1: usually oral infection, sometimes genital
HSV 2: more likely to be genital infection, can be oral

Classic Case

May have prodrome (i.e., itching, burning, tingling) on site. Sudden onset of groups of small vesicles sitting on an erythematous base. Easily ruptures and painful. Primary episode more severe and can last up to 2 weeks. Vesicle fluid and crust are contagious.

Treatment Plan

Diagnostic test: herpes viral culture. Usually diagnosed by clinical presentation.

Tzanck Smear
Initial Infection
Acyclovir (Zovirax) $5 \times$ /day $\times$ 10 days
Valacyclovir (Valtrex) BID $\times$ 10 days
Flare-up: Zovirax or Valtrex $\times$ 7 days. Treat as soon as possible: within first 48 hours

Suppressive Treatment
More than six flare-ups per year: consider prophylaxis.

Post-herpetic Neuralgia
Elderly and immunosuppressed at higher risk. Treat with low-dose TCAs (i.e., Elavil).

Complications

1) Post-herpetic neuralgia treated with TCAs (tricyclic antidepressants) such as amitriptyline (Elavil) at bedtime.
2) Infection of the trigeminal nerve ophthalmic branch (CN 5).
3) May cause corneal blindness.

Exam Tips

1) TCAs used to treat post-herpetic neuralgia (Elavil).
2) Acute episode treatment (Valtrex or Zovirax $\times$ 10 days).
3) CN 5 can damage the cornea, causing blindness.

*Treatment recommendations for this section adapted from the CDC *MMWR* (*Morbidity and Mortality Weekly Report*) Sexually Transmitted Disease Treatment Guidelines (2002).

LYMPHOGRANULOMA VENEREUM (LGV)

Also known as lymphogranuloma inguinale. Painless genital ulcer(s) with multiple enlarged tender inguinal nodes (or buboes). Rare infection.

Organism: *Chlamydia trachomatis*
Treatment: Doxycycline, tetracyclines

PHARMACOLOGY REVIEW

Fast Facts | Drug Categories

FDA Categories

Category A
Animal studies and studies in pregnant women have shown no risk to the fetus.

Category B
Animal studies fail to show risk to the fetus, but there are no adequate studies on pregnant women. The majority of drugs given to pregnant women are Category B.

Category C
Animal studies have shown adverse effects to the fetus, but there are no adequate studies in humans. The benefits may outweigh the risk.

Category D
Definite evidence of risk to human fetuses. The benefits may outweigh the risk.

Category X
Animal and human studies have shown fetal abnormalities. The risks outweigh the benefits.

Fast Facts | Pregnant Women and Drugs

1) For pain, use acetaminophen and not NSAIDs (i.e., ibuprofen, naproxen sodium).
2) Avoid laxatives (i.e., Ex-lax, Biscodyl) especially in the third trimester (may induce labor).
3) Most drugs used in pregnancy are in Category B (animal studies show no risk; no human data available). Penicillins and cephalosporins are considered safe in pregnancy (i.e., amoxicillin, cephalexin).

Table 3.9 | Category X Drugs

Drug	Purpose	Notes
Isotretinoin (Accutane) Vitamin A Derivative	Severe cystic and nodular acne (resistant to treatment)	Extremely teratogenic Use two methods reliable birth control D/C if pancreatitis, hypertriglyceremia, etc Only physicians with training can prescribe
Finasteride (Proscar) Alpha Reductase Inhibitor	Benign prostatic hypertrophy	Pregnant/childbearing women should avoid handling crushed or broken tablets
All Hormones Estrogen Progesterone Testesterone, etc	Oral contraceptives Loestrin, Desogen, etc. Polycystic ovaries Hypogonadism, etc	All hormones are contraindicated in pregnant women
Raloxifen (Evista) Selective Estrogen Blocker	Osteoporosis Bone disorders, etc	Not for use in premenopausal women Contraindicated if history of thromboembolism
Misoprostol Prostaglandin Analog	Prevents GI bleeds if on chronic NSAIDs Medical abortions	Prevents GI bleeds if on chronic NSAIDs (i.e., osteoarthritis, rheumatoid arthritis) Arthrotec is mixture of misoprostol and an NSAID (diclofenac sodium)
Leuprolide (Lupron) GnRH Analog	Endometriosis Infertility Precocious puberty Prostate cancer, etc	Gynecomastia Used for in vitro fertilization Hormone-dependent cancer
Methotrexate Antimetabolite	Rheumatoid arthritis Psoriasis, etc	Also used for cancer treatment

Note. Category X: Proven fetal risks outweigh its benefits.

Fast Facts | Immunizations

Mumps, Measles, and Rubella (MMR)
Varicella Vaccine

Live attenuated virus vaccines. If no reliable history of chickenpox, give anytime after the first birthday. Avoid salicylates × 6 weeks (theoretical risk of Reye's syndrome).

Table 3.10	Antibiotic Drug Class and Susceptible Organisms

Drug Class	Examples	Diseases Treated
Penicillins Category B	Pen Vee-K Dicloxacillin (Dynapen) Amoxicillin (Amoxil)	**Gram-positive bacteria** Cellulitis, erysipelas, impetigo Otitis media, strep throat Syphilis (spirochete)
Cephalosporins Category B	**First generation** Cephalexin (Keflex) **Second generation** Cefprozil (Cefzil) Cefaclor (Ceclor) **Third generation** Ceftriaxone (Rocephin)	**Gram-positive bacteria** Cellulitis, Strep throat **Both gram-positive and gram-negative** Pneumonia, Otitis media, Sinusitis **Gram-positive, gram-negative, and anaerobes** PID (pelvic inflammatory disease) Pneumonias, pyelonephritis, etc.
Macrolides Category B	Erythromycin Azithromycin (Zithromax) **Category C:** clarithromycin (Biaxin)	**Atypical bacteria, gram negatives** Atypical pneumonia Chlamydia infections Sinusitis, otitis media
Tetracyclines Category D	Tetracycline Minocycline (Minocin) Doxycycline (Vibramycin)	**Atypical bacteria/rickettsial/spirochete** Lyme's disease Mucopurulent cervicitis Rocky Mountain spotted fever
Fluoroquinolones Category C	Ciprofloxacin Ofloxacin **"New Quinolones"** Levafloxacin (Levaquin) Gemifloxacin (Factive)	**Gram negatives** UTIs, STDs, Pyelonephritis **Both gram-positive and gram-negative** Pneumonia (bacterial) Sinusitis, otitis media
Sulfa Drugs Category C	Sulfamethoxazole + trimethoprim (Bactrim, Septra)	**Gram negatives** Urinary tract infection (UTIs) Pyelonephritis
Antifungals Category C	Fluconazole (Diflucan) Terbinafine (Lamisil Tablets) Lamisil cream	Vaginitis (candida infections) Onychomycosis (tinea infections) Vaginitis

Note. Some of the drug classes listed are also effective against other types of organisms. This list is meant for review, and only pertinent information is included.

Higher risk of infection:
- Household contacts immunocompromised, health care workers
- Day care, elementary school, prisons

Influenza Vaccine (two types)

1) Live attenuated influenza virus vaccine (by nasal spray only). It is indicated only for healthy persons aged 5 to 49 years with no nasal abnormalities.
2) Live virus vaccines are contraindicated for pregnant women.
3) Inactivated influenza virus (injectable form) recommended for women if pregnant in the winter months.
4) It takes 2 weeks to produce antibodies after vaccination.
5) Do not give before age of 6 months because it is not effective (immature immune system).
6) After any live virus vaccine, advise reproductive-aged women to wait at least 3 months before becoming pregnant or to use birth control.

Two Types of Influenza Vaccines

1) Inactivated vaccine (killed virus). Indicated for pregnant women, persons aged 50 or older, chronic conditions (i.e., diabetics), persons living in nursing homes or long-term care facilities.
2) Live virus vaccine (live attenuated influenza vaccine or LAIV). Indicated only for healthy persons ages 5 to 49 years. Administered as a nasal spray.

Live Vaccines Contraindicated in Pregnancy/Severely Immunocompromised

1) Measles.
2) Mumps.
3) Rubella.
4) Varicella.
5) Live flu vaccine (nasal spray).

Fast Facts | Bacteria

Gram Positives

Staphylococcus aureus
Streptococcus

Recommended Drugs
Penicillins, first- to second-generation cephalosporins, broad-spectrum fluoroquinolones (i.e., Levaquin).

Gram Negatives

Haemophilus influenzae
Moraxella catarrhalis
Neisseria gonorrheae
Escherichia coli
Proteus mirabilis

Recommended Drugs
Second- to third-generation cephalosporins, Bactrim/Septra, macrolides, broad-spectrum fluoroquinolones (i.e., Levaquin).

Atypical Bacteria

Mycoplasma pneumoniae
Chlamydia trachomatis
Ureaplasma

Recommended Drugs
Tetracyclines, macrolides.

Spirochetes

Borrelia burgdoferi (Lyme disease)
Rickettsia rickettsii (Rocky Mountain spotted fever)
Treponema pallidum (syphilis)

Recommended Drugs
Doxycycline, amoxicillin/penicillin, third-generation cephalosporin.

MUSCULOSKELETAL SYSTEM

Fast Facts Danger Signals

Navicular Fracture

Acute wrist pain on deep palpation of the anatomical snuffbox that occurs after a history of trauma (i.e., falling forward with hyperextension of the wrist to break the fall).

Hip Fracture

History of slipping or falling. Anterior groin and thigh pain. Pain may radiate to the knee. Affected leg shorter. External rotation of the hip/leg (abduction). More common in elderly people with osteoporosis.

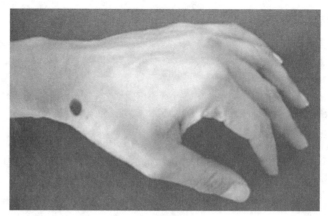

Figure 3.3. Navicular Space

Pelvic Fracture

History of significant or high-energy trauma such as a motor vehicle accident. Elderly with history of osteoporosis. Signs and symptoms depends on degree of injury to pelvis and other pelvic structures such as nerves, blood vessels, and pelvic organs. May complain of difficulty in ambulation, pain with hip movement, bladder and/or fecal incontinence. Severe hemorrhage can result in shock. May be life-threatening.

Fast Facts **Normal Findings**

Joint Anatomy

Synovial fluid: thick serous clear fluid that provides lubrication for the joint
■ Cloudy synovial fluid can be indicative of infection; order C&S
Synovial space: space between two bones (the joint) filled with synovial fluid
Articular cartilage: the cartilage lining the open surfaces of bones in a joint
Ligaments: help stabilize joints. Muscles attach to joints by their ligaments
Bursae: present on anterior and posterior areas of a joint and act as padding. Filled with synovial fluid. Cloudy fluid is abnormal and is indicative of infection

---

Fast Facts **Benign Variants**

Genu recurvatum: hyperextension or backward curvature of the knees
Genu valgum: knock-knees
Genu varum: bowlegs

Exam Tips

1) To remember valgum, think of "gum stuck between the knees" (knock-knees). Opposite is varus or bowlegs.

Fast Facts   Exercise and Injuries

Injuries and Exercise

Inflammation of the joints: injuries, exacerbations, inflammatory disorders
Within the first 48 hours, acutely inflamed joints should not be:
   ▪ Exercised in any form (not even isometric exercises)
No heat of any form is allowed (i.e., hot showers or tub baths, hot packs)
No active range of motion (ROM) exercises
   ▪ If done too early, will cause more inflammation and damage to the affected joints

RICE Mnemonic

Within the first 48 hours after musculoskeletal trauma, follow these rules:

Rest: avoid using injured joint or limb
Ice: cold packs on injured area (i.e., 20 minutes on, 10 minutes off) for first 48 hours
Compression: use an ACE bandage over joints to decrease swelling and provide support. Joints that are usually compressed are the ankles and the knees
Elevation: prevents or decreases swelling. Avoid weight-bearing on affected joint

Isometric Exercise

Useful during the early phase of recovery before regular active exercise is performed
Defined as the controlled and sustained contraction and relaxation of a muscle group
Less stressful on joints than regular exercise
Usually done first before active exercise post injury
Non-weight-bearing (does not work for osteoporosis)
   ▪ Only weight-bearing exercises work for osteoporosis (i.e., walking, biking)

Fast Facts   Orthopedic Maneuvers

Test both extremities. Use the normal limb as the "baseline" for comparison.

Drawer Sign

A test for knee stability (also can be done on ankles).

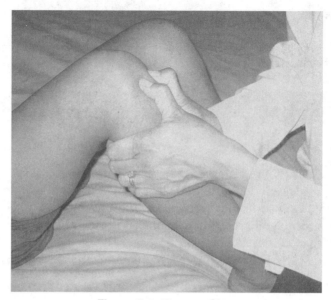

Figure 3.4. Drawer Sign

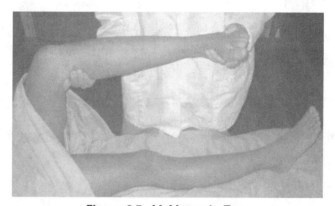

Figure 3.5. McMurray's Test

Finkelstein's Test

Positive: Pain over the dorsal thumb area. Suggests De Quervain's Tenosynovitis, an inflammation of the tendon and its sheath that is located at the base of the thumb.

McMurray's Test

Positive: Knee pain and a "click" sound. Suggests injury to the medial meniscus.

Lachman's Test

Positive: Knee joint laxity. Suggests anterior cruclate ligament (ACL) of the knee tear and instability.

MRI (magnetic resonance imaging)

Best for soft tissue injuries such as tendons and cartilage.

X-rays (radiographs)

Best for bone injuries such as fractures.

Orthopedic Terms

Abduction (varus): movement is going away from the body
Adduction (valgum): movement is going toward the body
Carpal (carpo): refers to the bones of the hands and the wrist
Tarsal (tarso): refers to bones of the feet or the ankle

Fast Facts | Disease Review

DEGENERATIVE JOINT DISEASE (DJD OR OSTEOARTHRITIS)

Arthritis occurs when the cartilage covering the articular surface of joints become damaged. Risk factors: older age, overuse of joints, and positive family history.

Goal of Treatment

1) Pain relief, preserve joint mobility, and function.
2) Strengthen supporting muscles (decreases stress over joints).
3) Decrease stress on the affected joint(s).

Classic Case

Early morning joint stiffness with inactivity of shorter duration compared to rheumatoid arthritis (RA) symptoms, which can last hours to days
Absence of systemic symptoms: not a systemic inflammatory illness like RA
Large weight-bearing joints such as hips and knees commonly affected

Heberdeen's Nodes (DIP)

Bony nodules on the distal interphalangeal joints (DIP).

Bouchard's Nodes (PIP)

Bony nodules on the proximal interphalangeal joints (PIP).

Treatment Plan

1) Mild analgesics if pain but no inflammation (i.e., acetaminophen/Tylenol).
2) If inflammation present: shorter-acting NSAIDS preferred (i.e., ibuprofen, naproxen).
3) If high-risk stomach ulcers: COX-2 inhibitors: celecoxib (Celebrex).
4) Exercises only after acute inflammation gone such as knee-strengthening (quadriceps) exercises to reduce stress on knees.

Exam Tips

1) Heberdeen's and/or Bouchard's nodes have appeared many times on the exam. Memorize the location of each. The following may help:
   ▪ Heberdeen's: the "-deen" ending on the word is the letter "D" for DIP joint
2) By the process of elimination, Bouchard's is on the PIP joint.
3) Types of treatment methods are used for DJD: analgesics, NSAIDS, steroid injection on inflamed joints (NO systemic/oral steroids), surgery (i.e., joint replacement).
4) Do not confuse DJD treatment with treatment for RA.
5) Treatment for RA includes all of DJD treatment methods plus systemic steroids, antimalarials (plaquinil), and antimetabolites (methotrexate).

RHEUMATOID ARTHRITIS (RA)

Systemic autoimmune disorder that is more common in women (8:1). Mainly manifested through multiple joint inflammation and damage. Patients are at higher risk for other autoimmune disorders Graves disease, pernicious anemia, others).

Classic Case

Adult female complains of gradual onset of symptoms over months with daily fatigue, low-grade fever, generalized body aches, and myalgia. Complain of generalized aching joints, which usually involves the fingers/hands and wrist. Morning stiffness last longer than DJD's with painful warm and swollen joints.

Objective

Joint involvement is symmetrical with more joints involved compared to DJD
Most common joints affected: hands, wrist, elbows, ankles, and shoulders
Morning stiffness last longer compared to osteoarthritis (DJD)
Rheumatoid nodules present (chronic disease)

Labs

Sedimentation rate: elevated
CBC: mild microcytic or normocytic anemia common
Rheumatoid factor: positive in 75% to 80% of patients
Radiographs: bony erosions, joint space narrowing, subluxations (or dislocation)

Treatment Plan

Refer to rheumatologist for aggressive management.

Medications

1) Analgesics (i.e., acetaminophen or narcotics such as hydrocodone).
2) NSAIDs (i.e., ibuprofen, naproxen sodium).
3) Steroids: systemic oral doses (i.e., methylprednisone or Medrol Dose Pack).
4) Plaquinil (an antimalarial), gold salts, and so forth.
5) Methotrexate (DMARD or disease modifying agent for rheumatoid disease).
6) Surgery: joint replacement such as the hip, knees.

Complications

1) Uveitis (ophthalmologist stat).
2) Scleritis, vasculitis, pericarditis, and so forth.

Exam Tips

1) Uveitis: refer to ophthalmologist for treatment (high-dose steroids).
2) Drug class question: Plaquinil is an antimalarial.

GOUT

Deposition of uric acid crystals inside joints and tendons due to genetic excess production or low excretion of purine crystals (by-product of protein metabolism). High levels of uric acid crystallizes in joints with predisposition for first joint of large toe. More common in middle-aged males >30 years.

Classic Case

Middle-aged male presents with painful hot, red, and swollen metatarsophalangeal joint of great toe (podagra). Patient is limping due to severe pain on weight-bearing on affected toe. History of previous attacks on the same site. Precipitated by alcohol, meats, or seafood. Chronic gout has tophi (small white nodules full of urates on ears and joints).

Labs

Uric acid level: elevated (>7 mg/dL). Acute phase: first goal is to provide pain relief

Only two types of NSAIDs most effective (narcotics do not work as well)

Acute Phase

1) Indomethacin (Indocin) BID or naproxen sodium (Anaprox DS) BID PRN.
2) If no relief, combine with colchicine 0.5 mg 1 tab every hour until relief or diarrhea occurs.

After acute phase over, wait at least 4 to 6 weeks before initiating maintenance treatment.

Maintenance

1) Allopurinol (Zyloprim) daily for years to lifetime. Check CBC (affects bone marrow).
2) Probenecid (a uricosuric) lowers uric acid.

ANKYLOSING SPONDYLITIS

Chronic inflammatory disease resulting in severe arthritic changes of the spine and sacroiliac joints. Other joints affected are the hips, feet, and shoulders. Associated with Reiter's syndrome, psoriasis, and IBS (irritable bowel syndrome). Also known as a "rheumatoid variant."

Classic Case

Middle-aged male complains of a chronic case of severe back pain (>3 months) that is not relieved by rest. Loss of full range of motion of the spine.

Treatment Plan

Spinal radiograph: classic "bamboo spine"
NSAIDS and narcotics for back pain
Sleep on firm mattress in supine position
Sit in erect position, avoid stooping (postural training)

Labs

Rheumatoid factor usually negative
Sedimentation rate and CRP (c-reactive protein): elevated

Complications

1) Fusing of the spine with significant loss of range of motion.
2) Spinal stenosis (narrowed spine).

LOW BACK PAIN

Very common disorder with a lifetime incidence of 85%. Usually due to soft tissue inflammation, sciatica, sprains, muscle spasms, or herniated discs (usually on L5–S1). Elderly with osteoporosis or chronic long-term steroids. Rule out fracture.

Further Evaluation Is Recommended

History of significant trauma
Suspect cancer metastases
Osteomyelitis
Fracture (elderly with osteoporosis, chronic steroid use)
Patient age >50 with new onset of back pain
History of spinal stenosis (ankylosing spondylitis)
Symptoms worsening despite usual treatment
Herniated disc: common site is at L5 to S1 (buttock/leg pain)

Labs

MRI: best method for diagnosing a herniated disc.

Treatment Plan

1) NSAIDS (naproxen sodium); warm packs.
2) Muscle relaxants if associated with muscle spasms (causes drowsiness; warn patient).
3) Abdominal and core strengthening exercises after acute phase.

No bedrest except for severe cases (24 hours).

Complications

Cauda Equina Syndrome
Acute pressure on a sacral nerve root results in inflammatory and ischemic changes to the nerve. Sacral nerves innervate pelvic structures such as the sphincters (anal and bladder). Considered a surgical emergency. Needs decompression. Refer to ER.

Signs
1) Bowel incontinence.
2) Bladder incontinence.
3) Saddle anesthesia.

Exam Tip

1) Recognize signs and symptoms so you are able to diagnose it on the exam.

Clinical Tips

1) The innervation of the bladder and anal sphincter comes from the sacral nerves.
2) The name *cauda equina* means "horse tail." Sacral nerves when spread out straight appear like a horse's tail.

ACUTE MUSCULOSKELETAL INJURIES

Treatment

RICE (acronym for rest, ice, compression, elevation)
1) Cold is best first 48 hours post injury:
   - 20 minutes per hour × several times/day (frequency varies)
2) Rest and elevate affected joint to help decrease swelling.
3) Compress joints as needed. Use ACE bandage (joints most commonly compressed are knees and ankles). Helps with swelling and provides stability.
4) NSAIDS (naproxen BID, ibuprofen QID) for pain and swelling PRN.

TENDINITIS (ALL CASES)

Microtears on a tendon(s) causes inflammation resulting in pain. Usually due to repetitive microtrauma, overuse, or strain. Follow RICE mnemonic for acute injuries.

SUPRASPINATUS TENDINITIS

Common cause of shoulder pain. Also called cuff tendinitis. Due to inflammation of the supraspinatus tendon.

Classic Case

Complains of shoulder pain with certain movements. The movements that aggravate the pain are arm elevation and abduction (i.e., reaching to the back pocket). There is local point tenderness over the tendon located on the anterior area of the shoulder.

EPICONDYLITIS

Common cause of elbow pain. Lateral epicondyle tendon pain (tennis elbow) or medial epicondyle tendon pain (golfer's elbow).

SPRAINS

Grade III (complete rupture of ligaments). Refer these patients to an orthopedic specialist:

1) Inability to ambulate.
2) Resists any foot motion.
3) Marked edema.
4) Severe pain.
5) Large amount of bruising.

MENISCUS TEAR (OF KNEES)

The meniscus is the cartilaginous lining between joints. Tears on the cartilage result from trauma and/or overuse.

Classic Case

Complains of locking of the knee(s). Patient may limp. Complains of knee pain and difficulty walking and bending the knee. Unable to fully extend affected knee.

Best test: MRI (magnetic resonance imaging). Refer to orthopedic specialist for repair.

RUPTURED BAKER'S CYST (BURSITIS)

Bursae are protective synovial sacs over joints that contain synovial fluid. When inflamed, synovial fluid production increases, causing swelling or bursitis.

Classic Case

Physically active patient (jogs or runs) complains of ball-like mass behind one knee that is soft and smooth. Pressure pain or asymptomatic. If cyst ruptures, will cause an inflammatory reaction resembling cellulitis on the area such as redness, swelling, and tenderness.

Objective

A Baker's cyst resembles a golf ball in the middle of the popliteal fossa. If it is ruptured, synovial fluid is released into the surrounding tissues, causing an inflammatory reaction. The area becomes red, inflamed and tender.

Treatment Plan

1) RICE (rest, ice, compression, and elevation).

2) Large bursa drained with syringe, 18-gauge needle. Synovial fluid a clear golden color.
3) If cloudy synovial fluid, order C&S to rule out infection.

Exam Tips

1) X-ray of knee does not show menisceal injury or any joint cartilage.
2) Best test for joint injuries is the MRI.
3) Remember the signs of a meniscus tear (joint locks up).
4) Carpals or carpo- (bones of the hand).
5) Tarsals or tarso- (bones of the foot).

NEUROLOGY

Fast Facts Danger Signals

Dangerous Headaches

1) Abrupt onset of severe headache ("thunderclap" headache).
2) "Worst HA of my life."
3) First onset of headache age 50 years.
4) Sudden onset of headache after coughing, exertion, straining or sex (exertional headache).
5) Sudden change in level of consciousness.
6) Focal neurological signs (such as unequal pupil size).
7) Headache with papilledema (increased ICP secondary to any of above).

Rule out the worst-case scenario with these patients, such as:

Subarachnoid hemorrhage
Leaking aneurysm
Bacterial meningitis
Increased ICP (intracranial pressure)
Brain abscess
Brain tumor

Temporal Arteritis (giant cell arteritis)

New onset of headaches on one temple that is accompanied by scalp tenderness. It is associated with visual disturbances or blindness of the eye from the affected side. An indurated, reddened and cordlike temporal artery that is tender to touch is found on the same side as the headache. Sedimentation rate is elevated. More common in older adults.

Acute Angle-Closure Glaucoma

Acute onset of headaches behind an eye or around one eye accompanied by eye pain, blurred vision, and nausea and/or vomiting. The cornea looks hazy and the affected pupil is dilated midway. More common in older adults.

Acute Bacterial Meningitis

Acute onset of high fever, severe headache, and stiff neck and meningismus. Meningococcal disease (discussed under Danger Signals section in Dermtology). Classic purple-colored petechial rashes. Accompanied by nausea, vomiting, and photophobia. Rapid worsening of symptoms progressing to lethargy, confusion, and finally coma. If not treated, fatal. Reportable disease.

Fast Facts | Neurological Testing

Neurological Exam

Mental Status (frontal lobes)

- Mini-Mental Exam (orientation, memory, logic, etc.), speech
- Cranial nerve exam

Cerebellar System

- Romberg test
- Tandem gait

Sensory System

- Vibration sense
- Pain sensation
- Touch
- Two-point recognition

Stereognosis (ability to recognize familiar object through sense of touch only):

- Place a familiar object (i.e., coin, pen) on the patient's palm (patient's eyes are closed).

Motor Exam

Gross and fine motor movements (hands). Walking, using hands, jumping, and so forth.

Reflexes

Both sides should be compared to each other and should be equal.

Grading Reflexes

0   No response

1+   Low response

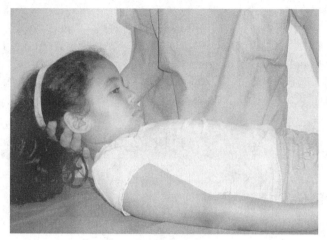

Figure 3.6. Brudzinski's Sign

2+ Normal or average response
3+ Brisker than average
4+ Very brisk response

Neurological Maneuvers

Both these tests are used to assess for meningeal irritation. Both tests are done with the patient in a supine position. More sensitive tests in children compared with adults.

Kernig's Sign
Flex patient's hip one at a time, then attempt to straighten the leg while keeping the hip flexed at 90 degrees.
    Positive: resistance to leg straightening because of painful hamstrings (due to inflammation on lumbar nerve roots).

Brudzinski Sign
Passively flex/bend the patient's neck toward the chest.
    Positive: patient reflexively flexes the hips and knee to relieve pressure and pain (due to inflammation of lumbar nerve roots).

Cranial Nerve Testing (CN)

Mnemonic: "On Old Olympus' Towering Tops, A Finn and German Viewed Some Hops." The first letter stands for the name of the cranial nerve. The word order corresponds to the sequential numbering of the cranial nerves.

CN 1:   On (olfactory)
CN 2:   Old (optic)

Table 3.11 — Cranial Nerve Testing

Number	Name	Technique
1	Olfactory	Sense of smell (coffee, lemon)
2	Optic	Distance vision Near vision
3, 4, and 6	Oculomotor Trochlear Abducens	EOMs (extraocular muscles) Visual fields of gaze
5	Trigeminal V1 (ophthalmic) V2 (maxillary) V3 (mandibular)	Motor: clench jaws Sensory: corneal reflex/facial sensation Contains three branches
7	Facial	Puff cheeks, raise eyebrows, smile
8	Acoustic	Hearing test Whisper test
9 and 10	Glossopharyngeal Vagus	Gag, symmetrical soft palate Uvula is midline, voice quality
11	Spinal accessory	Trapezius muscle atrophy Shoulder shrug
12	Hypoglossal	Tongue fasciculations Tongue atrophy

CN 3:   Olympus' (oculomotor)
CN 4:   Towering (trochlear)
CN 5:   Tops (trigeminal)
CN 6:   A (abducens)
CN 7:   Finn (facial)
CN 8:   And (acoustic)
CN 9:   German (glossopharyngeal)
CN 10: Viewed (vagus)
CN 11: Some (spinal accessory)
CN 12: Hops (hypoglossal)

Exam Tips

1) Memorization tips on cranial nerves:
   - CN 1: you have one nose
   - CN 2: you have two eyes
   - CN 8: the number 8 stands for two ears sitting on top of each other
   - CN 11: number 11 reminds you of two shoulders shrugging together

2) Because cranial nerves are listed only by number on the test (not by name), the correct chronological order is important. Memorize the mnemonic to guide you.
3) Herpes zoster infection (shingles) of CN 5 ophthalmic branch can result in blindness.
4) Rash at tip of nose and the temple area: rule out shingles infection.
5) Cranial nerves are listed by number only.
6) Memorize "On Old Olympus' Towering Tops, A Finn and German Viewed Some Hops."
7) Write down on scratch paper with corresponding cranial nerve "numbers."

Fast Facts   Benign Variants

Anisocoria

The iris of each eye is a different color (usually one eye is blue and the other is brown).

Benign Familial Tremor

A fine tremor of the hand with unknown cause. Tends to run in certain families.

Fast Facts   Disease Review

ACUTE BACTERIAL MENINGITIS

A serious and acute bacterial infection of the meninges resulting in increased intracranial pressure (ICP) and damage to the brain. The most common pathogen for all age groups is *Neisseria meningitides*. *H. influenzae* more common in infants and children <6 years of age. Higher risk with otitis media and sinusitis. Patients who recover commonly have some neurologic sequelae.

Classic Case

Described earlier under the Danger Signals section.

Labs

Lumbar puncture: CSF (cerebrospinal fluid) large numbers of WBCs (purulent).
    Elevated opening pressure
Gram stain and C&S of fluid
CBC with differential, electrolytes, and so on

Medications

Infants: ampicillin or third-generation cephalosporin
Adults: third-generation cephalosporin plus chloramphenicol
Older than age 50 years: amoxicillin plus third-generation cephalosporin
Prophylaxis of close contacts with rifampin or ceftriaxone. Reportable disease.

MIGRAINE HEADACHES (WITH OR WITHOUT AURA)

Migraine headache with aura (precedes the migraine headache) may present as scotomas (blind spots on visual field) or flashing lights that precedes the headache. A positive family history and being female puts one at higher risk (3:1). Migraine headaches can present as abdominal pains in small children.

Classic Case

A female patient complains of a gradual onset of a bad throbbing headache behind one eye along with some photophobia and phonophobia. It is accompanied by nausea and/or vomiting. She reports that resting in a dark and quiet room along with an ice pack on her forehead makes her feel better.

Treatment Plan

Neuro exam will be normal.

Rest in a quiet and darkened room with an ice pack to forehead
Nausea: drink ginger ale or chew dry toast. Avoid heavy fatty meals
Avoid precipitating foods or activities such as:
- MSG (monosodium glutamate) in Chinese food, chocolate
- Red wines, wine, beer, caffeine
- Menses, sleep changes, drinks, stress

Abortive Treatment
1) 5-HT-1 agonists: sumatriptan (Imitrex):
   - Do not start within 2 weeks of MAOI (monoamine oxidase inhibitor)
   - Do not combine with ergots (i.e., ergotamine/caffeine or Cafergot)
   - Over age 40, give first dose in office (theoretical risk of an acute MI)
2) NSAIDs, analgesics (i.e., Extra Strength Tylenol), or narcotics (codeine, hydrocodone).
3) Ergotamine/caffeine (Cafergot):
   - Potent vasoconstrictor
   - Do not mix with other vasoconstrictors (triptans, decongestants, etc.)
   - Common side effect is nausea
4) Antiemetics:
   - Trimethobenzamide (Tigan) IM, supp., po

Prophylactic Treatment
Beta-blockers: propranolol (Inderal) daily or BID
Tricyclic antidepressants (TCAs): amitriptylline (Elavil) at HS

Contraindications (vasoconstricting drugs)
1) Suspected or known CHD (coronary heart disease).
2) PVD (peripheral vascular disease).
3) Uncontrolled hypertension.
4) Complex migraine (i.e., basilar/hemiplegic migraine).

Focal Migraines

Also called basilar or hemiplegic migraines. Focal neuro findings with strokelike signs and symptoms. Resembles a transient ischemic attack (TIA). These patients are at higher risk of stroke. Avoid giving estrogens or any agents promoting clot formation.

Exam Tips

1) Distinguish the drugs used for abortive treatment versus chronic prophylaxis.
2) Answer options may list the drug class instead of the generic name.

TEMPORAL ARTERITIS (Giant Cell Arteritis)

A systemic inflammatory process (vasculitis) of the medium and large arteries of the body. If the temporal artery is involved, called temporal arteritis. More common in males 50 years of age of older.

Classic Case

An older male complains of headache on his temple along with marked scalp tenderness. Complains of visual disturbances over affected side. May have temporary blindness in affected eye (amaurosis fugax). Physical exam reveals indurated cordlike temporal artery that is tender. Sedimentation rate is elevated.

Treatment Plan

Refer to ophthalmologist stat (or refer to ER). Treated with high-dose prednisone. Carotid biopsy (gold standard).

Complications

Permanent blindness if not diagnosed early (ischemic optic neuropathy).

Exam Tips

1) Sed rate is screening test for temporal arteritis (elevated).
2) A common case scenario is the person complaining of "the worst headache of my life." Best plan is to refer to ER or call 911.

Clinical Tips

A high index of suspicion is necessary because of serious sequelae. Order the sed rate stat. Start prednisone in office if you suspect temporal arteritis. Refer to ER.

TRIGEMINAL NEURALGIA (TIC DOULOUREUX)

A unilateral headache caused by impingement (i.e., tumor) or inflammation of the trigeminal nerve (CN 5). Peaks in 60s (rare before age 35). More common in females.

Classic Case

Older female complains of an onset of severe and sharp shooting pains on one side of her face that are triggered by chewing, eating cold foods, and cold air. The severe lancinating pain lasts a few seconds and only stops when the offending activity ceases.

Treatment Plan

Carbamazepine (Tegretol) or phenytoin (Dilantin). MRI or CT scan. Avoid precipitating factors.

CLUSTER HEADACHE

A sudden onset of severe "ice-pick" (lancinating pain) headaches behind one eye that occur several times a day. Headache is accompanied by tearing, lacrimation, and rhinitis. The attacks happen at the same times daily. Cause is unknown. Resolves spontaneously, but may return in the future in some patients. More common in adult males in their 30s to 40s.

Classic Case

Middle-aged male complains of severe headaches that occur several times a day. He describes them as severe and stabbing "ice pick" pains behind one eye or one temple. Headache is accompanied by tearing, a clear runny nasal discharge (rhinitis), and a drooping eyelid (ptosis).

Treatment Plan

Sumatriptan (Imitrex) injection. 100% oxygen at 7 L/minute.

Complications

Higher risk of suicide (males) compared with the other types of chronic headaches.

MUSCLE TENSION HEADACHE

These headaches are secondary to an increase in life stressors that causes the muscles of the scalp to go into spasm. It is a bilateral headache.

Classic Case

An adult patient complains of a headache that is "bandlike" and feels like "someone is squeezing my head." The pain is described as dull in character. The patient admits to increased stress and denies blurred vision and nausea.

Treatment Plan

NSAIDs such as naproxen sodium (Anaprox DS) BID, acetaminophen (Tylenol) QID as needed (PRN). Stress reduction and relaxation techniques. Decrease stressors.

Exam Tips

1) With the exception of muscle tension headaches, which are bilateral, all of the headaches seen on the exam (and notes) are unilateral.
2) Muscle tension: bandlike head pain; may last for days
3) Migraine: throbbing, nausea, photophobia, phonophobia
4) Trigeminal neuralgia (tic douloureux): pain in one side of face/cheek is precipitated by talking, chewing, cold food or cold air on affected area.
5) Temporal arteritis: indurated temporal artery, pain behind eye/scalp
6) Cluster: only HA accompanied by tearing and nasal congestion; severe pain is behind one eye/one side of head. Occurs several times a day. Spontaneously resolves. Seen more in middle-aged males.

BELL'S PALSY

Abrupt onset of unilateral facial paralysis due to dysfunction of the motor branch of the facial nerve (CN 7). Facial paralysis can progress rapidly within 24 hours. Skin sensation remains intact, but tear production on the affected side may stop. Most cases spontaneously resolve. Prolonged cases (several weeks) may leave permanent neurological sequelae. Etiology ranges from viral infection of the nerve to an autoimmune process or pressure from a tumor.

Table 3.12 | Classic Signs and Symptoms: Headaches

Headache	Symptoms	Aggravating Factors
Migraine Without Aura *With Aura*	Throbbing pain behind one eye Photophobia, phonophobia Nausea/vomiting *Above plus scotoma, scintillating lights, halos, etc*	Foods. Red wine, MSG, menstruation, stress, etc Teenage to middle-aged females
Trigeminal Neuralgia (CN 5)	Intense and very brief Sharp stabbing pain One cheek (second branch CN 5)	Cold food, cold air, talking, touch, chewing Older, elderly
Cluster	Severe "ice-pick" piercing pain behind one eye and temple. With: *tearing, rhinorrhea, ptosis and miosis (Horner's syndrome)*	Occurs at same time daily in clusters × weeks to months Middle-aged males
Temporal Arteritis Giant-Cell Arteritis	Unilateral, temporal area With scalp tenderness. Skin over artery is indurated, tender, warm and reddened. Amaurosis fugax (temporary blindness) may be seen	Polymyalgia rheumatica common in these patients (up to 50%) Medical urgency Older, elderly
Muscle Tension	Bilateral "bandlike" pain, dull pain, may last days. May be accompanied by spasms of the trapezius muscles	Stress Adolescents, adults

Classic Case

An older adult complains of waking up that morning with one side of his face paralyzed. He has difficulty chewing and swallowing food on the same side and has noticed that he cannot fully close his eyelid.

Treatment Plan

Rule out stroke, TIA, mastoid infections, bone fracture, Lyme's disease, tumor
Corticosteroids at high doses × 10 days (wean)
Acyclovir (Zovirax) if herpes simplex suspected
Protect cornea from drying and ulceration with applications of an eye lubricant (a.m.) and lubricating ointment at bedtime. Patch eye if patient unable to fully close the eyelid

Complications

Corneal ulceration
Permanent facial weakness (up to 10%)

Table 3.13	Treatment of Headaches	
Headache	**Acute Treatment**	**Prophylaxis/Other**
Migraine	Ice pack forehead. Rest in quiet and dark room. Rx: NSAID, triptans, ergots, etc. Tigan supp. (for nausea)	Tricyclics (TCAs) Beta-blockers
Temporal Arteritis Also known as Giant Cell Arteritis	Refer to ER or stat ophthalmologist Lab: ESR ↑ (sed rate) (screening) Rx: high-dose prednisone	Permanent blindness can result. Temporal artery biopsy (gold standard)
Cluster	100% oxygen at 7 to 10 L/minute Use mask. Intranasal 4% lidocaine	May become suicidal
Trigeminal Neuralgia	Carbamazepine (Tegretol) or phenytoin (Dilantin). Check serum levels	Tegretol or Dilantin for several weeks to months
Muscle Tension	NSAIDS, Tylenol, hot bath/shower, massage, etc	Reduce stress, yoga, massage, biofeedback

Common Drugs: Headache Treatment
Acute Treatment (PRN only)
NSAIDs
Naprosyn sodium (Naprosyn, Aleve) BID or Ibuprofen (Advil, Motrin) TID to QID
SE: GI pain/bleeding/ulceration, renal damage, increased BP in HTN
Triptans
Sumatriptan (Imitrex) injection, nasal, po tabs or sublingual
SE: nausea, acute MI, etc.
Analgesics
Acetaminophen (Tylenol) QID PRN
SE: hepatic damage, etc.
Prophylaxis (must be taken daily to work)
Tricyclic Antidepressants (TCAs)
Amitriptyline (Elavil) at HS or imipramine (Tofranil) at HS
SE: sedation, dry mouth, confusion in elderly, etc.
Beta-Blockers
Propranolol (Inderal LA) or atenolol (Tenormin) daily
Contra: second- or third-degree AV block, asthma, COPD, bradycardia, etc.

CARPAL TUNNEL SYNDROME (CTS)

Median nerve compression due to swelling of the carpal tunnel. Commonly caused by activities that require repetitive wrist motion. Can also be due to hypothyroidism.

Classic Case

Adult patient who uses hands frequently for job (i.e., typing) complains of gradual onset (over weeks to months) of numbness and tingling (paresthesias) on the thumb, index finger, and middle finger areas. Hand grip of affected hand(s) weaker. May complain of problems lifting heavy objects. Chronic severe cases

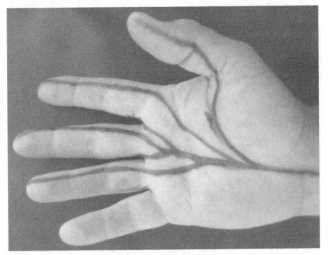

Figure 3.7. Median Nerve

involve atrophy of the thenar eminence (a late sign). History of an occupation or hobby that involves frequent wrist/hand movements.

Tinel's Sign

Tap anterior wrist briskly.
Positive finding: paresthesia or reproduction of symptoms.

Phalen's Sign

Full flexion of wrist for 60 seconds.
Positive finding: reproduction of symptoms.

Exam Tips

1) There is usually a question on either Tinel's or Phalen's sign.

MENTAL HEALTH

Fast Facts Danger Signals

High Risk of Suicide

History of attempted suicide
Family history of suicide
Plan to use a gun or other lethal weapon
History of mental illness such as depression, bipolar disorder

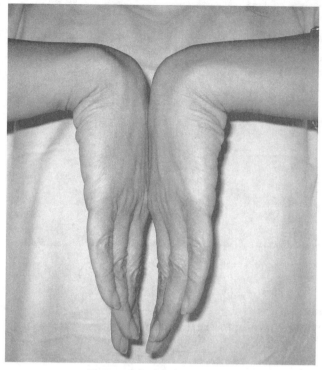

Figure 3.8. Phalen's Sign

Physical illness
Loss (family, social, financial)
Alcohol abuser
Females make more attempts compared to males, but males have a higher success
rate

Fast Facts Disease Review

MAJOR DEPRESSION

Also known as unipolar depression (vs. bipolar depression). Attributed to dysfunction of the neurotransmitters serotonin and norepinephrine. Strong genetic
component.

Diagnosis

Sad mood and diminished interest or pleasure (anhedonia) for a few weeks plus
following criteria (depressed mood plus four from below):

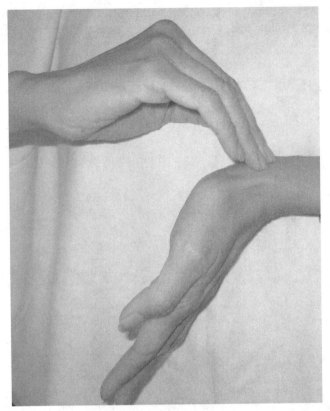

Figure 3.9. Tinel's Sign

Energy: fatigued or increased irritability, restlessness
Poor self-image and poor self-esteem
Feelings of guilt and hopelessness
Cognition: difficulty concentrating and thinking; poor short-term memory
Altered sleep (oversleeping or insomnia)
Appetite: altered appetite (anorexia or increased appetite)

Evaluation

Immediate Goal: assess for suicidal or homicidal ideation, Check history of previous suicide or homicidal attempts, illicit drugs, bipolar disorder (patient and family). Rule out organic causes such as hypothyroidism, anemia, autoimmune disorders.

Treatment Plan

1) First line: selective serotonin reuptake inhibitors (SSRIs).
2) Second line: tricyclic antidepressants (TCAs).

3) Psychotherapy plus antidepressants works better than either method alone.

4) After initiation, follow up 2 weeks to check for compliance and side effects.

ALCOHOLISM

Compulsive desire to drink alcohol despite personal, financial, social consequences.

Level >0.8% is illegal for driving. Females metabolize alcohol more slowly than do males.

Labs

GGT (gamma glutamyl transaminase):
- Lone elevation (or with ALT or AST) is a sign of occult alcohol abuse

AST/ALT ratio:
- Ratio of 2.0 or higher more likely with alcohol abuse

Cage Test

Quick screening test for identification of alcohol abuse/alcoholism.
Positive finding of at least 2 (out of 4) highly suggestive of alcoholism:

C: Do you feel the need to cut down?
A: Are you annoyed when your spouse/friend comments about your drinking?
G: Do you feel guilty about your drinking?
E: Do you need to drink early in the morning? (an eye-opener)

Examples of some quotes using CAGE:

C: "I would like to drink less on the weekends," "I only drink a lot on weekends"
A: "My wife always nags me about my drinking," "My best friend thinks I drink too much"
G: "I feel bad that I don't spend enough time with the kids because of my drinking"
E: "I need a drink to feel better when I wake up in the morning"

Delirium Tremens

Delirium, confusion, hallucinations, delusions, tachycardia, hypertension, grand mal seizures. Considered a medical emergency. Refer to ER.

Treatment Plan

1) Benzodiazepines (Librium, Valium), antipsychotics if needed (i.e., Haldol).

2) Vitamins: Thiamine 100 mg IV, folate and multivitamins with high-caloric diet.
3) Refer to Alcoholics Anonymous (12-step program), therapist.

Korsakoff's Syndrome

A complication of chronic alcohol abuse. A potentially permanent CNS (central nervous system) disorder due to chronic alcohol abuse causing dementia. May recover with intensive thiamine supplementation. Etiology: chronic thiamine deficiency damages the brain permanently.

Exam Tips

1) Alcoholics Anonymous (AA) is one of the most successful methods for recovering alcoholics. They are a group of people meeting on a regular basis to share issues.
2) AA is based on a 12 Step program or stages.
3) Support group for family is called Al-Anon.
4) Support group for teen children is called Ala-teen.
5) One glass of wine or one beer per day is not alcohol abuse.
6) Cirrhosis increases risk of liver cancer.

ANOREXIA NERVOSA

Onset usually during adolescence. Irrational preoccupation and intense fear of gaining weight. Severe food restriction or binge eating and purging. Some examples of purging are laxatives, vomiting, and excessive daily exercise (a method of "purging").

Complications

Marked weight loss (>15% of body weight)
Amenorrhea (no menses × 3 or more consecutive months) may cause osteopenia or osteoporosis
Lanugo (increased lanugo especially in the back and shoulders)
Osteoporosis: due to prolonged estrogen depletion and low calcium intake. Stress fractures
Cardiomyopathy. Death usually due to cardiac cause or suicide

Exam Tips

1) Recognize how anorexic patients present (i.e., lanugo, peripheral edema, amenorrhea, weight loss >10% of body weight).
2) Increased risk of osteoporosis or osteopenia.
3) Low albumin level.

Fast Facts | Psychotropic Drugs

Selective Serotonin Reuptake Inhibitors (SSRIs)

First-line treatment for:

- Major depression, OCD (obsessive-compulsive disorder),
- GAD (generalized anxiety disorder), panic disorder, social anxiety disorder
- Premenstrual dysphoric disorder (or PMS)

Fluoxetine (Prozac): longest half-life of all SSRIs (may last up to 4 weeks)

Sertraline (Zoloft), paroxetine (Paxil; has the shortest half-life)

Side Effects

Sexual dysfunction, loss of appetite, anxiety, insomnia, tremor, sexual dysfunction

Avoid with anorexic patients and undernourished elderly (depresses appetite more)

Contraindications

Avoid SSRIs within 14 days of a MAOI (serotonin syndrome)

Be careful in prescribing drug to patients with anorexia nervosa (can worsen anorexia)

Tricyclic Antidepressants (TCAs)

Not used as first-line treatment for depression.

- Fatal arrhythmia if patient overdoses (suicide attempt)

  Example: Imipramine (Tofranil), amitriptyline (Elavil), nortriptyline (Norpramine)

Monoamine Oxidase Inhibitors (MAOI)

Rarely used (for refractory depression not responsive to multiple drugs).
- Phenelzine (Nardil), tranylcypromine (Parnate)

Contraindications

- Do not combine with SSRI or tricyclic antidepressants
- Wait at least 2 weeks before initiating (high risk of serotonin syndrome)

Avoid foods with high tyramine: aged cheese, red wine, chocolate, fermented food such as beer, others.

Acute Serotonin Syndrome

Signs and symptoms include shivering, diaphoresis, hyperreflexia, fever, mental status changes, muscle spasms (myoclonus). Life-threatening. Caused by high levels of serotonin secondary to certain drugs. Higher risk if taking two types of drugs that block serotonin such as SSRIs and SNRIs (i.e., Effexor, triptans such as Imitrex, Maxalt).

Nicotine Patches

Do not use with other nicotine products (i.e., gum, inhaler); patient will overdose with nicotine. Nicotine overdose can cause acute MIs, hypertension, agitation in susceptible patients.

Benzodiazepines

Tranquilizer's action is potentiated by alcohol, psych drugs, hypnotics, others
For elderly patients, Xanax is a better choice because it has a shorter half-life
> *Examples*
> Alprazolam (Xanax) 0.25 to 6 mg TID (lasts about 4 hours)
> Diazepam (Valium) 2 to 40 mg BID (last about 12 hours)

Illicit Drugs

Cocaine (stimulant)
Nasal perforation if chronic use, tachycardia, euphoria, hyperactivity, hypertension
Chest pain (preexisting CAD, can have acute MI, CVA)

Amphetamines (stimulants)
Preferred treatment of ADHD (attention deficit hyperreactivity disorder) and ADD (attention deficit disorder).
> Signs of overdose:
- Tachycardia, euphoria, hyperactivity, hypertension
- Chest pain (preexisting CAD, can have acute MI, CVA)
> *Examples:* Adderall, dexedrine.

Marijuana
Feelings of well-being, very relaxed, sleepy
Nausea relief (some cancer patients). Wean if chronic user

Exam Tips

1) A list of drugs is given and you are asked to pick out the SSRI (suffix "-ine") such as fluoxetine, sertraline, fluvoxamine.
2) Diazepam is used for patients in acute alcohol withdrawal and/or delirium tremens.
3) Foods that interact with MAOIs are important to remember because it is a safety issue.
4) TCAs: herpetic neuralgia, migraine headache prophylaxis (not acute treatment).

Clinical Tips

a) Patients starting to recover from depression may commit suicide (from increase in psychic energy).

b) If potentially suicidal, be careful when refilling or prescribing certain medications that may be fatal if patient overdoses (i.e., benzodiazepines, hypnotics, narcotics, amphetamines, TCAs, etc.). Give the smallest amount and lowest dose possible.

c) SSRI overdose very rarely causes death (vs. TCAs)

d) TCAs such as Elavil are sedating. Give at bedtime.

ABUSE: ALL TYPES

Abusive behaviors are multifactorial. They may include physical, emotional, and sexual abuse and/or neglect. They can happen at any age and during pregnancy (higher risk).

A common finding is a delay in seeking medical treatment for the injury. The pattern of the injuries is inconsistent with the history. Elderly who are most likely to be abused are those >80 years old and/or frail. Children with mental, physical, or other disabilities and male children are more likely to be abused.

Factors That Increase Likelihood of Child Abuse

Increased financial strain
Job loss or job stress
Low educational attainment
Stepchild
Abuser has a history of being abused as a child

Physical Exam

1) Another health provider (witness) should be in the same room during the exam.
2) Interview victim without abuser in the same room.
3) Visual evidence of trauma via Polaroid camera to document all injuries.
4) Look for: spiral fractures (greenstick fracture), multiple healing fractures especially in rib area, burn marks with pattern, welts, and so forth.
5) Look for are signs of neglect (underweight, dirty clothes, dehydration, etc.).
6) STD testing:
   - Chlamydial and GC cultures (must use cultures in addition to the Gen Probe)
   - HIV, hepatitis B, syphilis, herpes type 2
   - Genital, throat, and anal area culture and testing must be done

Treatment Plan

1) Prophylactic treatment against several STDs (with parental consent for minors).
2) Health care professionals must report actual or suspected child abuse.

Good Communication Concepts

1) State things objectively. Do not be judgmental.

   Example: "You have bright red stripes on your back" instead of "It looks as if you have been whipped on the back."

2) Open-ended questions are preferred.

   Example: "How can I help you?" instead of "What type of object was used to hurt your back?"

3) Do not reassure patients (stops a patient from talking more about their problems).

   Example: "We will make sure you get help" instead of "Don't worry, everything will be fine."

4) Let the patient ventilate his/her feelings. Do not discourage patient from talking.

   Example: "Why don't you tell me why you feel so sad?"

5) Validate feelings,

   Example: "Why do you feel that way?" instead of "I would feel angry too if someone hit me."

Exam Tips

1) There will always be a few questions on abuse (especially the ANCC exam). The abuser is described as a controlling person who does not want the abused person out of sight; the abuser answers all the questions for the patient.
2) Abuse cases: interview couple separately (or the child from the parent).
3) Any answer choice that reassures patients is always wrong.
4) Judgmental responses are always wrong.
5) Delaying an action (i.e., waiting until the patient feels better, etc.) is always wrong.

ADOLESCENCE

| Fast Facts | Danger Signals |

Testicular Torsion

Sudden onset of unilateral testicular pain that increases in severity. Pain may radiate to the abdomen and the groin. Associated with severe nausea and vomiting. Ischemic changes result in a firm, reddened and swollen scrotal sac accompanied by testicular pain.

Urinalysis: negative for WBCs. Doppler ultrasound to check for blood flow to the affected testicle. Testicle not functional after 24 hours if not repaired. Repaired within the first 6 hours, about 80% are salvaged. Refer to ER. A surgical emergency.

Testicular Cancer

Teenage to young adult male complains of a sensation of heaviness in one scrotum or discomfort in the lower abdomen. Painless to slightly uncomfortable nodule or testicular enlargement. Gradual onset. May be asymptomatic until it has metastasized to the lungs or other distal sites.

Fast Facts | Normal Findings

Adolescence

Defined as the onset of puberty until sexual maturity.
Most common cause of death:
- Motor vehicle crashes

Puberty

The time period in life when secondary sexual characteristic start to develop because of hormonal stimulation. Girls' ovaries start producing estrogen and progesterone. Boys' testes start producing testosterone. All of these changes result in reproductive capability.

Girls
- Precocious puberty if puberty starts before age 8 years
- Delayed puberty if no breast development by age 13 years

Growth Spurt
Majority of somatic changes occur between the ages of 10 and 13 years.
- Majority of skeletal growth occurs before menses. Afterward, growth slows down
- Girls start their growth spurts one year earlier than boys

Growth Time Line in Girls
Breast development → peak growth acceleration → menarche.

Menarche
- Average age is 13 years (ranges from 10 to 15 years)
- After Tanner stage II starts (breast bud stage), girls start menses within 1 to 2 years

Boys
- Precocious puberty if starts before age 9 years
- Delayed puberty if no testicular/scrotal growth by age 14 years

Growth Spurt
■ Boys' growth spurts is 1 year later than girls'

Spermarche
■ Average age is 13.3 years

Tanner Stages

Boys
Stage I: prepuberty
Stage II: testis begins to enlarge/increased rugation of scrotum
Stage III: penis elongates
Stage IV: penis thickens. Spermarche begins
Stage V: adult pattern

Girls
Stage I: prepuberty
Stage II: breast bud (onset of thelarche or breast development)
Stage III: breast tissue and areola are in one mound
Stage IV: areola/nipples form a secondary mound
Stage V: adult pattern

Pubic Hair (both genders)
Stage I: prepuberty
Stage I: sparse growth of straight hair that is easily counted
Stage III: hair starts to curl and gets darker
Stage IV: hair curly but not on medial thigh yet as in adult. Hair is coarser.
Stage V: adult pattern, hair spreads to medial thigh and lower abdomen

Table 3.14	Tanner Stages		
Stage	**Girls**	**Boys**	**Pubic Hair**
I	Prepuberty	Prepuberty	None
II	Breast bud	Testes enlarges Scrotum rugae ↑	Few straight, fine hairs
III	Breast and areola One mound	Penis lengthens	Darker, coarse Starts to curl
VI	Breast and areola Secondary mound	Penis widens	Thicker, curly Darker, coarse
V	Adult pattern	Adult pattern	Adult pattern Inner thigh

| Table 3.15 | Immunizations: Age 10 Year and Older |

Vaccine	Immunizations
Hepatitis B	Total 3 doses over 6 months
MMR	Give second dose (if needs to catch up)
Varicella	If no reliable history of chickenpox after age 12 months After age 13 years, need 2 doses
Tetanus	Every 10 years (teens usually due for booster by age 14 to 16 years)
Hepatitis A	High-risk groups (homosexuals), endemic areas (certain areas of Southwest United States, Latin America, Africa, Asia)
Influenza	Annually if high-risk (congenital heart disease, asthma, etc.) 2 types: inactivated and live virus (nasal)
Polio	Catch up if did not receive total of 3 doses as an infant need 3 doses (lifetime)
Meningococcal	For all college freshmen living in dormitories Meningococcal conjugate vaccine (MCV4)

Note. Adapted from Centers for Disease Control Recommended Immunization Schedule (2006). This table is a simplified version and is designed for studying for the certification exams only. Do not use this table as a guideline for clinical practice.

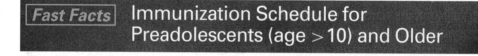

| Fast Facts | Immunization Schedule for Preadolescents (age > 10) and Older |

This schedule is for patients who did not complete immunization or were not immunized as infants.

Exam Tips

1) All college freshmen living in dormitories: high risk of meningococcal infection. Meningococcal conjugate vaccine (MCV4) is recommended by the CDC.

2) Live attenuated influenza virus (LAIV) nasal only: if indicated, use only on healthy persons from ages 5 to 49 years.

3) High risk for flu with vacinnation recommended: HIV, asthma, heart disease, sickle cell, cystic fibrosis, diabetes, others. Household members/health workers caring or living with any person with the above conditions and infants also need to be vaccinated.

4) Vaccine Adverse Event Reporting System (VAERS): governmental program to report clinically adverse events.

Fast Facts Laboratory Tests

Elevated Alkaline Phosphatase

Normally elevated from puberty to teenage years secondary to rapid growth spurts. Enzyme is produced by growing bone or patients healing from major fractures.

Fast Facts Legal Issues

Right to Consent and Confidentiality

Minors can give consent without a parent or guardian for the following:

- Contraception
- Diagnosis and management of pregnancy
- Treatment for STDs

Emancipated Minor Criteria

These minors may give full consent as an adult without parental involvement:

- Married
- Parent or pregnant
- Enlisted in the armed forces

Other Issues

Gunshot wounds, stab wounds and child abuse (actual or suspected abuse) must be reported to the authorities.

Exam Tips

1) Puberty starts at Tanner stage II (breast buds in girl testis and onset of testicular enlargement and increased rugation of scrotum in boys).
2) Puberty ends at Tanner stage V (adult stage).
3) Only Tanner stage II to stage IV needs to be memorized for the exam.
4) There is no need to memorize pubic hair changes for either gender. Memorize only the breast changes (girsl) and the genital changes (boys).

GYNECOMASTIA

Excessive growth of breast tissue. Most cases resolve spontaneously. Normal in up to 40% of pubertal boys (peaks at age 14). Seen in neonates because of maternal hormones; resolves when hormones are gone.

Classic Case

Pubertal to adolescent male is brought in for a visit by a parent for complaint of enlarged breasts (one may be larger) and tender breast. May be tender to palpation. Child is embarrassed and scared about breast changes.

Objective

Round, rubbery, and mobile mound (disclike) under the areola of both breasts
Skin has no dimpling, redness, or changes. If mass irregular, fixed, hard, order a sonogram

Treatment Plan

Evaluate for Tanner stage (check testicular size, pubic hair, axillary hair, body odor)
Rule out serious etiology (testicular or adrenal tumors, brain tumor, hypogonadism, etc.)
Check for drug use: both illicit and prescription (i.e., steroids, cimetidine, antipsychotics)

Pseudogynecomastia

Breast is adipose tissue (not gynecomastia)
Seen more in obese males

IDIOPATHIC SCOLIOSIS

Screening test: Adams forward bend test
Lateral curvature of the spine. More common in girls (80% of patients)
Painless and asymptomatic. Scoliosis is more likely to progress if it occurs in the beginning of the growth spurt

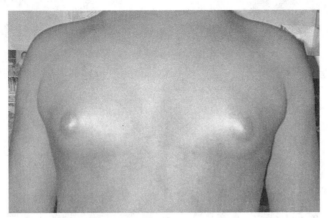

Figure 3.10. Gynecomastia

Classic Case

Pubertal to young teen complains that one hip or shoulder is higher than the other. No complaints of pain.

Adams Forward Bend Test

Bend forward with both arms hanging free. Look for asymmetry of spine, scapula, thoracic and lumbar curvature. Also known as the forward bend test.

Scoliosis Treatment Parameters

Curves less than 20 degrees:
- Observe and monitor for changes in spinal curvature

Curves of 20 to 40 degrees:
- Bracing (i.e., Milwaukee brace)

Curves greater than 40 degrees:
- Surgical correction with Harrington rod used on spine

Exam Tips

1) Curves less than 20 degrees are treated only by monitoring of the scoliosis for worsening.
2) Screening exam is the forward bend test.

OSGOOD-SCHLATTER DISEASE

Microtears of the patellar tendon due to overstress or overuse of the quadriceps muscles of the knees. Repetitive stress and trauma from excessive traction to the

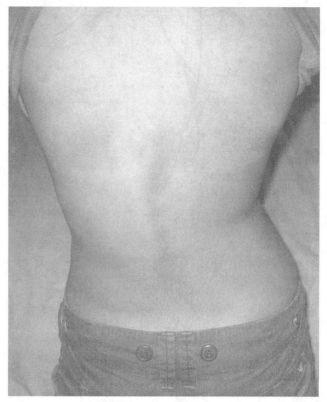

Figure 3.11. Scoliosis

patellar tendon. More common in boys from ages 10 to 17 years. More common during growth spurts, especially in males.

Classic Case

More common in teenage males who are physically active and play sports that stress the quadriceps muscle (i.e., basketball, soccer). Complaints of tender bony mass over the anterior tubercle of both (or one) knees. Aggravated by activities that stress knees such as jumping.

Medications

Tylenol or NSAID for pain; avoid sports, excessive exercise
Lateral x-rays of knees (optional). Diagnosed clinically
Avoid excessive stress or physical activity of the knees for 1 to 2 years
Spontaneous resolution from a few weeks to a few months. Casting, intralesional steroid injections rarely needed

Exam Tips

1) Scoliosis question on treating 10-degree curve (observe for worsening).

DELAYED PUBERTY

If a girl does not develop a breast bud (Tanner stage 2) by age 14 or if a boy does not have testicular development by age of 15 years, it is considered as delayed puberty.

Labs

Check hormone levels (i.e., gonadotropins, estrogen, progesterone, DHEA, FSH, TSH)

X-ray of the hand is used for estimating "bone age":

- When the long bone epiphyses (growth plates) fused, skeletal growth is finished
- Refer to pediatric endocrinologist

GERIATRICS

| Fast Facts | Danger Signals

Temporal Arteritis (giant cell arteritis)

Temporal headache (one sided) with tenderness or induration over temporal artery; may be accompanied by sudden visual loss on one eye (amaurasis fugax). Scalp tenderness of affected side. Screening test is the sedimentation rate which will be elevated.

Cerebrovascular Accident (CVA)

Sudden onset of neurological deficit which worsens within hours. Deficits can include changes such as blurred vision, slurred speech, one-sided upper and/or lower extremity weakness, confusion. Signs and symptoms dependent on location of infarct.

Actinic Keratosis (precursor of squamous cell carcinoma)

Small rough pink to reddish lesions that do not heal. Located in sun exposed areas such as the cheeks, nose, back of neck, arms, chest, etc. More common in light-skinned individuals. Squamous-cell precancer skin lesions. Diagnostic method of choice is the biopsy. Small number of lesions can by treated with cryo. Larger numbers with wider distribution treated with 5-FU cream.

Fractures of the Hip

Acute onset of limping and guarding affected limb. Inability or problems with bearing weight. Hip pain; may be referred to the knee. Unequal leg length. Affected leg is abducted (turned away from the body). History of osteoporosis or osteopenia. Fractures of the hip are a major cause of morbidity and mortality in the elderly. Up to 20% of elderly with hip fractures die from complications (i.e., pneumonia).

Exam Tips

1) Actinic keratosis: precursor of squamous cell cancer. Memory tip: the letter "C" in ACTINIC is a reminder for CANCER.
2) Do not confuse this with seborrheic keratosis, which is benign (common mistake).

Fast Facts   Normal Findings

Skin Findings

Thinner epidermis, dermis, and subcutaneous layers
Less fat, less elasticity (less collagen), slower wound healing
Sebaceous glands hypertrophy

Seborrheic Keratoses

Soft wartlike skin lesions that appear "pasted on." Mostly seen on the back/trunk. Benign.

Senile Purpura

Bright purple-colored patches with well-demarcated edges. Located on the dorsum of the forearms and hands. Lesions eventually resolved over several weeks. Benign.

Lentigines

Also known as "liver spots." Tan to brown-colored macules on the dorsum of the hands and forearms. Due to sun damage. More common in light skin. Benign.

Arcus Senilis (corneal arcus)

Opaque white ring at the periphery of the cornea. Develops gradually and not associated with visual changes.

Cataracts

Opacity and stiffening of the lens of the eye(s)
Test: Red reflex (reflection is opaque versus orange-red glow)

Presbyacusis (sensorineural hearing loss)

High-frequency hearing lost first (i.e., speaking voice is high-frequency). Degenerative changes of the ossicles, fewer auditory neurons, and atrophy of the hair cells resulting in sensorineural hearing loss.

Cardiac

Elongation and tortuosity (twisting) of the arteries. Thickened intimal layer of arteries resulting in Increased systolic BP due to increased vascular resistance (isolated systolic hypertension). Mild increase of left ventricular muscle is normal.

Baroreceptors less sensitive to changes in position. Decreased sensitivity of the autonomic nervous system. Blunted BP response.

■ Higher risk of orthostatic hypotension.

S4 heart sound a "normal finding" in the elderly if not associated with heart disease.

Lungs

Less elasticity and fewer cilia
Peak expiratory flow decreased. Residual volume increased
Total lung capacity remains unchanged

Liver

Liver size and function decreased. The enzyme systems (i.e., cytochrome P450) less active. Slower metabolism of drugs. Cholesterol levels increased.

Renal Function

GFR (glomerular filtration rate) starts to decrease starting at the age 40. By age of 70, up to 30% of renal function is lost. Decreased renal blood flow. Reduced clearance of drugs.

Musculoskeletal System

Kyphosis: compression fractures of vertebrae (osteoporosis)
Osteoporosis and osteopenia. Osteoarthritis (DJD)

Gastrointestinal System (GI)

Less hydrochloric acid, decreased sensitivity of taste buds. Decreased efficiency absorbing nutrients from the small intestines

Increased risk of colon cancer (age >50 years is strongest risk factor)

Endocrine

Increased levels of insulin along with mild peripheral insulin resistance. Fat is redistributed mostly in the abdomen and the thighs.

Sex Hormones

Testes active for the entire life cycle of males. Produce less testosterone

Females: estrogen and progesterone production cease due to ovarian failure (menopause)

Adipose tissue is able to synthesize very small amounts of estrogen

Hematology

Increased risk of iron and folate-deficiency anemia due to decrease efficiency of the GI tract.

Immune System

Immune system activity slightly decreased.

Fast Facts Risk Factors in the Elderly

Falls

1) Frailness, dementia, poor eyesight, and/or poor lighting.
2) Use of area rugs, poor fit to shoes or slippers.
3) Certain medications that cause sedation and/or confusion.

Drugs: Higher Risk of Adverse Effects

Diphenhydramine (Benadryl): sedation/confusion in elderly

Benzodiazepines: confusion, dizziness, ataxia resulting in falls, other accidents

Hypnotics: avoid long-acting (i.e., Halcion). Prefer shorter duration (i.e., Ambien)

Narcotics: start at lower doses; lasts longer in the elderly

Beta blockers: depression and slowing

Amitriptyline or Elavil (tricyclic antidepressants): confusion, delirium, hallucinations

Digoxin (warfarin sodium): high doses cause visual changes, fatigue, depression

Muscle relaxants (Soma, Skelaxin, Norflex): drowsiness, confusion, delirium

Exam Tips

1) Delirium is reversible; dementia is irreversible.
2) Reversible causes for delirium: high fever, infections, metabolic derangements, certain drugs, dehydration, others.
3) Irreversible causes for dementia: Alzheimer's disease, CVAs, severe chronic B12 deficiency, Parkinson's disease, others.
4) Do not confuse reversible versus irreversible causes of dementia/delirium on the exam.
5) The most common side effect from digoxin overdose are GI effects such as nausea, abdominal discomfort. Halos around lights are not an early symptom of overdose.

Clinical Tips

1) Try to prescribe shorter acting drugs. For example, for benzodiazepines, Xanax has a shorter effect (half-life of 4 hours) versus that of Valium (can last 12 hours).
2) Avoid using diphenhydramine (Benadryl) in elderly, especially those with dementia.

Fast Facts ° Screening for Dementia

Mini-Mental Exam (MME)

A brief screening exam to assess for dementia. Results: low scores are seen in dementia, delirium, schizophrenia. Five subject areas are tested.

1) Orientation:
   - Date, day of the week, state, county, home address, and so forth.
2) Attention and calculation:
   - Serial 7s (ask patient to subtract 7 from 100 and so on)
   - Spell "world" (or another word) backwards
3) Recall:
   - Name three objects. Ask patient to repeat names after 5 minutes (short-term memory)
4) Write a sentence:
   - Tell the patient to write a sentence such as "I am going to the doctor"
5) Copy a design:
   - Examiner draws a square or a triangle and tells the patient to copy the design

Clock Drawing Test

Quick method for assessing dementia. If abnormal, screen with MME.
Instruct patient to draw a clock and mark it with the hands showing a certain time.

Exam Tips

1) A question will ask you to identify the MME "activity" that is being performed. You are being tested for your ability to apply the concepts of the MME.

Sample Question

A nurse practitioner instructs a patient to copy a square (or spell *world* backwards, subtract 7 from 100, etc.). Which of the following tests is being performed:

a) MMPI (or Minnesota Multiphasic Personality Inventory; for personality testing)
b) CAGE (for alcohol abuse screening in primary care)
c) MME (correct answer)
d) Beck's Inventory (a depression screening tool)

The correct answer is option C or the MME.

Fast Facts Immunizations

Pneumovax vaccine

Start vaccinating healthy older adults at the age of 65 years (or older). The patient only needs only one dose per lifetime if healthy.

Annual flu vaccine

Given starting in November of each year. Vaccine strains changes every year due to the viral mutations. Immunity from the flu vaccine lasts only a few months.

Tetanus/diptheria (Td) vaccine

Given every 10 years for the entire lifetime. For contaminated wounds, give a booster if the last one was taken 5 years or more before the incident.

Fast Facts Disease Review

DEMENTIA

An irreversible disorder with gradual and insidious onset. Global intellectual decline. Short-term memory usually one of the early signs of the disorder. Terminal stage is about 10 years in Alzheimer's disease (most common cause). Patient is usually incoherent to nonverbal, unable to ambulate, eat or perform self-care.
Duration: lifetime.

Etiology

Alzheimer's disease (most common cause of dementia in this country)
Stroke or cerebrovascular accident (CVA)
Parkinson's disease (up to 20% become demented)
AIDS dementia

Medications

Start as early as possible on Cognex, Elderpryl, or Tacrine (hepatotoxicity risk)
Gingko biloba (increases CNS blood circulation). Antioxidants
Supportive. No cure, but medications can delay progression

DELIRIUM

A reversible process that has an acute and dramatic onset and is temporary. Duration is usually brief (hours to days). Acute decline in mental status. Excitable, irritable, and combative. Patient is incoherent and disoriented.

Etiology

Fever
Shock
Drugs, alcohol
Dehydration

Treatment Plan

Remove and/or treat illness, metabolic derangement, other.

"SUNDOWNING"

Seen in both delirium and dementia.
Starting at dusk/sundown, the patient becomes very agitated, confused, and combative. Symptoms resolve in the morning. Reoccurs commonly.

Treatment Plan

1) Avoid quiet and dark rooms.
2) Well-lighted room with a radio, TV, or clock.
3) Familiar surroundings important. Do not move furniture or change décor.
4) Avoid drugs that affect cognition (antihistamines, sedatives, hypnotics, narcotics).

ALZHEIMER'S DISEASE (AD)

Accumulation of neurofibrillary plaques/tangles cause permanent damage to brain.

The median survival time after diagnosis is 10 years. Three A's: aphasia, apraxia, agnosia.

Aphasia (difficulty verbalizing)
Apraxia (difficulty with gross motor movements such as walking)
Agnosia (inability to recognize familiar objects and people)

Classic Case

An early symptom is short-term memory loss that patient attempts to hide by confabulation.
After 10 years (terminal stage), the patient is usually nonverbal/incoherent, incontinent, wheelchair-bound, and needs total care.

Medications

Selegiline (Eldepryl): start early; slows down disease process
Gingko biloba: increases blood circulation of the brain and helps with memory
Tacrine (Cognex): start early; must monitor liver enzymes periodically

Treatment Plan

Most patients with dementia are taken care of at home by a family member or caregiver.
Fecal incontinence: a major reason a patient is placed in a nursing home by the family.

Complications

Death usually due to an overwhelming infection such as pneumonia and sepsis
Hip fractures are also a common cause of death (from complications)

PARKINSON'S DISEASE

Progressive neurodegenerative disease (marked decrease of dopamine receptors). More common after 60 years of age. Depression common (up to two-thirds of all patients).

Classic Signs

An elderly patient complains of a gradual onset of motor symptoms such as cogwheel rigidity, pill-rolling tremor with difficulty initiating voluntary movement.

Walks with slow shuffling gait. Generalized muscular rigidity with masked facies. Up to 20% have dementia.

Treatment Plan

Rule out other causes of dementia that are reversible (i.e., B12 deficient, heavy metals, neurosyphilis, drug effects, tumors that are resectable, etc.).

Medications

1) Levodopa-carbidopa (Symmetrel) BID.
2) Selegiline (Eldepryl) daily.

Complications

1) Frequent falls may result in fractures of the face, hips, and so forth.

IMMUNIZATIONS: GERIATRIC

Pneumovax Vaccine

Start vaccinating healthy older adults at the age of 65 years (or older). The patient only needs only one dose per lifetime if healthy.

Annual flu vaccine

Given starting in November of each year. Vaccine strains changes every year due to the viral mutations. Immunity from the flu vaccine lasts only a few months.

Exam Tips

1) If a case scenario presents a patient aged 65 years who is being seen for a wellness visit during November or the Fall, the patient needs to be vaccinated with the Pneumovax and flu vaccines.
2) If the patient is older than 65 years of age, then he only needs a flu vaccine.

Clinical Tip

1) Eldepryl is a specialized MAO inhibitor. Do not combine with an SSRI. Increases risk of serotonin syndrome (see Mental Health section).

NONCLINICAL TOPICS

NURSING PRACTICE

Reimbursement

Nurse practitioners (NPs) can be reimbursed directly by Medicare, Medicaid, Champus, and some insurance plans. Medicare reimburses NPs 85% of the usual and customary fee that is paid to a physician for the same visit.

Statutory Authority

Another term used for this concept is *legal authority*. Elected officials (legislature) vote on a bill (i.e., Nurse Practice Act). Bills that pass become law and have statutory authority and become law.

Nurse Practice Act

Each state has a Nurse Practice Act. The Nurse Practice Act gives nurses the legal right to practice. It has statutory authority and is legally enforceable.

Nurse Practitioner (NP) Practice

The legal authority for NP practice is granted through the Nurse Practice Act. The right to practice is not derived from the federal government, the AMA, or the Department of Health.

Board of Nursing (BON)

An official governmental agency whose main job is the enforcement of the Nurse Practice Act of the state. Another prominent role is the granting of licensure to nurses. Inversely, it can also revoke licenses and discipline nurses.

Standards of Practice (American Nurses Association; 1996)

This document lists nursing standards of practice in a generic manner and is meant to be used on a national level. It contains "authoritative statements" that are used to evaluate and measure the nursing "quality of practice, service, or education."

NURSE PRACTITIONER ROLE

Requirements for Nurse Practitioner Practice

A nurse practitioner must meet the *minimal* educational requirements as required by the Nurse Practice Act in the state of practice.

Collaborative Agreements

A written document between a physician and nurse practitioner outlining the nurse practitioner's role and responsibility to the clinical practice. It must be signed by both and is usually submitted to the board of nursing. Agreements must be reviewed periodically.

Title Protection

Professional designations such as registered nurse (RN) or nurse practitioner are protected by law and cannot be used by anyone who does not meet the educational criteria for a nurse. Laws such as this help protect the public from unlicensed "nurses."

Clinical Guidelines

Clinical guidelines are written by expert panels and/or specialty organizations (i.e., the American Heart Association or the American Cancer Society). They are evidence-based and act as treatment guidelines. A fo//ew examples of diseases with treatment guidelines include hypertension, hyperlipidemia, and pneumonia.

Nurse Practitioner Role

Loretta C. Ford, PhD, RN and Henry K. Silver, MD introduced the NP role in 1965. First nurse practitioners were pediatric NPs.

A huge shortage of primary care physicians in rural areas was one of the driving forces for the development of this role. The University of Colorado started its first class in 1978 and was the first one to develop and start a nurse practitioner (NP) program in the country.

Budget Reconciliation Act of 1989 (HR 3299)

The first time nurse practitioners were reimbursed directly by Medicare. Only board-certified pediatric and family nurse practitioners were allowed as primary providers as long as they practiced in designated "rural" areas.

MALPRACTICE INSURANCE

Occurrence-Based Policy

Covers claims against the NP not only during the active period, but also afterwards. The date that a claim is filed does not matter as long as the alleged event occurred during the period when the policy was active.

Example: malpractice policy active from January 2003 to January 2004. In June 2007, the NP stops carrying the insurance. If a lawsuit is filed in 2007 for an event that occurred during the time that the policy was active, the claim is still covered under an occurrence-based policy but not under a claims-based policy.

Claims-based Policy

Covers claims only if the NP is currently enrolled in the company's malpractice insurance program. Any claims filed in the future (even if the incident occurred during the time the policy was active) is not covered if the NP is no longer enrolled in the company's malpractice program.

CASE AND RISK MANAGEMENT

Case Management (case managers)

The process of monitoring the appropriateness and managing the health care of patients with high-cost and/or chronic medical conditions. This is done entitis such as insurance companies, health care organizations, hospitals, etc.

Risk Management

A system of monitoring and assessing for high-risk areas and procedures in an organization. If high-risk areas are identified, interventions are done to minimize the chances of the event happening in the future. Risk management helps to reduce the risk of adverse events within an organization.

Utilization Review (UR)

The process of evaluating the appropriateness of inpatient hospitalization. Proof of the medical necessity for the patient's hospitalization is done mainly through chart reviews.

Accreditation

Done by a nongovernmental entity. It is a voluntary process. A well-known accrediting organization is the JCAHO (Joint Commission for the Accreditation of Health Organizations). Accreditation demonstrates to the public that the health facility has gone beyond the normal requirements and has excelled in its class.

LEGAL HEALTH ISSUES

The following are legally binding documents. The patient must be mentally competent. The documents need to be witnessed and notarized in order to be valid.

Power of Attorney for Health

A person (or the proxy) is designated by the patient to make his future health care decisions in the event that he becomes mentally incompetent.

Power of Attorney

As above. This role is broader and encompasses not only health care decisions, but also in other areas of the patient's life such as financial affairs.

Living Will

Written instructions listing the patient's preferences for treatment or nontreatment. Ideally, nurses and other health providers should discuss the document when the patient is admitted (if mentally competent). Health care providers for the patient and family members ideally should be made aware of the patient's decision.

Informed Consent

Patient must be mentally competent to give informed consent (i.e., not on pain medications, no dementia, no drugs affecting cognition, etc.) and should be at least 18 years of age or an emancipated minor. A mentally competent patient has the right to refuse treatment or withdraw at anytime.

  The patient is informed of the following and given an opportunity to ask questions:

1) Purpose of the procedure/treatment/ research study
2) Success rate or failure for the suggested treatment or procedure.
3) Other alternative(s) to the suggested procedure/treatment for the medical condition.
4) Risk vs. benefits of the procedure such as adverse events, anesthesia risk, others.
5) Prognosis and success rate.

INSTITUTIONAL REVIEW BOARDS (IRB)

Reviews research studies and proposals. They have authority to review and approve research protocols for their instittution. Ensures that there is protection of human subjects, ethical treatment, and adequate informed consent obtained.

Some examples of ethical guidelines for protection of human subjects are: The HHS (Health and Human Services) Protection of Human Subjects and the Nursing.

Ethical Concepts

1) Beneficence (the duty to help others).
2) Nonmalfeasance (the duty to avoid harm to others).
3) Confidentiality (the right to keep records private).
4) Accountability (the nurse is responsible for her actions).
5) Respect for human dignity.
6) Compassion.
7) Right to privacy of records, including financial records (HIPPA or the Health Insurance Portability and Accountability Act).

PUBLIC HEALTH POLICY

Medicare Part A

Automatic at age 65 years if the patient paid Medicare taxes (deducted from paychecks or other forms of payment when younger).
Pays for:

1) Inpatient hospitalizations.
2) Skilled nursing facilities (not custodial, long-term care or nursing homes).

Medicare Part B

Patient must sign up and pay a monthly premium to become eligible for Part B.

1) Outpatient care.
2) Pays 80%, members pay 20%.

Medicare Part B: Medically Necessary Services or Supplies (outpatient)
1) Outpatient physician visits, labs, X-rays.
2) Durable medical equipment such as wheelchairs, walkers.
3) Skilled nursing visits.

4) Mammograms/colonoscopy after age 50.
5) Rehabilitation.

Medicare

Does not pay for:

1) Routine care (routine PE, glasses, dental, etc.).
2) Custodial nursing homes (do not confuse with skilled nursing facilities).

Title XIX of the Social Security Act (Medicaid)

A federal and state matching program (state must match what the federal government allocates for its Medicaid programs).

1) Medical assistance to low income persons, the disabled, blind, or members of families with dependent children.
2) Pays for health care, nursing home, prescription drugs.
3) Providers must agree to accept Medicaid payment in full and not collect from the patient or beneficiaries.

THEORETICAL CONCEPTS

Health Belief Model (Becker; 1972)

The person who feels susceptible to the disease and believes that he will benefit from changing his behavior is more likely to perform the healthier behavior.

Self-Efficacy Theory (Alfred Bandura; 1970s)

A person who believes that he can succeed in performing an action (or feelings of self-efficacy) that will result in a positive outcome is more likely to perform the healthier behavior.

Systems Theory

All parts of a system are interrelated and dependent on each other.
If one part of the system is damaged or dysfunctional, the rest of the system is also affected.

Family Systems Theory

Derived from systems theory. Families develop at a different rate. If one family member is dysfunctional, the rest of the family is affected negatively. For example, if a member has poor coping or communication skills, the entire family becomes dysfunctional.

HEALTH CARE ORGANIZATIONS

HMO (Health Maintenance Organization) and PPO (Preferred Provider Organization)

Health care providers are paid a monthly fee for each patient enrolled in their panel. This is called the *capitation fee.*

HMO (Health Maintenance Organization)

Patients are assigned to a primary care provider (PCP). Patients must get authorization for services, certain tests, procedures, or specialist visits from the PCP office.

PPO (Preferred Provider Organization)

Patient does not need authorization to visit specialists. Patients encouraged to utilize "preferred providers." Patients can see physicians who are "out of network," but the cost is higher for the patient.

Practice Questions

SECTION A

1

During a physical exam, the nurse practitioner instructs the patient to make a fist by folding his thumb and then covering the thumb with the other fingers. The patient complains of pain (positive Finkelstein's sign). Which of the following conditions is this test indicative of:

a) Depuytren's contracture
b) DeQuervain's tenosynovitis
c) a "trigger" finger
d) a severe case of Carpal tunnel syndrome

2

Which of the following statements is true regarding claims-based professional malpractice insurance:

a) all malpractice claims made are paid as long as the nurse practitioner is in active practice
b) claims made during the past insured periods are covered as long as the nurse practitioner is currently enrolled in the malpractice insurance program with the company
c) even though the nurse practitioner is no longer insured by the same insurance company, any claims made against her on the dates that her malpractice insurance was active is still eligible for coverage
d) malpractice insurance will pay claims that are eligible if the nurse practitioner is found to be not at fault

3

Which of the following is a true statement regarding the serum glycosylated hemoglobin test:

a) it is the average blood glucose level during the previous 3 months
b) it detects the fasting blood glucose level in the previous 3 months
c) it is a test used to detect the amount of glucose and lactose in the blood
d) the test is more sensitive in type 2 diabetes than in type 1 diabetes

4

A 21-year-old female who is complaining of random palpitations associated with dizziness is diagnosed with mitral valve prolapse (MVP) by the nurse practitioner. Her echocardiogram reveals redundant and thickened leaflets. On physical exam, a grade III/VI systolic murmur with an ejection click is noted. Which of the following is a true statement regarding this condition:

a) endocarditis prophylaxis is indicated for some dental, urologic, and gastrointestinal invasive procedures
b) no endocarditis prophylaxis is indicated for any gastrointestinal procedures
c) warfarin sodium (Coumadin) is always indicated for older patients
d) endocarditis prophylaxis is necessary for dental procedures only

5

All of the following services are covered under Medicare Part A except:

a) inpatient hospitalizations
b) medicines administered to a patient while hospitalized
c) nursing home care
d) radiology tests done in a hospital

6

The nurse practitioner would test the obturator and iliopsoas muscles to evaluate a possible case of which of the following conditions:

a) acute cholecystitis
b) acute appendicitis
c) inguinal hernia
d) gastric ulcer

7

The Dawn Phenomenon is best described as which of the following:

a) it is due to abnormally low levels of serum glucose very early in the morning which stimulates the liver to secrete glucagon
b) it is an increase in the blood glucose levels early in the morning due to the physiologic spike of growth hormone
c) it is an autoimmune disorder resulting in very high fasting blood glucose levels
d) it is a rare phenomenon that only occurs in diabetics

8

An 18-year-old male is brought in by his mother to an urgent care center. She tells the nurse practitioner that he returned from a camping trip 3 days ago and now has a high fever, severe headache, myalgias, and neck discomfort. She reports that her son started to break out with rashes; some of them which are turning into dark red to purple-colored lesions. On physical examination, the temperature is 103.0°F, the pulse is 110 beats/minute, and the respiratory rate is at 22/minute. The blood pressure is 90/50 mm Hg. Which of the conditions is most likely:

a) Stevens-Johnson syndrome
b) meningococcemia
c) Rocky Mountain spotted fever
d) erythema multiforme

9

A 22-year-old student is seen in the college health clinic with complaints of fatigue, rhinitis, and a cough for 2 weeks. The cough is productive of small amounts of sputum. The patient has a negative health history, is not on any prescription medications, and denies a history of allergies. The physical exam reveals a temperature of 99.9°F, respirations of 18 per minute, and a pulse of 100 beats per minute. Lung exam reveals fine crackles on the left lower lobe of the lung. A chest radiograph (x-ray) shows diffuse infiltrates on the same lobe. What is the most likely diagnosis:

a) streptococcal pneumonia
b) mycoplasma pneumonia
c) allergic rhinitis
d) Legionnaire's disease

10

Which of the following antihypertensive medications should the nurse practitioner avoid when treating patients with emphysema:

a) calcium channel blockers
b) ACE inhibitors
c) beta blockers
d) diuretics

11

Linda B., a 30-year-old chef, complains of a sudden onset of hives that started to break out all over her body after she came back from lunch. It is accompanied by chest tightness and a dry cough. She tells a coworker that she has a history of eczema and had mild asthma during childhood. She appears anxious and is not sure of what to do next. Which of the following is the best intervention to follow for this patient:

a) immediately give a treatment of nebulized albuterol mixed with saline and repeat in 10 minutes if the patient's symptoms are not better

b) administer an injection of cimetidine (Tagamet) and an antihistamine as soon as possible

c) give an injection of epinephrine 1:1,000 intramuscularly immediately

d) immediately give the patient an injection of prednisone and epinephrine 1:1,000 intramuscularly and call for emergency assistance

12

In which of the following conditions would the cremasteric reflex be absent:

a) acute epididymitis

b) testicular torsion

c) acute prostatitis

d) it is always present

13

Which of the following is not associated with B12-deficiency anemia:

a) spoon-shaped nails and pica

b) a red and swollen tongue (glossitis) and a vegan diet

c) macrocytes and multisegmented neutrophils

d) tingling and numbness in both feet

14

A diabetic patient has a urinalysis ordered. The results are: 4+ ketones, trace leukocytes, negative nitrites, and negative red blood cells. Which of the following would the nurse practitioner do next:

a) order an ultrasound of the kidneys to rule out subacute renal failure

b) advise the patient to check his blood glucose QID daily and return to the clinic for a follow-up in 48 hours

c) order a 24-hour urine for microalbumin

d) assess for a history of illicit drug or alcohol use

15

All of the following are true statements about diverticula except:

a) diverticula are located in the colon

b) a low-fiber diet is associated with the condition

c) diverticula in the colon are colonized with bacteria

d) supplementing with fiber such as psyllium (Metamucil) is never recommended

16

Patients who are diagnosed with gonorrhea are also treated for the following because of high rates of coinfection:

a) *Mycoplasma pneumoniae*

b) *Chlamydia trachomatis*

c) syphilis

d) pelvic inflammatory disease

17

An older woman complains to the nurse practitioner that she has leakage of urine when she sneezes or is laughing. The patient thinks that it is getting worse. Which of the following would be appropriate initial intervention:

a) educate the patient about Kegel exercises

b) recommend that she limit her fluid intake to less than 1 L per day

c) refer the patient to a urologist for a cystoscopy

d) advise the patient that she will be given medicine to help her with bladder control

18

A 15-year-old high school student who is going through a growth spurt has a baseline laboratory test done during a routine physical exam. The serum alkaline phosphatase level is expected to be:

a) normal

b) higher than normal

c) lower than normal

d) none of the above

19

Which of the following antihypertensive medications has beneficial effects to an elderly white female with osteoporosis:

a) calcium channel blockers

b) ace inhibitors

c) beta blockers

d) diuretics

20

The Lachman maneuver is used to detect which of the following:

a) instability of the knee due to anterior cruciate ligament damage

b) nerve damage of the knee due to past injury

c) the integrity of the patellar tendon

d) tears on the meniscus of the knee

21

When an adolescent male's penis grows in length more than in width, which of the following Tanner stage is he classified:

a) Tanner stage II

b) Tanner stage III

c) Tanner stage IV
d) Tanner stage V

22

An obese patient who is being discharged from the local hospital for DVT (deep vein thrombosis) wants to know if there is anything he can do to minimize recurrence of the disorder. Which of the following is a false statement:

a) use thromboembolic stockings as much as possible
b) avoid prolonged inactivity
c) report any bleeding in the gums and excessive bruising
d) start exercising vigorously as soon as possible so that the circulation in the affected lower extremitiy improves

23

Human papilloma virus (HPV) infection of the larynx has been associated with:

a) laryngeal cancer
b) esophageal stricture
c) cervical cancer
d) metaplasia of the squamous cells

24

Mr. Brown is a 65-year-old carpenter complaining of morning stiffness and pain in both his hands and right knee on awakening. He feels some relief after warming up. On exam, the nurse notices the presence of Heberdeen's nodes. Which of the following is most likely:

a) osteoporosis
b) rheumatoid arthritis
c) osteoarthritis
d) Reiter's syndrome

25

A positive posterior drawer sign in a soccer player signifies:

a) an abnormal knee
b) instability of the knee
c) a large amount of swelling on the knee
d) an injury of the meniscus

26

Valgus stress means:

a) the force is being directed toward the midline of the body
b) the force is being directed away from the body

c) the patient is emotionally distressed

d) the vagal nerve is inflamed

27

Healthy People 2010 has several focus areas. All of the following are focus areas except:

a) mental health disorders

b) injury prevention

c) diabetes and HIV (human immunodeficiency virus)

d) sexual abstinence

28

What is the most common laboratory test used in primary care to evaluate for the glomerular filtration rate (GFR) in a patient with diabetes mellitus:

a) electrolyte panel

b) creatinine

c) alkaline phosphatase

d) BUN-to-creatinine ratio

29

All of the following are false statements regarding acute gastritis except:

a) chronic intake of nonsteroidal analgesics (NSAIDs) can cause the disorder

b) chronic lack of dietary fiber is the main cause of the disorder

c) the screening test for the disorder is the barium swallow test

d) the gold standard to evaluate the disorder is a colonoscopy

30

Signs and symptoms of depression include all of the following except:

a) anhedonia

b) low self-esteem

c) apathy

d) apraxia

31

Which of the following is an accurate description of eliciting for Murphy's sign:

a) on deep inspiration by the patient, palpate firmly in the right upper quadrant of the abdomen below the costovertebral angle

b) bend patient's hips and knees at 90 degrees, then passively rotate hip externally, then internally

c) ask the patient to squat, then place the stethoscope on apical area

d) press into the abdomen deeply, then release it suddenly

32

A pregnant woman complains of a painful right knee after playing with her 3-year-old son. She wants to be treated for the pain because it is keeping her awake at night. Which of the following is the most appropriate drug to give this patient:

a) low-dose ibuprofen (Advil)
b) acetaminophen (Tylenol)
c) naproxen sodium (Aleve)
d) baby aspirin (Bayer)

33

Epidemiologic studies show that Hashimoto's disease occurs most commonly in:

a) middle-aged to older women
b) smokers
c) obese individuals
d) older men

34

A 48-year-old woman is told by her physician that she is starting menopause. All of the following are possible findings in premenopausal women except:

a) hot flashes that may interfere with sleep
b) irregular menstrual periods
c) severe vaginal atrophic changes
d) cyclic mood swings

35

A 63-year-old patient with a 10-year history of poorly controlled hypertension presents with a cluster of physical exam findings. Which of the following indicate target organ damage commonly seen in hypertensive patients:

a) pedal edema, hepatomegaly, and enlarged kidneys
b) hepatomegaly, AV (arteriovenous) nicking, bibasilar crackles
c) renal infection, S3, neuromuscular abnormalities
d) glaucoma, jugular vein atrophy, heart failure

36

The following skin lesions are found more commonly in the elderly except:

a) actinic keratosis
b) solar lentigines
c) tinea cruris
d) seborrheic keratosis

37

A 30-year-old female who is sexually active complains of a large amount of milklike vaginal discharge. A microscopy slide reveals squamous epithelial cells with blurred margins. The vaginal pH is at 6.0. Which of the following is most likely:

a) trichomonas infection
b) bacterial vaginosis
c) candidal infection
d) a normal finding

38

The Pap smear result on a 20-year-old sexually active student who uses condoms inconsistently shows a large amount of inflammation. Which of the following is the best follow-up:

a) call the patient to return to the clinic so she can get tested for a possible cervical infection
b) treat the patient with metronidazole vaginal cream over the phone
c) call the patient and tell her she needs a repeat Pap smear in 6 months
d) advise her to use a Betadine douche at HS × 3 days

39

During a routine Pap smear done on a 53-year-old, several areas of flat white skin lesions are found on the patient's vulva. The skin lesions look thin and atrophic. The patient reports that the area is sometimes itchy and has been present for several years. Which condition is best described:

a) chronic scabies infection
b) lichen sclerosus
c) chronic candidal vaginitis
d) a physiologic variant

40

The heart sound S2 is caused by:

a) closure of the atrioventricular valves
b) closure of the semilunar valves
c) opening of the atrioventricular valves
d) opening of the semilunar valves

41

Diabetes mellitus is the leading cause of:

a) lower limb amputations
b) decubitus ulcers

c) dementia

d) heart attacks

42

All of the following are covered under Medicare Part B except:

a) persons aged 65 years or older

b) durable medical equipment

c) mammograms annually starting at age 50

d) anesthesiologists' services

43

All of the following patients are at higher risk for suicide except:

a) 66-year-old white male whose wife of 40 years recently died

b) a high school student who binges on alcoholic drinks but only on weekends

c) a depressed 45-year-old female with family history of suicide

d) a grandmother who has recently been diagnosed with both hypertension and hypothyroidism

44

A 70-year-old male patient complains of a bright red-colored spot in his left eye for 2 days. He denies eye pain, visual changes, or headaches. He has a new onset of cough from a recent viral upper respiratory infection. The only medicine he is on is Bayer aspirin, one tablet a day. Which of the following is most likely:

a) corneal abrasion

b) acute bacterial conjunctivitis

c) acute uveitis

d) subconjunctival hemorrhage

45

Which of the following is appropriate follow-up for this 70-year-old patient:

a) referral to an optometrist

b) referral to an ophthalmologist

c) advise the patient that it is a benign condition and will resolve spontaneously

d) prescribe an ophthalmic antibiotic solution

46

Jason, a type 1 diabetic, is being seen for a 3-day history of frequency and nocturia. He denies flank pain and is afebrile. The urinalysis result shows negative ketones, trace amount of blood, negative nitrites, and 3+ leukocytes. He has a trace amount of protein. Which of the following is the best test to order initially:

a) urine for culture and sensitivity
b) 24-hour urine for protein and creatinine clearance
c) 24-hour urine for microalbumin
d) an intravenous pyelogram (IVP)

47

During an episodic visit, a blood pressure of 172/90 is found on a woman with a 10-year history of controlled stage I hypertension and osteoarthritis. Her knees are slightly deformed and she is currently complaining of severe pain on her left knee. She has been self-treating with over-the-counter naproxen sodium (Aleve) two tablets twice a day (BID) for the past 2 months. How do NSAIDS (nonsteroidal anti-inflammatory drugs) affect hypertension:

a) they increase the drug level of diuretics in the body
b) they affect the kidneys and can elevate blood pressure
c) a drug–drug interaction is common finding in these patients
d) they are not associated with adverse effects for patients with hypertension

48

Which of the following pharmacologic agents is used to treat nicotine dependence (smoking cessation):

a) sertraline (Zoloft)
b) bupropion (Zyban)
c) multivitamins
d) diazepam (Valium)

49

Rocky Mountain spotted fever is caused by the bite of which of the following:

a) mosquito
b) tick
c) flying insect
d) flea

50

All of the following are false statements about atopic dermatitis except:

a) contact with cold objects may exacerbate the condition
b) it does not have a linear distribution
c) it is associated with bullae
d) it is not pruritic

SECTION B

51

A 65-year-old grandmother tells the nurse practitioner that on waking up in the morning, she noticed that her left eye was very painful and tearing profusely. She had noticed crusty small round rashes on the side of her left forehead along with a few on the tip of her nose. Which of the following conditions is most likely:

a) varicella zoster virus infection of the cornea
b) corneal ulcer
c) viral conjunctivitis
d) bacterial conjunctivitis

52

An 22-year-old sexually active woman is complaining of amenorrhea and vaginal spotting. On exam, her left adnexa is tender and cervical motion tenderness is positive. Which test should the nurse practitioner initially order:

a) flat plate of the abdomen
b) CBC (complete blood count) with white cell differentials
c) pregnancy test
d) pelvic ultrasound

53

Which of the following heart sounds is associated with heart failure:

a) S3
b) S1, S2, and S3
c) S1, S2, and S4
d) Still's murmur and S4

54

A crossing guard complains of twisting his right knee while walking that morning. The knee is swollen and tender to palpation. The nurse practitioner suspects a grade II sprain. The initial treatment plan includes which of the following:

a) intermittent application of cold packs during the first 24 hours followed by applications of low heat at bedtime
b) elevation of the affected limb with episodic applications of cold packs for the next 48 hours
c) rechecking the knee in 24 hours and isometric exercises

d) the application of an ACE bandage to the affected knee and a warm shower

55

Trimethoprim sulfamethazole (Bactrim) is contraindicated in which of the following conditions:

a) G6PD-deficiency anemia
b) lead poisoning
c) beta thalassemia minor
d) B12-deficiency anemia

56

An 18-year-old male with a history of sickle cell anemia calls the nurse practitioner on the phone complaining that he woke up with a painful penile erection four hours ago. The nurse practitioner would follow which of the following treatment plans:

a) Insert a Foley catheter and measure the patient's intake and output for the next 24 hours
b) Insert a small Foley catheter to obtain a specimen for a urinalysis and urine for culture and sensitivity
c) recommend an increase in the fluid intake up to 2 L per day and warm packs
d) recommend immediate referral to the emergency room

57

A patient is being given a physical exam for an elective surgical procedure. The patient reports taking a herbal substance. The nurse practitioner is well aware that the patient should be educated to stop taking the substance a few days before surgery. Which of the following herbs should be stopped a few days before surgery to minimize the risk for an adverse drug interaction between the herb and anesthetics:

a) St. John's wort
b) Echinachea
c) Saw Palmetto
d) Mint tea

58

Folic acid supplementation is recommended for women who are planning pregnancy in order to:

a) prevent renal agenesis
b) prevent anencephaly
c) prevent kidney defects
d) prevent heart defects

59

All of the following are possible etiologies for secondary hypertension except:

a) acute pyelonephritis
b) pheochromocytoma
c) renovascular stenosis
d) coarctation of the aorta

60

Fitz-Hugh-Curtis syndrome is associated with which of the following infections:

a) syphilis
b) *Chlamydia trachomatis*
c) herpes genitalis
d) lymphogranuloma venereum

61

A nursing home resident's previous roommate is started on treatment for tuberculosis. They shared the same room for 3 months. What is the minimum size of induration considered positive for this patient:

a) 3 mm
b) 5 mm
c) 10 mm
d) 15 mm

62

A patient with AIDS (acquired immunodeficiency syndrome) wants to be vaccinated. Which of the following vaccines is contraindicated for this patient:

a) diphtheria and tetanus
b) hepatitis A and hepatitis B
c) varicella and nasal flu vaccine (FluMist)
d) influenza and mumps

63

A 40-year-old woman who is undergoing treatment for infertility complains of not having a menstrual period for several weeks. The night before, she started spotting and is now having pain in her lower abdomen. Her blood pressure is 160/80, the pulse rate is 110 beats per minute, and her temperature is 99.0 °F. All of the following are differential diagnosis to consider in this patient except:

a) irritable bowel syndrome (IBS)
b) threatened abortion
c) ectopic pregnancy
d) PID (acute pelvic inflammatory disease)

64

A 13-year-old adolescent who is not sexually active is brought in by her mother for an immunization update and physical exam. According to the mother, her daughter had two doses of hepatitis B vaccine 1 year ago. All of the following are indicated for this visit except:

a) Hepatitis B vaccine
b) Tetanus vaccine
c) screen for depression
d) HIV test

65

Rh-negative pregnant women with negative rubella titers should be vaccinated at what time period in pregnancy:

a) she can be vaccinated at any time in her pregnancy
b) during the second trimester
c) during the third trimester
d) during the postpartum period

66

Medicare Part B will pay for all of the following services except:

a) outpatient physician visits
b) durable medical equipment
c) outpatient laboratory tests
d) eyeglasses and routine dental care

67

A 38-year-old women with a history of rheumatoid arthritis and systemic lupus erythematosus (SLE) is being seen for a routine follow-up visit. The results of the CBC (complete blood count) are the following: hemoglobin of 11.0 mg/dL, hematocrit of 34%, and an MCV of 85 fL. The serum ferritin level is mildly elevated, and the transferrin and TIBC (total iron binding capacity) are within normal range. Which of the following is most likely:

a) microcytic anemia
b) normocytic anemia
c) macrocytic anemia
d) hemolytic anemia

68

A 67-year-old retired clerk presents with complaints of shortness of breath and weight gain over a 2-week period. A nonproductive cough accompanies her symptoms. The lung exam is positive for fine crackles and egophony on both bases. Which of the following conditions is most likely:

a) acute exacerbation of asthma
b) left heart failure
c) right heart failure
d) chronic obstructive pulmonary disease (COPD)

69

Which of the following drugs is most likely to relieve the cause of this patient's symptoms:

a) captopril (Capoten)
b) trimethoprim/sulfamethazole (Bactrim DS)
c) furosemide (Lasix)
d) hydrocodone/guaifenesin syrup (Hycotuss)

70

A 20-year-old patient has recently been diagnosed with migraine headache. The nurse practitioner is educating the patient about factors that are known to trigger migraine headaches. Which of the following is incorrect advice:

a) avoid foods with high tyramine content
b) avoid foods with high potassium content
c) get enough sleep
d) avoid fermented foods

71

A 21-year-old female with a history of mitral valve prolapse (MVP) is requesting prophylaxis before her dental surgery. Which of the following would you prescribe this patient:

a) amoxicillin 2.5 gm 30 minutes before and repeat 2 hours after the procedure
b) amoxicillin 2 gm 60 minutes before the procedure
c) amoxicillin 3 gm 1 hour before and 3 hours after the procedure
d) amoxicillin 3.5 mg within 1 to 2 hours before the procedure

72

Small bluish-white spots which are located in the buccal mucosa by the upper molars are called:

a) buccal cysts
b) Koplik's spots
c) lentigenes
d) Fordyce spots

73

Stella, a 21-year-old mother, complains to you that she has been feeling irritable and jittery almost daily for the past few months. She complains of frequent palpitations and more frequent bowel movements along with weight loss. Her BP is 160/70, her pulse is 110, and she is afebrile. All of the following conditions should be considered in the differential diagnosis except:

a) Hashimoto's disease
b) Graves disease
c) generalized anxiety disorder
d) illicit drug use

74

An elderly patient with a productive cough and fever is diagnosed with pneumonia. All of the following organisms are capable of causing community-acquired pneumonia except:

a) *Haemophilus influenzae*
b) *Mycoplasma pneumoniae*
c) *Treponema pallidum*
d) *Moxarella catarrhalis*

75

The "blue dot" sign, which is not considered a true surgical emergency, is usually located on the upper pole of the testicle. It is caused by:

a) a testicular torsion
b) blood underneath the scrotal skin
c) an acute infection with either chlamydia or gonorrhea
d) torsion of a testicular appendage

76

A triglyceride level of 800 mg/dL is noted the laboratory report. Which of the following conditions is a serious complication from high triglyceride levels:

a) acute renal failure
b) acute appendicitis
c) acute pancreatitis
d) familial hypertriglyceremia

77

An emergency room nurse presents to the employee health clinic 10 hours after a needlestick incident while starting an intravenous line on a patient. She tells the nurse practitioner in the clinic that she had forgotten to write up the incident because she was too busy the night before. All of the following are appropriate interventions except:

a) tetanus vaccine
b) Western blot test
c) hepatitis B testing
d) an ELISA test

78

An elderly woman has been on digoxin (Lanoxin) for 10 years. Her EKG is showing a new onset of atrial fibrillation. Her pulse is 60 beats per minute. She complains of gastrointestinal upset. Which of the following interventions is most appropriate:

a) order an electrolyte panel and a digoxin level
b) order a serum TSH, a digoxin level, and an electrolyte panel
c) order a serum digoxin level and cut her digoxin dose in half while you wait for results
d) discontinue the digoxin and order another 12-lead EKG

79

Which of the following maneuvers may be positive in a patient who is complaining of an acute onset of high fever, chills, severe headache, photophobia, and nausea that is accompanied by limited range of motion of the neck:

a) anterior drawer sign
b) Kernig's sign
c) Cullen's sign
d) Lachman's sign

80

Which is a true statement regarding occurrence-based malpractice insurance policies:

a) if the insurance company's lawyer finds the nurse practitioner negligent, it is the nurse's responsibility to pay for the claim
b) claims against the nurse practitioner are covered as long as she had an active malpractice policy at the time of the incident
c) claims against the nurse practitioner are usually paid if she is found not to be negligent
d) claims against the nurse practitioner are covered even if she had paid her premiums at the time of the incident

81

The most common pathogen found in acute epididymitis in younger males is:

a) E. coli
b) *Chlamydia trachomatis*
c) *Staphylococcus aureus*
d) Ureaplasma

82

An asthmatic patient who was seen for a viral upper respiratory infection presents to the nurse practitioner's office complaining of a recent onset of shortness of breath, inspiratory and expiratory wheezing, and chest tightness. He has been using his inhaler from 4 to 6 times a day. When the nurse practitioner quickly evaluates the patient, he notices that the patient is diaphoretic and tachypneic. Which of the following interventions is not indicated:

a) administer oxygen by nasal cannula at 7 L/minute
b) give the patient an injection of epinephrine subcutaneously immediately
c) quickly assess the patient's blood pressure and pulse
d) initiate CPR (cardiopulmonary resuscitation) immediately

83

A 35-year-old male walks into an urgent care clinic complaining of extremely painful headaches that started recently over the past week. The headaches occur daily several times a day in brief attacks of severe lancinating-type pain. The patient has noticed that the headache pain causes ipsilateral ptosis (drooping eyelid) and lacrimation accompanied by clear rhinorrhea. The patient is pacing and appears distressed. Which of the following conditions is being described:

a) cluster headache
b) migraine headache with aura
c) trigeminal neuralgia
d) basilar migraine

84

A 21-year-old male college student has recently been informed that he has a human papilloma virus (HPV) infection on the shaft of his penis. Which of the following methods can be used to visualize subclinical HPV lesions on the penile skin:

a) perform a KOH (potassium hydroxide) exam
b) scrape off some of the affected skin and send it for a culture and sensitivity
c) apply acetic acid to the penile shaft and look for acetowhite changes
d) order a serum herpes virus titer

85

Carol M. is a 40-year-old bank teller who has recently been diagnosed with obsessive-compulsive disorder by her therapist. Her symptoms would include:

a) ritualistic behaviors that the patient feels compelled to repeat
b) attempts to ignore or suppress the repetitive behaviors increases anxiety
c) frequent intrusive and repetitive thoughts and impulses
d) all of the above

86

Which of the following medications is indicated for the treatment of obsessive-compulsive disorder:

a) paroxetine (Paxil CR)
b) haloperidol (Haldol)

c) alprazolam (Xanax)
d) imipramine (Elavil)

87

You would advise an 18-year-old female student who has been given a booster dose of MMR at the college health clinic that:

a) she might have a low-grade fever during the first 24 to 48 hours
b) she should not get pregnant within the next 3 months
c) her arm will be very sore on the injection site in 24 to 48 hours
d) her arm will have some induration on the injection site in 24 to 48 hours

88

Jean, a 68-year-old female, is suspected of having Alzheimer's disease. Which of the following is the best initial method for assessing the condition:

a) CT scan of the brain
b) Mini Mental Exam
c) obtain the history from the patient, friends, and family members
d) EEG

89

A 55-year-old woman who has type 2 diabetes is concerned about her kidneys. She has a history of three urinary tract infections within the past 8 months but is currently asymptomatic. Which of the following is the best course to follow:

a) recheck the patient's urine during the visit and then refer her to the nephrologist
b) order a monthly urinalysis test
c) order a nuclear scan of the kidney
d) refer the patient to a urologist

90

A nurse practitioner is giving dietary counseling to a 30-year-old male alcoholic who has recently been diagnosed with folic acid deficiency anemia. Which of the following foods should the nurse practitioner recommend to this patient:

a) tomatoes, oranges, and bananas
b) cheese, yogurt, and milk
c) lettuce, beef, and dairy products
d) spinach, liver, and whole wheat bread

91

The ELISA and Western blot test are both used to test for the HIV virus. Which of the following statements is correct:

a) they are both tests to detect viral RNA

b) they are both tests to detect for antibodies against HIV (human immunodeficiency virus)
c) they are both tests used to detect for antibodies against HIV (human immunodeficiency virus)
d) they are both the best diagnostic tests for HIV (human immunodeficiency virus)

92

All of the following conditions are contraindications for metformin (Glucophage) except:

a) renal disease
b) gross obesity
c) alcoholism
d) liver disease

93

Terazosin (Hytrin) is classified under which of the following drug class:

a) alpha blockers
b) beta blockers
c) calcium channel blockers
d) tricyclic blockers

94

A 67-year-old female with a 50-pack-per-year history of smoking presents for a routine annual physical examination. She complains of becoming easily short of breath and of fatigue. Physical examination reveals diminished breath sounds, Hyperresonance, and hypertrophied respiratory accessory muscles. Her complete blood count (CBC) results reveals that her hematocrit level is slightly elevated. Her pulmonary function test (PFT) results show increased total lung capacity. What is the most likely diagnosis for this patient:

a) bronchogenic carcinoma
b) chronic obstructive lung disease
c) chronic bronchitis
d) congestive heart failure

95

Your patient of 10 years, Mrs. Leman, is concerned about her most recent diagnosis. She was told by her dermatologist that she has an advanced case of actinic keratosis. Which of the following is the best explanation for this patient:

a) it is a benign condition
b) it is a precancerous lesion and needs to be followed up with her dermatologist
c) apply hydrocortisone cream 1% BID for 2 weeks and most of it will go away
d) it is important for her to follow up with an oncologist

96

The Nursing Code of Ethics contains how many provisions:

a) 7 provisions
b) 8 provisions
c) 9 provisions
d) 10 provisions

97

Which of the following laboratory exams is most commonly used to measure the size of red blood cells in a sample of blood:

a) TIBC (total iron binding capacity)
b) MHC (mean hemoglobin concentration)
c) MCV (mean corpuscular volume)
d) hemoglobin electrophoresis

98

A 55-year-old male patient describes to you an episode of chest tightness in his substernal area that radiated to his back while he was jogging. It was relieved immediately when he stopped. Which of the following conditions does this best describe:

a) angina pectoris
b) acute myocardial infarction
c) gastroesophageal reflux disease
d) acute costochondritis

99

Which of the following would you recommend to this 55-year-old patient:

a) start an exercise program by starting with walking instead of jogging
b) consult with a cardiologist for further evaluation
c) consult with a gastroenterologist to rule out acute cholecystitis
d) take ibuprofen (Advil) 600 mg for pain every 4 to 6 hours as needed

100

An 83-year-old male with a history of hypertension complains to the nurse practitioner of some weakness in his left arm that slowly progressed to his left leg. It is accompanied by dizziness and slightly blurred vision. He has had the symptoms for the past 24 hours. Which of the following conditions is most likely:

a) cerebrovascular accident (CVA)
b) acute vertigo
c) multiple sclerosis (MS)
d) transient ischemic attack (TIA)

SECTION C

101

All of the following measures have been found to help lower the risk of osteoporosis except:

a) drinking organic juice
b) eating low-fat dairy foods
c) performing weight-bearing exercises
d) vitamin D supplementation

102

A 28-year-old male nurse of Hispanic descent with hypertension complains of a sore throat and nasal congestion that started 1 week ago. He tells the nurse practitioner at the employee health office that his other symptoms have resolved except for a dry cough that started a few days afterward. The patient denies allergies. His vital signs are stable and he is afebrile. Which of the following medications is best initiated at this visit:

a) clarithromycin (Biaxin) 500 mg po BID (twice a day) for 10 days
b) dextromethorphan and guaifenesin (Robitussin DM) 1 to 2 teaspoons every 4 hours
c) pseudoephedrine (Sudafed) 30 mg QID (four times a day)
d) diphenhydramine (Benadryl) 25 mg at bedtime

103

Which of the following has orchitis as a possible complication:

a) rubella
b) mumps
c) varicella
d) hepatitis B

104

The Jarisch-Herxheimer reaction is best described as:

a) an immune-mediated reaction precipitated by the destruction of a large number of spirochetes due to an antibiotic injection
b) severe chills and elevated blood pressures
c) caused either by infection with *Chlamydia trachomatis* or gonorrheal infection of the liver capsule
d) associated with certain viral illnesses

105

During breast exam of a 30-year-old nulliparous female, the nurse practitioner palpates several rubbery mobile areas of breast tissue. They are slightly tender to palpation and are present in both breasts. There are no skin changes and no nipple discharge. The patient is expecting her menstrual period in 5 days. Which of the following interventions is the best choice:

a) referral to a gynecologist for further evaluation
b) tell her to return 1 week after her period so her breasts can be rechecked
c) advise the patient to return in 6 months so that you can recheck her breasts
d) schedule the patient for a mammogram

106

Pulsus paradoxus is more likely to be seen in all of the following conditions except:

a) status asthmaticus
b) pleural effusion
c) acute myocardial infarction
d) cardiac tamponade

107

Which of the following should you expect to find on a wet mount slide of a patient diagnosed with bacterial vaginosis:

a) Tzanck cells
b) a large number of leukocytes and epithelial cells
c) a large number of squamous epithelial cells whose surfaces and edges are coated with large numbers of bacteria along with a few leukocytes
d) epithelial cells and a small amount of blood

108

A 30-year-old female is in the office complaining of palpitations and some light-headedness for the past 6 months. These are random episodes. The nurse practitioner notices a midsystolic click with a late systolic murmur that is best heard in the apical area during auscultation of the chest. You would suspect:

a) atrial fibrillation
b) sinus arrhythmia
c) mitral stenosis
d) mitral valve prolapse (MVP)

109

Your 35-year-old patient is being worked up for microscopic hematuria. The following are differential diagnosis of microscopic hematuria except:

a) kidney stones
b) bladder cancer
c) acute pyelonephritis
d) renal artery stenosis

110

During a routine physical exam of a 60-year-old Black woman, the nurse practitioner notices a triangular thickening of the bulbar conjunctiva on the temporal side of the patient's face. It is encroaching on the cornea. The patient denies pain and visual changes. Which of the following is most likely:

a) corneal arcus
b) pterygium
c) pinguecula
d) chalazion

111

Mr. J. has been on pravastatin (Pravachol) 20 mg HS for the past three months. He complains of feeling very fatigued lately and denies lack of sleep. He has noticed that his urine is a darker color the past 2 weeks. You would:

a) discontinue his pravastatin and order a liver function profile
b) continue the pravastatin but on half the dose
c) schedule him for a complete physical exam
d) schedule him for a liver function profile

112

Which of the following conditions is a contraindication for pioglitazone (Actos):

a) severe congestive heart failure
b) chronic infections
c) underweight patients
d) patients with severe depression

113

A teenage girl complains that she has never had a period. On examination, the nurse practitioner notes that she is at Tanner stage II. What are the physical exam findings during this stage:

a) breast buds and some straight pubic hair
b) fully developed breast and curly pubic hair
c) breast tissue with the areola on a separate mound with curly pubic hair
d) no breast tissue and no pubic hair

114

The Phalen test is used to evaluate for:

a) inflammation of the median nerve
b) rheumatoid arthritis
c) degenerative joint changes
d) chronic tenosynovitis

115

Which of the following treatment regimens is recommended to treat a *Helicobacter pylori* infection:

a) metronidazole (Flagyl) BID, doxycycline BID and omeprazole (Prilosec) daily
b) bismuth subsalicylate (Pepto-Bismol) tablets QID, metronidazole (Flagyl) QID, azithromycin (Zithromax), and cimetidine (Tagamet) daily
c) Amoxicillin BID, sulfamethazole trimethoprim (Bactrim DS) BID and ranitidine (Zantac) daily
d) clarithromycin (Biaxin) BID, amoxicillin BID, and omeprazole (Prilosec) QD daily

116

All of the following are known to cause chronic cough except:

a) chronic bronchitis
b) allergic rhinitis
c) acute viral upper respiratory infection (URI)
d) gastroesophageal reflux disease (GERD)

117

The following are true statements about aspirin and its action on platelets except:

a) its effects on platelets is irreversible
b) its effects on platelets may last up to 3 weeks
c) it is used for prophylaxis against strokes and acute myocardial infarctions
d) its effects only last 2 weeks and are reversible

118

All of the following agents are used to control the inflammatory changes seen in the lungs of asthmatics except:

a) albuterol inhaler (Proventil)
b) triamcinolone (Azmacort)
c) montelukast (Singulair)
d) cromolyn sodium inhaler (Intal)

119

All of the following antibiotics area contraindicated for children younger than 18 years of age except:

a) minocycline (Minocin)
b) ciprofloxacin (Cipro)
c) ceftriaxone (Rocephin)
d) levofloxacin (Levaquin)

120

All of the following are useful in treating allergic rhinitis except:

a) allergy injections
b) oral antihistamines
c) systemic steroids
d) oral decongestants

121

Erysipelas is cause by which of the following organisms:

a) *E. coli*
b) *Haemophilus influenzae*
c) Group A beta-hemolytic streptococcus
d) *Staphylococcus aureus*

122

A 62-year-old female with a 10 year history of severe low back pain reports to the nurse practitioner of a new onset of difficulty controlling her urine that is associated with numbness on her perineal area. She denies trauma. You would suspect which of the following:

a) fracture of the lower spine
b) a herniated disc
c) cauda equina syndrome
d) ankylosing spondylitis

123

A 38-year-old White female with a BMI of 32 complains of colicky pain on the right upper quadrant of her abdomen that gets worse if she eats fried food. During the physical exam, the nurse practitioner presses deeply on the left lower quadrant of the abdomen. After releasing her hand, the patient complained of pain on the right side of the lower abdomen. What is the name of this exam:

a) Rebound tenderness
b) Rovsing's sign
c) Murphy's sign
d) Psoas test

124

Which of the following viral infections is associated with possible abnormal lymphocytes that resolve a few weeks after the acute infection:

a) CMV (cytomegalovirus)
b) EBV (Epstein-Barr virus)
c) HPV (human papilloma virus)
d) Coxsackie virus

125

The following is a screening test for scoliosis:

a) straight leg raising test
b) Adams forward bend test
c) growth hormone titers
d) serum alkaline phosphatase

126

Jenny, who is a Type 1 diabetic complains of a 1-week episode of dysuria, frequency and a strong odor to her urine. She denies fever and chills. This is her second episode of the year. What is the best treatment option for this patient during this visit:

a) treat the patient with a 7 day course of antibiotics and order a urine for culture and sensitivity (C&S) before and after treatment
b) order a urine C&S and hold treatment until you get the results of the test from the lab
c) treat the patient with antibiotis and encourage her to drink more fluids and cranberry juice
d) treat the patient with a 3 day course of antibiotics and order a urine for C&S after treatment to document the complete resolution of the infection

127

All of the following are infections affecting the labia and vagina except:

a) bacterial vaginosis
b) candidiasis
c) trichomoniasis
d) *Chlamydia trachomatis*

128

During the eye exam of a 50-year-old hypertensive patient complaining of a severe headache, the nurse practitioner finds that the borders of the disc margins of both eyes are slightly blurred. The veins are larger than the arteries and there is no AV (arteriovenous) nicking. What is the significance of this clinical finding:

a) they are all normal findings
b) the patient has hypertensive retinopathy
c) the ICP (intracranial pressure) of the brain is increased
d) the patient has acute closed-angle glaucoma

129

A 30-year-old overweight high school teacher complains of a dry cough that has been present for 3 months. The cough worsens when he is supine. He complains of a few episodes of a sour taste in the back of his throat. The patient's cough may be caused by:

a) asthma
b) GERD (gastroesophageal reflux disease)
c) pneumonia
d) chronic postnasal drip

130

The red reflex is elicited by shining a light on the eyes at an angle with the light about 15 inches away. The nurse practitioner is screening for:

a) cataracts
b) strabismus
c) blindness
d) the blinking response

131

A 44-year-old patient with Down's syndrome develops impaired memory and difficulty with his usual daily life routines. He is having problems functioning at his job which he has been doing for 10 years. The physical exam and routine labs are all negative. The vital signs are normal. His appetite is normal. The most likely diagnosis is:

a) Tic douloureux
b) a stroke
c) Alzheimer's disease
d) delirium

132

Which of the following findings is associated with the chronic use of chewing tobacco:

a) cheilosis
b) glossitis
c) a geographic tongue
d) leukoplakia of the tongue

133

Which of the following is recommended treatment for erythema migrans (or early Lyme's disease):

a) doxycycline (Vibramycin) 100 mg po BID × 21 days
b) ciprofloxacin (Cipro) 250 mg po BID × 14 days
c) erythromycin (E-Mycin) 333 mg po TID × 10 days
d) dicloxacillin 500 mg po BID × 10 days

134

Nurse practitioners and clinical nurse specialists derived their legal right to practice from:

a) the Nurse Practice Act of the state where they practice
b) the laws of the state where they practice
c) the Medicare Bill
d) the Board of Nursing from the state where they practice

135

You are checking a 67-year-old female's breast during an annual gynecological exam. The left nipple and surrounding areolar skin are scaly and reddened. The patient denies pain and pruritis. She has noticed this scaliness on her left nipple for many months. Her dermatologist gave her a topical steroid that she used on the rash twice a day for 1 month. The patient never went back for the follow-up. She still has the rash and wants an evaluation. The nurse practitioner suspects Paget's disease of the breast. Which of the following is the best treatment plan for this patient:

a) prescribe another potent topical steroid and tell the patient to use it twice a day for 4 weeks
b) order a mammogram and refer the patient to a breast surgeon
c) advise her to stop using soap on both breasts when she bathes to avoid drying up the skin on her areola and nipples
d) order a sonogram of the breast and fine needle biopsy of the breast

136

The following are considered at higher risk for tuberculosis except:

a) teenager recently diagnosed with leukemia
b) nurse who works in a community clinic in the inner city
c) 60-year-old male working in a homeless shelter
d) a 22-year-old female recently diagnosed with asthma

137

During a sports physical exam of a 20-year-old athlete, the nurse practitioner notices a split of the S2 component of the heart sound during deep inspiration. She notes that it disappears on expiration. The heart rate is regular and no murmurs are auscultated. Which of the following is correct:

a) this is an abnormal finding and should be evaluated further by a cardiologist
b) a stress test should be ordered
c) this is a normal finding in some young athletes
d) an echocardiogram should be ordered

138

Mrs. J.L. is a 55-year-old female with a BMI of 30 with a history of asthma. She has hypertension that has been under control with hydrochlorothiazide 12.5 mg po daily. Her total cholesterol is 230 g/dL. How many risk factors for coronary heart disease (CAD) does she have:

a) one risk factor
b) two risk factors
c) three risk factors
d) four risk factors

139

A common side effect of metformin (Glucophage) therapy is:

a) weight gain
b) lactic acidosis
c) hypoglycemic episodes
d) gastrointestinal upset

140

While doing a cardiac exam on a 75-year-old male, the nurse practitioner notices an irregularly irregular rhythm with a pulse rate of 110 beats per minute. The patient is alert and is not in distress. Which of the following is most likely:

a) atrial fibrillation
b) ventricular fibrillation
c) cardiac arrhythmia
d) first-degree right bundle branch block

141

The following are patients who are at high risk for complications due to urinary tract infections. Who of the following does not belong in this category:

a) a 38-year-old diabetic patient with a HgbA1C of 6.0%
b) a woman with a history of rheumatoid arthritis who is currently being treated with a regimen of methotrexate and low-dose steroids
c) a 21-year-old woman who is under treatment for a sexually transmitted infection
d) pregnant women

142

A 68-year-old woman with hypertension and diabetes is seen by the nurse practitioner for a dry cough that worsens at night when she lies in bed. She has shortness of breath that worsens when she exerts herself. The patient's pulse rate is 90/min and regular. The patient has gained 6 pounds over the past 2 months. She is on a nitroglycerine patch and furosemide daily. The best explanation for her symptoms is:

a) kidney failure
b) congestive heart failure
c) ACE inhibitor induced coughing
d) thyroid disease

143

A nurse practitioner is doing a funduscopic exam on a 35-year-old female during a routine physical exam. He notices that she has sharp disc margins and a yellowish-orange color to her optic disc. The ratio of veins to arteries is 3:2. What is the next most appropriate action:

a) advise the patient that she had a normal exam
b) advise the patient that she had an abnormal exam
c) refer the patient to the emergency room
d) refer the patient to an ophthalmologist

144

During a sports physical, the nurse practitioner records a vision of 20/30. Which of the following statements below is true:

a) the patient can see at 20 feet what a person with normal vision can see at 30 feet
b) the patient can see at 30 feet what a person with normal vision can see at 20 feet
c) the patient cannot engage in contact sports
d) the patient needs to be referred to an ophthalmologist

145

Carol, a 30-year-old type 1 diabetic, is on regular and NPH insulin in the morning and in the evening. She recently started attending aerobic classes in the afternoon. Because of her workouts, her blood sugars have dipped below 50 mg/dL very early in the morning. The hypoglycemia is stimulating her liver into secreting glucagon. As a result, the patient's fasting blood sugar levels in the morning have been elevated above normal. Which of the following is being described correctly:

a) Somogyi phenomenon
b) Dawn phenomenon
c) Raynaud's phenomenon
d) insulin resistance

146

A 40-year-old female is positive for anti-HCV. Which test is appropriate for follow-up:

a) HCV RNA
b) HCV antibodies
c) HCV core antigen
d) hepatitis C surface antigen

147

To evaluate a 55-year-old male patient who is a smoker and has peripheral vascular disease (PVD), the nurse practitioner would initially start with the following intervention:

a) order a venogram
b) order TED hose
c) check the apical pulse
d) check the pedal and posterior tibial pulses

148

All of the following drugs can interact with theophylline (Theo-24) except:

a) erythromycin
b) montelukast (Singulair)
c) phenytoin sodium (Dilantin)
d) cimetidine (Tagamet)

149

You note a high-pitched and blowing pansystolic murmur on a 50-year-old male. It is grade II/VI and is best heard at the apical area. Which of the following is most likely:

a) ventricular septal defect (VSD)
b) tricuspid regurgitation
c) mitral regurgitation
d) mitral stenosis

150

Which of the following drugs is the preferred treatment for a skin infection with the organism called *Bacillus anthracis* (anthrax):

a) amoxicillin/clavulanic acid (Augmentin)
b) ciprofloxacin (Cipro)

c) ceftriaxone (Rocephin) injections
d) erythromycin

SECTION D

151

An 18-year-old female with a history of hypothyroidism presents to an urgent care clinic complaining of numbness and tingling on the fingertips on both her hands for several hours. On examination, both radial pulses are at +2 and equal bilaterally. The patient reports a history over the past several months of identical episodes that last several hours. The skin color changes range from blue to white, and then a dark red. Eventually the skin returns to normal and the tingling and numbness disappear. Which of the following conditions is best described:

a) Hashimoto's disease
b) Raynaud's disease
c) peripheral neuropathy
d) vitamin B12 deficiency anemia

152

Which of the following clinical findings is associated with a measles (rubeola) infection:

a) multiple crops of papules that evolve into vesicles and pustules
b) small red spots with bluish centers located by the posterior molaris
c) fever
d) myalgias

153

You are reviewing a Pap smear report on a 25-year-old female. Which of the following cells should be on a Pap smear to be classified as a satisfactory specimen:

a) clue cells and endometrial cells
b) vaginal cells and cervical cells
c) squamous epithelial cells and endocervical cells
d) leukocytes and red blood cells

154

Which of the following T-scores derived during the dual x-ray absorptiometry (DXA) test of an 80-year-old woman's bones is indicative of osteoporosis:

a) T score of less than –2.50
b) T score of less than –2.00
c) T score of above –1.00
d) T score of above 1.50

155

A 56-year-old man complains of several episodes of severe lancinating pain that shoots up to his right cheek and is precipitated by drinking cold drinks or chewing. These episodes start suddenly and end spontaneously after a few seconds with several episodes per day. He denies any trauma, facial weakness, or difficulty swallowing. He has stopped drinking cold drinks because of the pain. Which of the following is most likely:

a) trigeminal neuralgia
b) cluster headache
c) acute sinusitis
d) sinus headache

156

The KOH (potassium hydroxide) prep is helpful in helping with the diagnosis of all the following conditions except:

a) tinea infections
b) *Candida albicans* infections on the skin
c) bacterial vaginosis
d) atypical bacterial infections

157

Which of the following is classified as an atypical antidepressant:

a) amitriptyline (Elavil)
b) lorazepam (Ativan)
c) sertraline (Zoloft)
d) bupropion hydrochloride (Wellbutrin)

158

All of the following pulmonary tests require the patient's voice to perform correctly except:

a) egophony
b) tactile fremitus
c) whispered pectoriloquy
d) auscultation

159

Which of the following interventions is not indicated for an acute case of DVT (deep vein thrombosis) in a 35-year-old female who was on oral contraceptive pills:

a) special support stockings
b) gentle exercises of the lower extremities
c) elevation of the affected limb
d) anticoagulation therapy

160

All of the following infections are reportable diseases except:

a) Lyme's disease
b) Gonorrhea
c) Nongonococcal urethritis
d) Syphilis

161

A menopausal woman with osteopenia is attending a dietary education class. Which of the following foods are recommended:

a) yogurt and sardines
b) spinach and red meat
c) cheese and red meat
d) low-fat cheese and whole grain

162

All of the following dietary factors should be avoided by patients on oral anticoagulation therapy with warfarin sodium (Coumadin) because:

a) green leafy vegetables have high levels of vitamin K that can bind with the blood clotting cascade and increase bleeding time
b) yellow and green-colored vegetables have high amounts of beta carotene that can inactivate the active metabolite of the drug
c) food with high potassium content because of increased risk for cardiac arrhythmias
d) currently, no food restrictions are indicated because research has shown that it has minimal effect on the bleeding time

163

You are following up a 65-year-old male who has been on a new prescription of fluvastatin (Lescol) for 6 weeks. During a follow-up visit, he reports feeling extremely fatigued and having dark-colored urine. He denies any generalized muscle soreness. Which of the following is the most appropriate treatment plan:

a) order a CBC with differential
b) order a liver function profile
c) recommend an increase in fluid intake and rest
d) order a urine for culture and sensitivity

164

What would you advise him regarding his fluvastatin (Lescol) prescription:

a) Continue taking the medicine until the lab results are available
b) Take half the usual daily dose until the lab results are available

c) Take the medicine every other day instead of daily until the lab results are available

d) stop taking the medicine until the lab results are available

165

A 56-year-old male presents to the nurse practitioner complaining of a history of back pain for the past 4 months. On examination, the range of motion of the patient's spine is mildly limited while bending forward. The other joints in the patients body are normal. Only the spine seems to be affected. The patient reports that a lab test from a previous doctor showed increased ESR (sedimentation rate), a negative ANA (antinuclear antigen), and a negative rheumatoid factor. Which of the following is best described:

a) rheumatoid arthritis

b) lupus erythematosus

c) degenerative joint disease of the spine

d) ankylosing spondylitis

166

A post-menopausal woman who has been on low-dose estrogen and progesterone replacement hormone therapy for her severe vasomotor symptoms complains to the nurse practitioner that she has had a few episodes of small amounts of vaginal bleeding that seem to occur at random over the past 4 months. She denies uterine cramping and dyspareunia. Which of the following is the best treatment plan for this patient:

a) recommend to the patient that a D&C (dilatation and curettage) procedure is very helpful in cases of postmenopausal bleeding

b) schedule the patient for a uterine ultrasound and uterine biopsy

c) prescribe a 13-day course of progesterone pills to induce uterine shedding of the thickened endometrial lining at the end of the month

d) refer the patient to the gynecologist for further evaluation

167

Which of the following drug classes is useful in the management of chronic COPD (chronic obstructive pulmonary disease) symptoms:

a) anticholinergics

b) antibiotics

c) systemic corticosteroids

d) antimalarial drugs

168

All of the following statements are correct regarding the Td vaccine except:

a) fever occurs in up to 80% of the patients

b) a possible side effect is induration on the injection site

c) the Td is given every 10 years

d) the DPT and DT should not be given beyond the 7th birthday

169

Which of the following is recommended by the Joint National Committee on Prevention, Detection, Evaluation, and Treatment of High Blood Pressure (JNC 7) as first-line treatment for hypertension for patients with microalbuminuria:

a) ACE (angiotensin converting enzyme) inhibitors

b) diuretics

c) calcium channel blockers

d) beta blockers

170

A 20-year-old woman who is sexually active complains of copious milklike vaginal discharge. On microscopy, the slide reveals a large number of mature squamous epithelial cells. The vaginal pH is 5.0. There are very few leukocytes and no red blood cells seen on the wet smear. Which of the following is most likely:

a) atrophic vaginitis

b) bacterial vaginosis

c) trichomoniasis

d) this is a normal finding

171

A test called the visual fields by confrontation is used to evaluate for:

a) peripheral vision

b) central vision

c) visual acuity

d) accommodation

172

The following skin findings are considered macules except:

a) freckles

b) petechiae

c) acne

d) a flat 0.5-cm brown-colored birthmark

173

Clara is a 20-year-old college student who reports to the student health clinic with a laceration in her left hand. She tells the nurse practitioner that she cut her hand while working in her garden. Her last tetanus booster was $5\frac{1}{2}$ years ago. Which of the following is the best treatment plan:

a) administer a booster dose of the Td vaccine

b) administer the Td vaccine and the tetanus immune globulin (HyperTet)
c) administer tetanus immune globulin (HyperTet) only
d) she does not need any tetanus immune globulin (HyperTet) or a Td booster

174

The apex of the heart is located at:

a) second ICS to the right of the sternal border
b) second ICS to the left of the sternal border
c) the left lower sternal border
d) the left side of the sternum at the fifth ICS by the midclavicular line

175

A middle-age female with blonde hair and blue eyes complains of small acnelike papules on the sides of her mouth and on her chin that do not seem to respond to topical acne medicine. It is not pruritic. She complains of flushing easily, especially when she drinks beer and wine. Her mother has a history of the same lesions. Which of the following is most likely:

a) adult-onset acne
b) rosacea
c) atopic dermatitis
d) perioral folliculitis

176

Koilonychia is associated with which of the following conditions:

a) lead poisoning
b) beta thalassemia trait
c) B12-deficiency anemia
d) iron-deficiency anemia

177

What causes the highest cancer mortality in women:

a) breast cancer
b) lung cancer
c) colon cancer
d) uterine cancer

178

All of the following are correct statements regarding the S3 component of the heart sound except:

a) it occurs very early in diastole and is sometimes called an opening snap
b) it is a normal finding in some children, healthy young adults, and athletes

c) it can be a normal variant if heard on a person aged 40 or older
d) it signifies congestive heart failure

179

A positive straight leg raising test is indicative of which of the following conditions:

a) myasthenia gravis
b) inflammation of the sciatic nerve
c) multiple sclerosis
d) Parkinson's disease

180

Which of the following would you recommend on an annual basis for an elderly patient with type 2 diabetes:

a) an eye exam with an ophthalmologist
b) follow-up visit with a urologist
c) periodic visits to an optometrist
d) colonoscopy

181

A 72-year-old White female complains to you of a crusty and nonhealing small ulcer on her upper lip that she has had for several months. She also has light red-colored lesions with a roughened texture on both her upper cheeks. Which of the following would be the most appropriate intervention for this patient:

a) triamcinolone acetonide (Kenalog) cream BID for 2 weeks
b) triple antibiotic ointment BID × 2 weeks
c) hydrocortisone 1% cream BID for 2 weeks
d) she needs to be evaluated by a dermatologist

182

Which of the following drugs is considered a "rescue" drug for asthmatics:

a) formoterol (Foradil) inhalers
b) albuterol (Ventolin) inhalers
c) montelukast (Singulair) tablets
d) triamcinolone (AeroBid) inhalers

183

Bouchardis nodule is found in which of the following:

a) rheumatoid arthritis
b) degenerative joint disease
c) psoriatic arthritis
d) septic arthritis

184

The red blood cell (RBC) peripheral smear in pernicious anemia will show:

a) microcytic and hypochromic cells
b) microcytic and normochromic cells
c) macrocytic and normochromic cells
d) macrocytic and hypochromic cells

185

You notice a medium-pitched harsh systolic murmur during an episodic exam on a 37-year-old woman. It is best heard at the right upper border of the sternum. Which of the following is most likely:

a) mitral stenosis
b) aortic stenosis
c) pulmonic stenosis
d) tricuspid regurgitation

186

A small abscess on a hair follicle of the eyelid is called:

a) hordeolum
b) pterygium
c) pinguecula
d) ptosis

187

Which of the following is indicated for the prophylactic treatment of migraine headache:

a) ibuprofen (Motrin)
b) naproxen sodium (Anaprox)
c) propranolol (Inderal)
d) sumatriptan (Imitrex)

188

A 40-year-old male complains to the nurse practitioner of severe episodic lancinating pains behind his left eye for the past 2 weeks. The pain does not seem to affect his vision. It is always accompanied by some nasal congestion and rhinitis. He complains that it is so painful that sometimes he feels like he wants to die. The patient's temperature is 98.8°F, the pulse is 92 beats per minute, and the respiratory rate is 14 per minute. The neurological exam is within normal limits. Which of the following conditions is most likely:

a) migraine headache with aura
b) cluster headache
c) tic douloureux
d) cranial neuralgia

189

Which of the following drugs is most likely to cause abdominal side effects:

a) sucralfate (Carafate)
b) acetaminophen (Tylenol)
c) clarithromycin (Biaxin)
d) penicillin

190

All of the following statements are true regarding domestic abuse except:

a) There is no delay in seeking medical treatment
b) The pattern of injuries is inconsistent with the history reported
c) Injuries are usually in the "central" area of the body instead of the extremities
d) Pregnant women have a higher risk of domestic abuse

191

Which of the following patients is least likely to become an alcohol abuser:

a) a 50-year-old construction worker who drinks one beer nightly while watching sports programs on television
b) A 30-year-old nurse who complains to her coworker that her mother's comments about her recreational drinking are starting to annoy her and her spouse
c) a 19-year-old college student who binges on alcoholic drinks but only on the weekend
d) a 70-year-old male who feels better after drinking rum in the morning

192

Alpha thalassemia minor is considered a:

a) macrocytic anemia and normochromic
b) normocytic and hyperchromic anemia
c) microcytic and hypochromic anemia
d) hemolytic anemia

193

Potential complications of mitral valve prolapse (MVP) include all of the following except:

a) severe mitral regurgitation
b) endocarditis
c) increased risk of stroke and TIA
d) mitral stenosis

194

A new patient is complaining of severe pruritis that is worse at night. Several family members also have the same symptoms. On examination, areas of excoriated papules are noted on some of the interdigital webs of both hands and on the axillae. This finding is most consistent with:

a) contact dermatitis
b) impetigo
c) larva migrans
d) scabies

195

An elderly woman with a history of rheumatoid arthritis reports to the nurse practitioner that she has been taking ibuprofen BID for many years. Which of the following organ systems has the highest risk of damage from chronic nonsteroidal anti-inflammatory drug (NSAIDS) use:

a) cardiovascular system
b) neurological system
c) gastrointestinal system
d) renal system

196

Ted, who is 15 years old, has just moved into the community and is staying in a foster home temporarily. There is no record of his immunizations. His foster mother wants him to be checked before he enters the local high school. Which of the following does this patient need:

a) Mantoux test
b) MMR
c) Td
d) all of the above

197

Which cranial nerve is being evaluated when a patient is instructed to shrug his shoulders:

a) CN 9
b) CN 10
c) CN 11
d) CN 12

198

A laboratory technician has a 10.5-millimeter area of redness and induration in his left forearm after getting a Mantoux test 48 hours before from the employee health nurse. The Mantoux test done by the same nurse 12 months ago was at

5 millimeters of induration. The technician denies cough, night sweats, and weight loss. Which of the following is a true statement:

a) the patient is at higher risk for active tuberculosis disease within the next 2 years
b) a chest radiograph and sputum culture are indicated
c) a sputum for culture and sensitivity and referral to an infectious disease specialist are indicated
d) the lab technician should not be allowed to draw blood from immunosuppressed patients

199

Learning how to drive with a therapist after a stroke is considered:

a) primary prevention
b) secondary prevention
c) tertiary prevention
d) health prevention

200

Which of the following individuals is at higher risk for osteoporosis:

a) 70-year-old female of African ancestry who walks daily for exercise
b) 42-year-old obese woman taking prednisone 10 mg daily for severe asthma for 2 years
c) 55-year-old White female who is an aerobics instructor
d) 45-year-old Asian female who has been on high-dose steroids for 1 week

SECTION E

201

Patients with celiac sprue should avoid which of the following in their diets:

a) organ meats
b) lactose
c) phenylalanine
d) gluten

202

Which of the following eye findings are seen in patients with diabetic neuropathy:

a) AV nicking
b) copper wire arterioles
c) flame hemorrhages
d) microaneurysms

203

The following conditions are absolute contraindications for the use of oral contraceptives except:

a) a benign hepatoma
b) history of emboli that resolved with heparin therapy 15 years ago
c) migraine headache with aura
d) a history of gallbladder disease during pregnancy

204

The most common cause of cancer mortality in this country is:

a) lung cancer
b) prostate cancer
c) colon cancer
d) skin cancer

205

Which of the following findings are seen on a patient with folate-deficiency anemia:

a) microcytic and hypochromic red blood cells
b) microcytic and normochromic red blood cells
c) normal size and color of the red blood cells
d) macrocytic and normocytic red blood cells

206

When confirming a case of temporal arteritis, the sedimentation rate (ESR) is expected to be:

a) normal
b) lower than normal
c) elevated
d) indeterminate result

207

Mrs. Green, age 45, is complaining of generalized morning stiffness especially on both her wrists and hands. It is much worse in the morning after she wakes up and lasts for a few hours. She also complains of fatigue and generalized body aches that have been present for the past few months. Which of the following is most likely:

a) osteoporosis
b) rheumatoid arthritis
c) osteoarthritis
d) gout

208

All of the following may cause delirium in susceptible individuals except:

a) severe infection
b) metabolic derangement
c) intoxication with certain substances
d) Creutzfeldt-Jakob disease

209

Which of the following drugs is effective therapy in a middle-aged African American male who is having an acute exacerbation of gout on his right great toe:

a) acetaminophen (Tylenol)
b) systemic steroids
c) indomethacin (Indocin)
d) allopurinol (Zyloprim)

210

The complications of untreated gout include:

a) loss of joint mobility and renal failure
b) loss of joint mobility and liver failure
c) an increased risk of urinary tract infections
d) bladder cancer

211

According to the document, Healthy People 2010, all of the following are considered leading health indicators except:

a) weight and obesity
b) immunizations
c) access to health care
d) international health promotion programs

212

You note bony nodules located at the proximal interphalangeal joints on both the hands of your 65-year-old female patient. Which of the following is most likely:

a) Bouchard's node
b) Heberdeen's node
c) osteoarthritic nodules
d) deposits of uric acid crystals

213

Which chronic illness disproportionately affects the Hispanic population:

a) diabetes mellitus

b) hypertension
c) alcohol abuse
d) skin cancer

214

A lipid profile done on a newly diagnosed hypertensive patient shows a triglyceride level of 950 mg/dL, total cholesterol 240 mg/dL, LDL 145 mg/dL, and an HDL of 35 mg/dL. What is the next best intervention for this patient:

a) educate the patient about lifestyle changes that will help lower his or her cholesterol levels
b) initiate a prescription of pravastatin (Pravachol) as soon as possible
c) recommend that the patient avoid eating fatty or fried foods
d) initiate a prescription of nicotinic acid (niacin, Niaspan)

215

The McMurray test is useful for evaluating the stability of an injured knee. Which of the following is being evaluated:

a) anterior cruciate ligament of the knee
b) posterior cruciate ligament of the knee
c) the patellar tendon
d) the meniscus of the knee

216

The "gold standard" for the diagnosis of active *Helicobacter pylori* infection of the stomach or duodenum is:

a) an *H. pylori* titer
b) an endoscopy with tissue biopsy
c) an upper GI series
d) a urea breath test

217

On which of the following dates did the American Nurses Association (ANA) House of Delegates and the board vote to accept all of the major provisions of the revised Code of Ethics:

a) April 1999
b) May 2000
c) June 2001
d) July 2002

218

A Hispanic middle-aged woman with a BMI of 29 complains of chronic tiredness and feeling thirsty despite drinking up to 10 glasses of water a day. The nurse practitioner wants to rule out type 2 diabetes mellitus. All of the following tests are acceptable methods for diagnosing diabetes according to the American Diabetes Association (ADA) except:

a) HgbA1c
b) fasting blood glucose
c) postprandial serum blood glucose
d) oral glucose tolerance testing with 75 gram glucose load (OGTT)

219

A bulla is defined as:

a) a solid nodule less than 1 cm in size
b) a superficial vesicle filled with serous fluid greater than 1 cm in size
c) a maculopapular lesion
d) a shallow ulcer

220

A 30-year-old nurse from the emergency room is shown to have a positive result in the Mantoux test. According to the nurse, she has always had negative results. Which of the following is not true:

a) the highest risk of having tuberculosis disease is within the next 2 years after seroconversion
b) isoniazid (INH) prophylaxis is not recommended for persons ages 30 years or older because of the higher risk of hepatic injury
c) a chest x-ray is recommended
d) the nurse should be asked about the signs and symptoms of active tuberculosis disease

221

Which of the following is the confirmatory test for the human immunodeficiency virus (HIV):

a) ELISA test for HIV
b) Western blot
c) HIV polymerase chain reaction (PCR) test
d) HIV antibody

222

All of the following clinical findings are associated with syphilis except:

a) condyloma lata
b) condyloma acuminata
c) painless chancre
d) rashes on the palms of the hands and the soles of the feet

223

All of the following are mechanical barrier methods of contraception except:

a) diaphragm with spermicidal gel
b) the sponge
c) condoms
d) Depo-Provera injections

224

Women with a history of pelvic inflammatory disease (PID) have an increased risk for all of the following complication(s) except:

a) ectopic pregnancy
b) scarring of the fallopian tube(s)
c) infertility
d) ovarian cysts

225

The differential diagnosis for genital ulceration includes all of the following except:

a) syphilis
b) genital herpes
c) chancroid
d) molluscum contagiosum

226

Lead poisoning can cause which type of anemia:

a) macrocytic anemia
b) normocytic anemia
c) microcytic anemia
d) hemolytic anemia

227

Hypovolemic shock would most likely occur with fractures of the:

a) spine
b) pelvis
c) femur
d) humerus

228

Podagra is associated with which of the following:

a) rheumatoid arthritis
b) gout

c) osteoarthritis
d) septic arthritis

229

While assessing for a cardiac murmur, the first time that a thrill can be palpated is at:

a) grade II
b) grade III
c) grade IV
d) grade V

230

A medium-pitched harsh midsystolic murmur is best heard at the right second intercostal space (ICS) of the chest. It radiates into the neck. Which of the following is best described:

a) aortic stenosis
b) pulmonic stenosis
c) aortic regurgitation
d) mitral stenosis

231

Which type of hepatitis virus infection is more likely to result in cirrhosis of the liver and an increased risk of developing hepatocellular carcinoma:

a) hepatitis A virus
b) hepatitis B virus
c) hepatitis C virus
d) hepatitis D virus

232

Which of the following cranial nerves is involved in Bell's palsy:

a) CN 9 & 10
b) CN 8
c) CN 7
d) CN 5

234

A 19-year-old male has recently been diagnosed with acute hepatitis B. He is sexually active and is monogamous and reports using condoms inconsistently. Which of the following is recommended for his male sexual partner, who was also tested for hepatitis with the following results: HBsAg (–), anti-HBs (–), anti-HCV (–), anti-HAV (+):

a) a hepatitis B vaccination

b) hepatitis B immune globulin
c) hepatitis B vaccination and hepatitis B immune globulin
d) no vaccination is needed at this time

235

All of the following conditions are associated with an increased risk for normocytic anemia except:

a) rheumatoid arthritis
b) discoid lupus
c) chronic autoimmune disorders
d) pregnancy

236

You can determine a pulse deficit by counting the:

a) apical and radial pulses at the same time, then subtracting the difference between the two
b) apical pulse first, then the radial pulse, and subtracting the difference between the two
c) apical pulse and the femoral pulse at the same time and subtracting the difference between the two
d) radial pulse first, then counting the femoral pulse, and subtracting the difference between the two

237

Which of the following is recommended treatment for a woman with a bacterial vaginosis:

a) azithromycin (Zithromax)
b) doxycycline (Dynapen)
c) ceftriaxone (Rocephin)
d) metronidazole (Flagyl)

238

Patients who are being screened for tuberculosis (Tb) and are immunocompromised should be evaluated for anergy. Which of the following is the best description of anergy testing:

a) apply candida or mumps antigen to the right forearm and the PPD on the left forearm and read results in 48 to 72 hours
b) apply candida or mumps antigen and PPD on left forearm only and check for a reaction in 24 hours
c) mix the candida or mumps antigen with the PPD apply it to both forearms
d) apply the candida or mumps antigen 24 hours before the PPD on the left forearm

239

A nurse practitioner is evaluating an 85-year-old male from a nursing home. He instructs the patient to remember the words *orange, street,* and *tiger.* The patient is instructed to recite back these words to the nurse practitioner in 10 minutes. Which of the tests is being described:

a) Becker Inventory
b) Mini-Mental exam
c) MMPI (Minnesota Multiphasic Personality Inventory)
d) the CAGE test

240

Patients younger than the age of 18 years may give consent to a health care provider without the prior knowledge of a parent or legal guardian in all of the following cases except:

a) treatment of chlamydia cervicitis
b) treatment for mild acne
c) pregnancy testing
d) STD (sexually transmitted disease) testing

241

A hypertensive middle-aged man who is Native American has recently been diagnosed with mild renal insufficiency. He has been on lisinopril (Accupril) for many years. Which of the following laboratory values should be carefully monitored:

a) hemoglobin, hematocrit, and MCV
b) serum creatinine and potassium level
c) AST and ALT
d) serum sodium, potassium, and magnesium

242

All of the following are correct statements regarding the durable power of attorney's role except:

a) their decisions are considered as legally binding
b) they can be used in other areas of the patient's life such as financial issues
c) they can decide for the patient who is on life support when it can be terminated
d) the patient's spouse has a right to override the durable power of attorney's decisions

243

What is the most common cause of left ventricular hypertrophy in the United States:

a) chronic atrial fibrillation

b) chronic hypertension
c) mitral valve prolapse
d) pulmonary hypertension

244

Asthmatics may have all of the following symptoms during an acute exacerbation except:

a) tachycardia
b) severe wheezing
c) chronic coughing
d) tachypnea

245

A nurse practitioner's right to practice is regulated under:

a) Medicare regulations
b) the board of medicine
c) the federal government
d) the board of Nursing

246

An athlete with history of exercise-induced asthma wants to know when he should take his albuterol inhaler. The nurse practitioner should advise the patient to:

a) premedicate himself 20 to 30 minutes prior to starting exercise
b) wait until he starts to exercise before using the inhaler
c) premedicate 60 minutes before starting exercise
d) wait until he finishes his exercises before using his inhaler

247

Atrophic macular degeneration (AMD) of the aged is the leading cause of blindness in the elderly in the United States. Which of the following statements is correct:

a) it is a slow or sudden painless loss of central vision
b) it is a slow or sudden painless loss of peripheral vision
c) it is an occlusion of the central retinal vein causing degeneration of the macular area
d) it is commonly caused by diabetic retinopathy

248

A 20-year-old woman is complaining of a 2-week history of facial pressure that worsens when she bends over. She complains of tooth pain on her upper molars. She notices that over-the-counter decongestants are not giving her relief. On physical exam, her lungs and heart sounds are normal. Which of the following is most likely:

a) an acute dental abscess
b) chronic sinusitis
c) acute sinusitis
d) severe allergic rhinitis

249

Which of the following conditions is potentially a life-threatening disorder:

a) Hashimoto's disease
b) higher than normal levels of TSH (thyroid stimulating hormone)
c) a thyroid storm
d) myxedema

250

What is the best procedure for evaluating a corneal abrasion:

a) tonometry
b) fluorescein stain
c) visual field test
d) funduscopy

SECTION F

251

You are examining a patient who has just been diagnosed with Bell's palsy. Bell's palsy is characterized by all of the following except:

a) drooling
b) inability to swallow
c) inability to close the eye on the affected side
d) drooping of the corner of the mouth on the affected side

252

Which of the following agents is preferred treatment for a diabetic with stage II hypertension:

a) ACE (angiotensin converting enzyme) inhibitor
b) calcium channel blockers
c) loop diuretics
d) alpha blockers

253

A peak expiratory flow (PEF) result of 60% to 80% of predicted range with 30% variability of symptoms is classified as which of the following:

a) mild intermittent asthma
b) mild persistent asthma
c) moderate persistent asthma
d) severe asthma

254

Which of the following conditions is associated with Auspitz's sign:

a) contact dermatitis
b) seborrheic dermatitis
c) systemic lupus erythematosus
d) psoriasis

255

Which of the following is used to confirm a diagnosis of Hashimoto's thyroiditis:

a) thyroid needle biopsy
b) TSH
c) antimicrosomal antibody test
d) complement-fixation test

256

Which of the following conditions is most likely to cause cupping of the optic disc:

a) brain tumor
b) brain abscess
c) acute glaucoma
d) acute intracranial bleeding

257

A patient is suing a local physician for malpractice. Which of the following is a false statement:

a) the nurse practitioner, hospital, and other personnel who have taken care of the patient can be included in the lawsuit by the plaintiff's lawyer
b) the nurse practitioner may be exempted from the lawsuit if documentation is thorough and can be verified
c) an expert witness should be from the same area of practice
d) the nurse practitioner's documentation can be subpoenaed by the plaintiff's lawyer

258

The best screening test for detecting hyperthyroidism and hypothyroidism is:

a) the total T3
b) thyroid stimulating hormone (TSH)
c) thyroid profile
d) palpation of the thyroid gland

259

A patient who recently returned from a vacation in Latin America complains of a severe headache and stiff neck that is accompanied by a high fever for the past 12 hours. While examining the patient, the nurse practitioner flexes the patient's neck while observing the patient's hips and legs for a reaction. The name of this test is:

a) Kernig's maneuver
b) Brudzinski's maneuver
c) Murphy's sign
d) Homan's sign

260

Which of the following groups has been recommended to be screened for thyroid disease:

a) women aged 50 years or older
b) adolescent females
c) elderly males
d) school-aged children

261

A 65-year-old Hispanic woman has a history of type 2 diabetes. A routine urinalysis results reveal a few epithelial cells and is negative for leukocytes, nitrites, and protein. Which of the following would you recommend next:

a) order a urine for culture and sensitivity
b) order a 24-hour urine for microalbumin
c) since it is negative, no further tests are necessary
d) recommend a screening IVP (intravenous pyelogram)

262

RhoGAM's mechanism of action is:

a) the destruction of Rh-positive fetal red blood cells that are present in the mother's circulatory system
b) the destruction of maternal antibodies against Rh-positive fetal red blood cells

c) the stimulation of maternal antibodies so that there is a decreased risk of hemolysis
d) the destruction of maternal antibodies against fetal red blood cells

263

A chest radiograph shows an area of consolidation on the left lower lobe. Which of the following conditions is most likely:

a) bacterial pneumonia
b) acute bronchitis
c) COPD (chronic obstructive pulmonary disease)
d) atypical pneumonia

264

What type of breath sounds are best heard over the base of the lungs:

a) fine breath sounds
b) vesicular breath sounds
c) bronchial sounds
d) tracheal breath sounds

265

The Joint National Committee on Prevention, Detection, Evaluation, and Treatment of High Blood Pressure's (JNC 7) most current recommendation for blood pressure goals in diabetics and for patients with coronary heart disease is:

a) <140/90
b) <130/85
c) <130/80
d) <125/75

266

Which of the following is considered as a mast cell stabilizer:

a) nedocromil sodium (Tilade)
b) albuterol (Ventolin) inhalers
c) a long-acting oral theophylline (Theo-Dur)
d) fluticasone inhaler (Flovent)

267

All of the following clinical findings are considered benign oral findings except:

a) a patch of leukoplakia
b) Fordyce spots
c) torus palatinus
d) fishtail uvula

268

Which of the following interventions is most appropriate to follow if a professional nurse is suspected of being impaired due to a possible addiction to narcotics:

a) document the nurse coworker's behavior and file an incident report
b) refer the nurse to a special rehabilitation program for impaired health professionals
c) report the nurse directly to the state's Board of Nursing
d) refer the nurse to a psychiatrist for further evaluation

269

During a routine physical exam of a 90-year-old woman, a low-pitched diastolic murmur grade II/VI is auscultated. It is located on the fifth intercostal space (ICS) on the left side of the midclavicular line. Which of the following is correct:

a) aortic regurgitation
b) mitral stenosis
c) mitral regurgitation
d) tricuspid regurgitation

270

Which of the following situations is considered emergent:

a) a laceration on the lower leg of a patient on aspirin (Bayer) 81 mg every other day
b) rapid breathing and tachycardia in a patient with a fever
c) an elderly man with abdominal pain whose vital signs appear stable
d) a 37-year-old male biker with a concussion due to a fall who appears agitated and does not appear to understand instructions given by the medical assistant checking his vital signs

271

Which of the following is considered an objective finding in patients who have a case of suppurative otitis media:

a) erythema of the tympanic membrane
b) decreased mobility of the tympanic membrane as measured by tympanogram
c) displacement of the light reflex
d) bulging of the tympanic membrane

272

Pulsus paradoxus is more likely to be associated with:

a) sarcoidosis
b) acute bronchitis
c) status asthmaticus
d) bacterial pneumonia

273

An older adult male complains of feeling something on his left scrotum. On palpation, soft and moveable blood vessels that feel like a "bag of worms" are noted underneath the scrotal skin. The testicle is not swollen or reddened. The most likely diagnosis is:

a) chronic orchitis
b) chronic epididymitis
c) testicular torsion
d) varicocele

274

All of the following are true statements regarding elderly abuse except:

a) the elderly aged 80 years or older are at the highest risk for abuse
b) a delay in medical care is a common finding
c) a new onset of a sexually transmitted disease (STD) in an elderly patient may signal sexual abuse
d) decreased anxiety and depression are common symptoms of the abuse in the elderly

275

The S1 heart sound is caused by:

a) closure of the atrioventricular valves
b) closure of the semilunar valves
c) opening of the atrioventricular valves
d) opening of the semilunar valves

276

Patients with Down's syndrome are at higher risk for all of the following except:

a) atlantoaxial instability
b) congenital heart disease
c) early onset of Alzheimer's disease
d) melanoma

277

Duvall and Miller used developmental theory to describe the family. Which of the following statements is true:

a) each family is developmentally unique in comparison to another family
b) families demonstrate common forms of membership across developmental stages
c) families complete each developmental task separately
d) families change over time because of the influence of environmental factors

278

The following abnormal lab results may be seen in patients with acute mononucleosis except:

a) lymphocytosis and/or atypical lymphocytes
b) positive EBV titers for IgM and IgG
c) elevated liver function tests
d) elevated creatinine and BUN

279

Which of the following is considered an abnormal result on a Weber test:

a) lateralization to one ear
b) no lateralization in either ear
c) air conduction lasts longer than bone conduction
d) bone conduction lasts longer than air conduction

280

All of the following are considered benign physiologic variants except:

a) xerosis (dry skin)
b) supernumerary nipples
c) split uvula
d) cheilosis

281

A 65-year-old woman's bone density result shows severe demineralization of cortical bone. All of the following pharmacologic agents are useful in treating this condition except:

a) raloxifene (Evista)
b) calcitonin (Miacalcin)
c) medroxyprogesterone (Depo-Provera)
d) conjugated estrogen (Premarin)

282

A fracture on the navicular area of the wrist is usually caused by falling forward and landing on the hands. The affected wrist is hyperextended to break the fall. The NP is well aware that all of the following statements are true regarding a fracture of the scaphoid bone of the wrist except:

a) it has higher rate of nonunion compared with the other bones on the wrist when it is fractured
b) the fracture frequently does not show up on an x-ray film when it is taken after the injury
c) the x-ray film will become positive if it is repeated in a few weeks
d) these fractures always need surgical intervention in order to stabilize the joint

283

John, a 21-year-old, has type 1 diabetes. His late afternoon blood sugars over the past 2 weeks are averaging about 220 mg/dL. He is on 10 units of regular and 15 units of NPH in the morning and the same dose in the afternoon. Which of the following is the best course to follow:

a) increase both doses of insulin
b) increase only the NPH insulin in the morning
c) decrease the afternoon dose of NPH insulin
d) decrease both NPH and regular insulin doses in the morning

284

The mother of an adult male with Down's syndrome is in the nurse practitioner's office and wants a sports physical done for her son. She reports that he wants to join the football team at his school. Which of the following is the best advice for this patient's mother:

a) her son can play a regular football game as long as he wears maximum protective football gear
b) her son cannot participate in any contact sports because of an increased risk of cervical spine injury
c) her son can participate in some sports after he has been checked for cervical instability
d) none of the above

285

The nurse practitioner is performing a physical exam on a 20-year-old male. The patient complains of a single nonpruritic and red-colored maculopapular rash that is round in shape. The rash has been slowly enlarging over time and some areas in the center of the rash have already cleared. It is starting to resemble a target. The patient reports that he went hunting 4 weeks ago. Which of the following is most likely:

a) erythema migrans
b) Rocky Mountain spotted fever
c) Stevens-Johnson syndrome
d) larva migrans

286

Some pharmacologic agents may cause confusion in the elderly. Which of the following pharmacologic agents is most likely to cause confusion in this population:

a) cimetidine (Tagamet), digoxin (Lanoxin), diphenhydramine (Benadryl)
b) acetaminophen (Tylenol), aspirin (Bayer), indomethacin (Indocin)
c) sucralfate (Carafate), docusate sodium (Surfak), psyllium (Metamucil)
d) cephalexin (Keflex), amoxicillin (Amoxil), clarithromycin (Biaxin)

287

A 55-year-old female with a history of migraine headaches has recently been diagnosed with stage II hypertension. Her EKG strips reveal second-degree heart block. The chest x-ray is normal. All of the following drug classes are contraindicated in this patient with the exception of:

a) ARBs (angiotensin receptor blockers)
b) beta-blockers
c) alpha blockers
d) calcium channel blockers

288

Which of the following cranial nerves is evaluated when a wisp of cotton is lightly brushed against the corner of the eye:

a) CN 2
b) CN 3
c) CN 4
d) CN 5

289

A nurse practitioner suspects that a new patient who is an alcoholic may have an acute case of pancreatitis. All of the following laboratory tests are more likely to demonstrate pancreatic injury except:

a) lipase
b) amylase
c) serum blood glucose
d) GGT (gamma glutamyl transpeptidase)

290

Which of the following is a possible side effect from ACE inhibitor therapy:

a) acute onset of dry cough
b) mild wheezing
c) hypokalemia
d) increased serum uric acid level

291

All of the following statements are false regarding the rehabilitation of alcoholics except:

a) Al-Anon is not designed for family members of alcoholics
b) disulfiram (Antabuse) is always effective
c) Alcoholics Anonymous is not an effective method for treating this condition
d) Avoid foods or drinks that contain alcohol such as cough syrups

292

A 35-year-old soccer player presents at an urgent care clinic with a complaint of swelling and pain on the medial aspect of the right knee. The patient reports that the soccer ball hit him on the other side of the same knee. On examination, the knee is swollen with tenderness on the joint line of the medial side of the knee. To assess for possible injury to the meniscus, which maneuver will yield the best information to the nurse practitioner:

a) anterior drawer test
b) posterior drawer test
c) Lachman test
d) McMurray's test

293

All of the following are incorrect statements regarding the Healthy People 2010 objectives except:

a) the document's objectives are applicable not only nationally, but also internationally
b) one of the objectives of the document is help people achieve not only physical health, but social and emotional health as well
c) the document's objectives are applicable only to people of the United States of America
d) the document is formulated by a special committee formed by an alliance of all the state health departments

294

The Pap smear result on a 20-year-old sexually active student who uses condoms inconsistently shows a large amount of white blood cells on the wet smear. During the speculum exam, the patient's cervix bled easily (friable) and a small amount of purulent discharge was found on the surface of the cervix. What is the next appropriate action:

a) call the patient and tell her to return for further testing with a Gen-Probe to rule out infection by chlamydia and gonorrhea
b) treat the patient with metronidazole vaginal cream over the phone
c) call the patient and tell her she needs a repeat Pap smear in 6 months
d) advise her to use a Betadine douche at bedtime × 3 days

295

All of the following are covered under the provisions under the ANA's Code of Ethics except:

a) advocacy for civil rights
b) acceptance of accountability and responsibility
c) preservation of patients' dignity
d) social reform

296

Which of the following is an absolute contraindication for oral contraceptive pills:

a) smoking under age 35 years of age and history of DVT (deep venous thrombosis)
b) basilar migraine headaches and a recent history of jaundice 6 months ago
c) depression and a history of gallbladder disease during pregnancy
d) controlled hypertension controlled and diabetes mellitus with vascular changes

297

Which of the following is the most common cause of cancer deaths for males in the United States:

a) prostate cancer
b) lung cancer
c) colon cancer
d) heart disease

298

Human papilloma virus infection in women has been associated with the development of:

a) ectopic pregnancy
b) infertility
c) cervical cancer
d) pelvic inflammatory disease

299

All of the following criteria are included in the diagnosis of patients with AIDS (acquired immunodeficiency syndrome) except:

a) reactivation of an EBV (Epstein-Barr virus) infection
b) oral thrush
c) Kaposi's sarcoma
d) hairy leukoplakia of the tongue

300

Which of the following conditions is the most common cause of sudden death among athletes:

a) brain aneurysm
b) hypertrophic cardiomyopathy
c) left ventricular hypertrophy
d) aortic stenosis

SECTION G

301

The span of the normal adult liver is:

a) 6 to 12 cm in the right midclavicular line
b) 12 to 16 cm in the right midclavicular line
c) 2 to 6 cm in the midsternal line
d) 4 to 8 cm in the midsternal line

302

The tandem gait is used to test which of the following:

a) cerebellum
b) sacral nerves
c) motor movements
d) sensory input

303

A neighbor's 18-year-old son, who is active in basketball, complains of pain and swelling on both knees. On physical exam, there is tenderness over the anterior tubercle of both knees. Which of the following is most likely:

a) chondromalacia patella
b) left knee sprain
c) Osgood-Schlatter disease
d) tear of the medial ligament

304

A 27-year-old kindergarten teacher presents with a severe sore throat accompanied by a pink generalized rash with sandpaper-like texture. She is currently treated with amoxicillin 500 mg three times a day for 10 days. Which of the following conditions is best described:

a) scarlatina
b) rash due to an allergic reaction to amoxicillin
c) reactivated mononucleosis
d) pityriasis rosea

305

During a physical exam, a 40-year-old patient who has hypertension is noted to have a few beats of horizontal nystagmus on extreme lateral gaze that disappeared when the patient's eyes returned back towards midline. Which statement below best describes this clinical finding:

a) it is caused by occult bleeding of the retinal artery
b) this is a normal finding

c) it is a sign of a possible brain mass

d) this is a borderline result and needs further evaluation

306

An urgent care nurse practitioner is assessing a 45-year-old White woman with a BMI of 32 for complaints of intermittent right upper quadrant pain that is precipitated by fatty meals over the past few weeks. On exam, the patient's heart and lungs are normal. There is no pain over the costovertebral angle (CVA). During abdominal exam, the bowel sounds are hyperactive. Murphy's sign is positive. Which of the following is best described:

a) acute cholecystitis

b) acute appendicitis

c) acute gastroenteritis

d) acute diverticulitis

307

Which of the following drugs is recommended by the CDC (Centers for Disease Control) as first line treatment for infections caused by *Bacillus anthracis* (anthrax):

a) clindamycin (Cleocin)

b) doxycycline (Vibramycin)

c) penicillin G injection

d) ciprofloxacin (Cipro)

308

Cullen's sign is associated with:

a) severe appendicitis

b) acute pancreatitis

c) hemorrhage

d) acute hepatitis

309

Which of the following activities is considered as non-weight-bearing exercise:

a) swimming

b) isometric exercises

c) passive range of motion

d) yoga

310

Mary, who is 65 years of age, comes into the clinic on the first week of November for her annual visit. Her last Td booster was 9 years ago. Which immunization(s) would you recommend:

a) Influenza vaccine only
b) Td and influenza vaccine
c) pneumococcal (Pneumovax) and influenza vaccines
d) she does not need any vaccinations to be administered in this visit

311

Acute bronchitis is characterized by:

a) high fever
b) purulent sputum
c) paroxysms of coughing that is dry or productive of mucoid sputum
d) slow onset

312

The nurse practitioner notices a gray ring on the edge of both irises of an 80-year-old male. He denies visual changes or pain and reports that he has had the "ring" for many years. Which of the following is most likely:

a) arcus senilis (senile arcus)
b) pinguecula
c) peripheral cataracts
d) macular degeneration

313

Which of the following is not indicated for treatment of psoriasis:

a) psoralens
b) Goeckerman's regimen (coal tar followed by UVB phototherapy)
c) oral and topical steroids
d) gold salt injections

314

The cones in the retina of the eye are responsible for:

a) central vision
b) peripheral vision
c) night vision
d) double vision

315

The nurse practitioner would refer all of the following below to a physician except:

a) severe facial burns
b) electrical burns
c) burns that involve the cartilage of the ear
d) second-degree burns on the lower arm

316

On auscultation of the chest, a split S2 is best heard at:

a) second intercostal space, right sternal border
b) second intercostal space, left sternal border
c) fifth intercostal space, midclavicular line
d) fourth intercostal space, left sternal border

317

According to the guidelines outlined in the Joint National Committee on Prevention, Detection, Evaluation, and Treatment of High Blood Pressure (JNC 7), the normal blood pressure is defined as:

a) <140/90
b) <130/85
c) <120/80
d) <110/75

318

Which of the following would be classified as a second-degree burn:

a) a severe sunburn with blistering
b) burns that involve the subcutaneous layer of skin
c) a reddened finger after touching a hot iron
d) burns that involved eschar

319

The mother of a 17-year-old boy is concerned that her son is not developing normally. On physical exam, the patient is noted to have small testes with no pubic or facial hair. You would advise the mother:

a) her son is developing normally
b) her son's physical development is delayed and needs to be evaluated by a pediatric endocrinologist
c) her son should be rechecked in 3 months; if he still does not have secondary sexual characteristics, a thorough hormonal workup would be initiated
d) her son's physiological development is slower than normal but is within the lower limits for his age group

320

Robert, who is 65 years of age, complains of a new onset of a headache on the right temple accompanied by skin sensitivity in the scalp and blurred vision of the right eye. The patient denies nausea or vomitting. The patient, who is a smoker with a history of glaucoma, also complains of a flare-up of his allergies. During the physical examination, there is an indurated area that is tender to touch on the right temple. The pupils are equal in size. The patient's nasal turbinates are swollen and have a bluish tinge. Which one of the following conditions is the top priority for the nurse practitioner to treat:

a) temporal arteritis (giant cell arteritis)
b) glaucoma
c) allergic rhinitis
d) nicotine dependence

321

All of the following sexually transmitted infections can become disseminated if not treated with the exception of:

a) *Neisseria gonorrheae*
b) *Treponema pallidum*
c) HIV (human immunodeficiency virus)
d) *Chlamydia trachomatis*

322

Which of the following cranial nerves is evaluated by the Rinne test:

a) CN 7
b) CN 8
c) CN 9 and 10
d) CN 11

323

Robert, a homeless man with an extensive history of alcohol abuse, is confused and combative when he arrives at the clinic. Friends report Robert hasn't consumed alcohol in 2 days and has progressively become uncontrollable. Likely causes for Robert's behavior would include all except:

a) subdural hematoma
b) acute delirium related to alcohol withdrawal
c) thiamine intoxication
d) gastrointestinal hemorrhage

324

Laura, who has adult-onset acne, is being followed up for acne by the nurse practitioner. During the facial exam, papules and pustules are seen mostly on the forehead, cheeks, and chin areas. The patient has been using medicated soap and other over-the-counter acne medications without much improvement. The nurse practitioner advises the patient that she has moderate acne. Which of the following would you recommend next:

a) isotretinoin (Accutane)
b) oral tetracycline
c) erythromycin topical solution
d) Retin-A 0.25% gel

325

The following statements are all true regarding herpes zoster except:

a) it is due to reactivation of latent varicella virus
b) the typical lesions are bullae
c) it is usually more severe in immunocompromised individuals
d) infection of the trigeminal nerve ophthalmic branch can cause corneal blindness

326

A 45-year-old construction worker complains of recurrent episodes of painful large dark red nodules, pustules, and abscesses on both his axillae that resolve with antibiotic treatment. The nodules are tender to palpation. Several pustules and abscess have started to drain purulent green dsicharge. In addition, severe scarring and sinus tracts are noted on the axillary area. The nurse practitioner explains to the patient that it is caused by bacterial infection of the sweat glands in his axillae. Which of the following conditions is best described:

a) hidradenitis suppurativa
b) severe nodular cystic acne
c) granuloma inguinale
d) cat scratch fever

327

A possible side effect from the use of nifedipine (Procardia XL) is:

a) hypokalemia
b) hyperkalemia and tetany
c) edema of the ankles and headaches
d) dry hacking cough and hyperuricemia

328

Which of the following is contraindicated in patients with acute prostatitis:

a) vigorous massage of the prostate
b) serial urine samples
c) rectal exams
d) gentle palpation of the epididymis

329

All of the following conditions are recommended screening for 25-year-old males except:

a) PSA (prostate specific antigen)
b) substance abuse
c) seatbelt use
d) safe sex practice

330

What is the first-line antibiotic recommended by the American Thoracic Society (ATS) for patients younger than 60 years of age who are diagnosed with uncomplicated community-acquired pneumonia:

a) first-generation cephalosporins
b) second-generation cephalosporins
c) macrolides
d) beta-lactam antibiotics

331

All of the following are eye findings found in patients with chronic uncontrolled hypertension. Which of the following eye findings is not associated with the disorder:

a) AV nicking and silver wire arterioles
b) copper wire arterioles
c) flame-shaped hemorrhages and cotton-wool spots
d) neovascularization and microaneurysms

332

While reviewing some lab reports, the nurse practitioner notices that one of her teenage male patient's labs are abnormal. The alkaline phosphatase level is elevated. The liver function tests are all within normal limits. The patient is a member of a soccer team with no history of recent injury. Which of the following statements is true:

a) it is an indication of possible liver damage from alcohol; order a liver ultrasound to rule out fatty liver
b) this is a normal finding due to the skeletal growth spurt in this age group
c) the patient needs to be evaluated further for pancreatic disease
d) the patient needs an ultrasound of the liver to rule out fatty liver and referral to a pediatric rheumatologist

333

Which of the following would be appropriate initial management of a second-degree burn:

a) irrigate with hydrogen peroxide and apply Silvadene cream BID
b) irrigate with normal saline and apply Silvadene cream BID
c) irrigate with tap water and apply Neosporin ointment BID
d) unroof all intact blisters and apply antibiotic ointment BID

334

A male patient is positive for the anti-HCV (hepatitis C antibody) test. All of the following are included in the patient's treatment plan except:

a) advise the patient that he is immune to hepatitis C and no further testing is indicated
b) order an ALT (alanine aminotransferase) test
c) obtain a subjective history to find factors for the disease
d) order an HCV RNA test

335

An 80-year-old woman complains about her "thin" skin. You explain that it is caused by all of the following except:

a) lower collagen content
b) loss of subcutaneous fat
c) atrophy of the sebaceous glands
d) damage from chronic sun exposure

336

All of the following statements are correct regarding licensure for nurse practitioners except:

a) it ensures a minimum level of professional competency
b) it grants permission for an individual to practice in a profession
c) it requires verification of educational training from an accredited graduate program
d) it reviews information via a nongovernmental agency

337

Which of the following is the correct statement regarding the size of the arterioles and veins on the fundi of the eye:

a) the veins are larger than the arterioles
b) the arterioles are larger than the veins
c) the arterioles are half the size of the veins
d) the veins and the arterioles are equal in size

338

All of the following factors have been found to increase the risk of atrial fibrillation in predisposed individuals except:

a) hypertension and hyperthyroidism
b) too much alcohol intake in predisposed patients
c) theophylline and stimulants
d) ovarian hormonal imbalance

339

A homeless middle-aged male complains of a migratory arthritis and dysuria. Currently, his right knee is swollen and painful. On examination, green-colored purulent penile discharge is noted. Which of the following is most likely:

a) gonorrhea
b) chlamydia
c) nongonococcal urethritis
d) acute epididymitis

340

You would associate a positive iliopsoas muscle test result with the following condition:

a) cerebral vascular accident (CVA)
b) urinary tract infection (UTI)
c) autoimmune diseases
d) acute abdomen

341

Which cranial nerves innervate the extraocular muscles (EOMs) of the eyes:

a) CN 2, CN 3, and CN 6
b) CN 3, CN 4, and CN 6
c) CN 4, CN 5, and CN 7
d) CN 5, CN 6, and CN V8

342

The most sensitive and specific diagnostic test for both sickle cell anemia and thalassemia is:

a) hemoglobin electrophoresis
b) a bone marrow biopsy
c) a blood peripheral smear
d) reticulocyte count

343

All of the following patients have an increased risk of developing adverse effects from metformin (Glucophage) except:

a) patients with renal disease
b) patients who are dehydrated
c) overweight patients
d) patients who are alcoholics

344

A 65-year-old homeless male presents to a public health clinic with complaints of an acute onset of chills and cough that started 2 days previously. The cough is productive of rust-colored sputum. The patient complains of sharp chest pain whenever he coughs. He denies pressure or radiation of the pain to his arms, neck, and jaw. His vital signs are the following: temperature: 102 °F, pulse of 100/minute, and a blood pressure of 130/80. The urinalysis shows a few epithelial cells and no leukocytes. Which of the following is most likely:

a) atypical pneumonia
b) viral pneumonia
c) bacterial pneumonia
d) acute bronchitis

345

Which of the following drugs would you recommend for this patient:

a) doxycycline (Dynapen) BID × 10 days
b) cefuroxime (Ceftin) TID × 10 days
c) trimethoprim sulfamethazole (Bactrim DS) BID × 10 days
d) erythromycin BID × 10 days

346

Which of the following antihypertensive agents should be weaned off in patients who have taken the drug for many years before the drug is discontinued:

a) diuretics
b) beta blockers
c) ACE inhibitors
d) calcium channel blockers

347

A 70-year-old male with open-angle glaucoma is prescribed Betimol (timolol) ophthalmic drops. All of the following are contraindications to Betimol ophthalmic drops except:

a) overt heart failure or sinus bradycardia
b) asthmatic patients
c) second- or third-degree AV block
d) migraine headaches

348

The side effects of antihistamines are mostly due to their:

a) anticholinergic effects
b) sedating effects
c) anti-inflammatory effects
d) immune system effects

349

"Sundowning" is sometimes seen in elderly patients with dementia. Which of the following is the best description of this phenomenon:

a) the patient becomes very agitated, confused, and aggressive after sunset and throughout the night with resolution of symptoms in the morning
b) the patient becomes less disoriented and less fearful after sunset
c) the patient starts hallucinating before sundown with resolution of symptoms in the morning
d) the patient becomes more forgetful and anxious during the night

350

A 30-year-old male patient with a history of Bipolar I disorder refuses to take his afternoon dose of pills. The nurse tells him of the possible consequences of his action, but the patient still refuses to cooperate. Which of the following is the best course for the nurse to follow:

a) document in the patient's record behaviors and the action taken by the nurse
b) reassure the patient that he will be fine after taking the medicine
c) document only the patient behavior
d) document only the nurse's action

SECTION H

351

While performing a sports physical on young adult, the nurse practitioner notes a split S2 during inspiration that disappears during expiration. The patient denies chest pain and dyspnea. The mother is with the patient and is concerned. What is the best advice for this patient's mother:

a) the patient needs to be referred to a cardiologist
b) educate the mother that it is a benign finding
c) advise the mother that because the patient is an athlete, he should have stress EKG as soon as possible
d) the patient should avoid strenuous physical exertion until further evaluation

352

Patients who are considered mentally competent need to be advised about their recommended treatment or procedure. This is called:

a) informed consent
b) durable power of attorney
c) competence
d) advanced directives

353

The following lifestyle modifications are an important aspect in the treatment of hypertension. Which of the following is incorrect:

a) reduce intake of potassium because of its cardiac effects
b) reduce intake of sodium and saturated fats
c) exercise at least three to four times per week
d) maintain an adequate intake of potassium, magnesium, and calcium

354

At what level of prevention is art therapy considered for patients who have history of a stroke:

a) primary prevention
b) secondary prevention
c) tertiary prevention
d) health prevention

355

Kyphosis is a late sign of:

a) old age
b) osteopenia
c) osteoporosis
d) osteoarthritis

356

Which of the following methods is used to diagnose gonorrheal proctitis:

a) serum chlamydia titer
b) Gen-Probe
c) Thayer-Martin culture
d) RPR and VDRL

357

The first nurse practitioner program was started by:

a) Alfred Bandura
b) President John F. Kennedy
c) the federal government
d) Loretta Ford, PhD

358

Terazosin (Hytrin) is used to treat which of the following conditions:

a) benign prostatic hypertrophy (BPH) and hypertension

b) chronic prostatitis and atrial fibrillation
c) urinary tract infections and arrhythmias
d) benign prostatic hypertrophy (BPH) and chronic prostatitis

359

All of the following are possible etiology for papilledema except:

a) intracranial abscess
b) ruptured aneurysm
c) basilar migraine headaches
d) cerebral edema

360

Which of the following clinical findings can mimic a case of testicular torsion:

a) the blue dot sign
b) Cullen's sign
c) Phrens sign
d) Murphy's sign

361

Paroxysmal nocturnal dyspnea is found predominantly in patients with which type of heart failure:

a) left heart failure
b) right heart failure
c) both left and right heart failure
d) partial heart failure

362

All of the following factors increase the risk of mortality for patients diagnosed with bacterial pneumonia except:

a) alcoholism
b) very young age or the elderly
c) multiple lobar involvement
d) hypertension

363

The bacteria responsible for the highest mortality in patients with community-acquired pneumonia is:

a) *Streptococcus pneumoniae*
b) *Mycoplasma pneumoniae*
c) *Moxarella catarrhalis*
d) *Haemophilus influenzae*

364

Mr. R. J. is a 40-year-old asthmatic male with hypertension. For the past 6 months, he has been following a low-fat, low-sodium diet and walking three times a week. His BP readings from the past two visits were 160/95 and 170/100. On this visit, it is 160/90. What is the most appropriate action for the nurse practitioner to follow at this visit:

a) continue the lifestyle modifications and recheck his blood pressure again in 4 weeks
b) initiate a prescription of hydrochlorothiazide 12.5 mg po daily
c) initiate a prescription of atenolol (Tenormin) 25 mg po daily
d) refer the patient to a cardiologist for a stress EKG

365

When initially treating an adult for acute bronchitis, which of the following should the nurse practitioner be least likely to order:

a) expectorants
b) antibiotics
c) bronchodilators
d) antitussives

366

According to JNC 7 criteria, which of the following are considered as cardiac risk equivalents:

a) microalbuminuria and diabetes
b) congestive heart failure
c) acute renal failure and chronic bronchitis
d) patients on anticoagulation therapy

367

Which of the following is one of the best screening tools to rule out alcohol abuse:

a) Alcoholics Anonymous
b) The Becker Depression Inventory
c) Mini-Mental Exam
d) CAGE test

368

Mrs. Nottam, who has a BMI of 29, has a 20-year history of essential hypertension. She has been on hydrochlorothiazide 25 mg po daily with excellent results. On this visit, she is complaining of feeling thirsty all the time even though she drinks more than 10 glasses of water per day. She reports to the nurse practitioner that she been having this problem for about 6 months. On reading the chart, the nurse practitioner notes that the last two fasting blood glucose levels have been 140 mg/dL and 168 mg/dL. A random blood glucose is at 210 mg/dL. Which of the following is the best treatment plan to follow at this visit:

a) order another random blood sugar test in 2 weeks
b) initiate a prescription of metformin (Glucophage) 500 mg po BID
c) order a 3-hour glucose tolerance test (GTT)
d) order a HgbA1c level

369

A newly diagnosed middle-aged type 2 diabetic wants to start an exercise program. All of the following statements are true except:

a) if the patient is unable to eat due to illness, antidiabetic agents should not be taken until the patient is able to eat again.
b) strenuous exercise is contraindicated for most type 1 diabetics because of a higher risk of hypoglycemic episodes
c) exercise increases the body's ability to metabolize glucose
d) patients who exercise vigorously in the afternoon may have hypoglycemic episodes in the evening or at night if they don't eat

370

What is the most common pathogen found in community-acquired atypical pneumonia:

a) *Chlamydia pneumoniae*
b) *Streptococcus pneumoniae*
c) *Moxarella catarrhalis*
d) *Mycoplasma pneumoniae*

371

All of the following are considered as target organs that are more likely to become damaged due to chronic hypertension except:

a) eyes
b) heart
c) adrenal glands
d) kidneys

372

A 56-year-old mechanic is brought to your office complaining of heavy pressure in the substernal area of his chest that is radiating to his jaw. The pain began while he was lifting up a tire. He now appears pale and is diaphoretic. His blood pressure is 100/60 mm Hg, and his pulse rate 50. What is the most appropriate action:

a) perform a 12-lead EKG
b) dial 911

c) administer a morphine injection for pain
d) observe the patient in the office

373

Which of the following is indicated for initial treatment of an uncomplicated case of *H. pylori* negative peptic ulcer disease (PUD):

a) omeprazole (Prilosec)
b) metoclopramide (Reglan)
c) ranitidine (Zantac)
d) Pepto-Bismol tablets

374

Erythromycin inhibits the cytochrome P-450 system. The following drugs should be avoided because of a potential for a drug interaction except:

a) theophylline (Theo-Dur)
b) warfarin (Coumadin)
c) diazepam (Valium)
d) furosemide (Lasix)

375

If left untreated, Zollinger-Ellison syndrome can cause which of the following:

a) severe ulcers in the stomach or duodenum
b) toxic megacolon
c) chronic diarrhea
d) malabsorption of fat-soluble vitamins

376

All of the following are classified as FDA category X drugs except:

a) misoprostol (Cytotec)
b) ciprofloxacin (Cipro)
c) finasteride (Proscar)
d) isotretinoin (Accutane)

377

You note during a physical exam pitting on the fingernails. This finding is best correlated with:

a) iron-deficiency anemia
b) psoriasis
c) onychomycosis
d) vitamin C deficiency

378

Which of the following is correct regarding the best site to listen for mitral regurgitation:

a) the apical area during S2
b) it is best heard at the base at S1
c) it is best heard at the apex at S1
d) it is best heard at the base at S2

379

Extreme tenderness and involuntary guarding at McBurney's point is a significant finding for possible:

a) acute cholecystitis
b) acute appendicitis
c) acute gastroenteritis
d) acute diverticulitis

380

All of the following can help relieve the symptom(s) of GERD except:

a) losing weight
b) stopping caffeine intake
c) chewing breath mints
d) stopping alcohol intake

381

A 34-year-old female is diagnosed with pelvic inflammatory disease (PID). The cervical Gen-Probe result is positive for *Neisseria gonorrheae* and negative for *Chlamydia trachomatis*. All of the following statements are true regarding the management of this patient except:

a) this patient should be treated for chlamydia even though the Gen-Probe for chlamydia is negative
b) ceftriaxone (Rocephin) 250 mg IM and doxycycline 100 mg po BID × 14 days is appropriate treatment for this patient
c) advise the patient to return to the clinic for a repeat pelvic exam in 48 hours
d) repeat the Gen-Probe test for *Chlamydia trachomatis* to ensure that the previous test was not a false-negative result

382

What Tanner stage is a girl at when her breasts have a secondary mound:

a) Tanner stage II
b) Tanner stage III
c) Tanner stage IV
d) Tanner stage V

383

A 36-year-old smoker is being evaluated for birth control choices. The patient has a history of chlamydial cervicitis. She has two small children. The best contraceptive method for this patient is:

a) Depo-Provera injections
b) oral contraceptives
c) IUD (intrauterine device)
d) estrogen patches

384

Which of the following antibiotics can interact with theophylline:

a) clarithromycin (Biaxin)
b) metronidazole (Flagyl)
c) amoxicillin (Amoxil)
d) trimethoprim sulfazole (Bactrim DS)

385

You would recommend the pneumococcal vaccine (Pneumovax) to patients with all of the following conditions except:

a) sickle cell anemia
b) splenectomy
c) patients infected with HIV
d) G6PD-deficiency anemia

386

A 40-year-old cashier complains of random episodes of dizziness and palpitations that have a sudden onset. The EKG shows p waves before each QRS complex and a heart rate of 170 beats/minute. A carotid massage decreases the heart rate to 80 beats/minute. This best describes:

a) ventricular tachycardia
b) paroxysmal atrial tachycardia
c) atrial fibrillation
d) ventricular fibrillation

387

A 25-year-old woman complains of dysuria, pruritis, and purulent vaginal discharge. Pelvic examination reveals a cervix with punctate superficial petecchia ("strawberry cervix"), an irritated and reddened vulvar area, and frothy discharge. Microscopic exam of the discharge reveals unicellular organisms. The correct pharmacologic therapy for the condition is:

a) oral metronidazole (Flagyl)
b) ceftriaxone sodium (Rocephin) injection
c) doxycycline hyclate (Vibramycin)
d) clotrimazole (Gyne-Lotrimin) cream or suppositories

388

All of the following conditions can cause secondary hypertension except:

a) adrenal tumors
b) renal artery stenosis
c) mitral regurgitation
d) sleep apnea

389

Metronidazole (Flagyl) produces the disulfuram (Antabuse) effect when combined with alcoholic drinks or medicine. You would educate the patient that:

a) she should avoid alcoholic drinks during the time she takes the medicine
b) she should avoid alcoholic drinks one day before, during therapy, and a few days after therapy
c) she should avoid alcoholic drinks after she takes the medicine
d) there is no need to avoid any food or drink

390

The treatment plan of patients with AIDS (acquired immunodeficiency syndrome) who have CD4 counts of <200/mm should emphasize:

a) administering an MMR vaccine
b) preventative therapy for toxoplasmosis
c) preventative therapy for *Pneumocystis carinii* pneumonia (PCP)
d) evaluation of the home environment

391

A positive obturator sign might signify which of the following conditions:

a) acute appendicitis
b) acute pancreatitis
c) acute cholecystitis
d) acute hepatitis

392

Where does spermatogenesis occur:

a) epididymitis
b) vas deferens

c) seminal vesicles
d) testes

393

Prophylaxis for *Pneumocystis carinii* pneumonia includes all of the following drugs except:

a) trimethoprim-sulfamethazole (Bactrim)
b) dapsone
c) aerosolized pentamidine
d) nedocromil sodium (Tilade)

394

All of the following findings are associated with acute labyrinthitis or acute vestibular neuritis except:

a) hearing loss and tinnitus
b) symptoms are provoked by changes in head position
c) vertigo with nausea
d) nystagmus

395

While performing a routine physical exam on a 60-year-old hypertensive male, the nurse practitioner notices a bruit over the carotid area on the left side of the neck. There is no induration on the skin. This patient is at higher risk for:

a) temporal arteritis and brain aneurysms
b) dizziness and headaches
c) abdominal aneurysm and congestive heart failure
d) stroke and coronary heart disease

396

A 46-year-old kindergarten teacher was recently treated for an episode of acute otitis media (AOM) of the right ear. During her follow-up visit, she reports that she is on the fifth day of her menstrual cycle. During the physical examination, the patient's throat is a bright red color with no purulent discharge. The Quick Strep test is negative. The result of her urine dipstick shows a large amount of blood, 3+ leukocytes, and is positive for nitrites. On further questioning, the patient denies flank pain and fever, but is positive for dysuria and urinary frequency. The patient reports that she has a sulfa allergy and may also be allergic to penicillins. Which of the following is the best initial intervention:

a) send a urine specimen for culture and sensitivity to the laboratory and treat the patient for a urinary tract infection (UTI)
b) recheck the urine by sending another specimen to the laboratory and evaluate the patient further for strep throat

c) treat the patient for acute otitis media (AOM) and an acute urinary tract infection (UTI)

d) advise the patient that she needs further evaluation

397

Which of the following is the most common skin cancer in the country:

a) basal skin cancer
b) squamous skin cancer
c) melanoma
d) none of the above

398

When starting an elderly patient on a new prescription of levothyroxine (Synthroid), the nurse practitioner should keep in mind that the rationale for starting an elderly patient on a lower dose is because of the following:

a) CNS (central nervous system) effects
b) cardiac effects
c) renal effects
d) hepatic effects

399

All of the following are useful in treating patients with COPD (chronic obstructive lung disease) except:

a) anticholinergics
b) short-acting B2 agonist
c) oral steroids
d) antihistamines

400

All of the following drugs interfere with the metabolism of oral contraceptives except:

a) tetracycline
b) rifampin
c) phenytoin (Dilantin)
d) corticosteroids

SECTION I

401

Which of the following is a recommended treatment by the CDC (Centers of Disease Control) for a case of uncomplicated gonorrheal and chlamydial infection:

a) metronidazole (Flagyl) 250 mg PO three times a day for 7 days
b) valacyclovir (Valtrex) 500 mg PO twice daily for 10 days
c) ceftriaxone sodium (Rocephin) 125 mg IM and doxycycline 100 mg two times day for 7 days
d) one dose of oral fluconazole (Diflucan) 150 mg

402

Which of the following factors is a relative contraindication for oral contraceptive pills:

a) active hepatitis A infection
b) history of an embolic episode that resolved with treatment
c) undiagnosed vaginal bleeding
d) migraine headache without focal aura

403

A nurse practitioner is taking part in a community outreach program for a local hospital. Most of her audience has a diagnosis of hypertension. They are all interested in learning more about a proper diet. When discussing potential sources of potassium and magnesium, which of the following is the best advice:

a) fruits, vegetables, and whole grains
b) fruits, whole grains, and sausages
c) bananas, beef, and yogurt
d) mushrooms, fermented foods, and vegetables

404

A 35-year-old sexually active male presents with a 1-week history of fever and pain on his left scrotum along with frequency and dysuria. On examination of the genitals, the nurse practitioner notices that the scrotum is reddened, swollen, and tender to touch. The CVA (costovertebral) exam is negative and the patient denies nausea and vomiting. When the affected testicle is elevated toward the patient's body or when the patient uses his old football support brief, the pain is lessened. The urinalysis shows 2+ blood and a large amount of leukocytes. What is the most likely diagnosis:

a) acute urinary tract infection
b) acute pyelonephritis
c) acute orchitis
d) acute epididymitis

405

Julia M., a 16-year-old patient, is being treated for her first urinary tract infection. Which of the following antibiotics would be contraindicated:

a) cephalexin (Keflex)
b) ampicillin (Amoxil)
c) ofloxacin (Floxin)
d) nitrofurantoin crystals (Macrobid)

406

All of the following are considered as risk factors for breast cancer except:

a) nulliparity
b) early menarche
c) polycystic ovaries
d) premature menopause

407

The following statements about benign prostatic hypertrophy (BPH) are correct except:

a) it is seen in up to 50% of males older than 50 years old
b) dribbling and nocturia are common patient complaints
c) saw palmetto is always effective in reducing symptoms
d) the PSA value is usually slightly elevated

408

The normal hemoglobin A1C level is:

a) 3% to 4.5%
b) 4% to 5.9%
c) 6% to 7%
d) below 8%

409

At what Tanner stage does puberty start:

a) Tanner stage I
b) Tanner stage II
c) Tanner stage III
d) Tanner stage IV

410

All of the following conditions are recommended screening for a 40-year-old Black male except:

a) obesity
b) heart disease
c) prostate cancer
d) lung cancer

411

Acute prostatitis can present with all of the following signs and symptoms except:

a) fever and chills

b) tenderness of the scrotum on the affected side
c) perineal pain
d) slow onset of symptoms

412

Which of the following is the most common etiology of nongonococcal urethritis (NGU):

a) *Escherichia coli*
b) *Chlamydia trachomatis*
c) *Neisseria gonorrheae*
d) *Mycoplasma*

413

Which of the following factors is considered a relative contraindication for combined oral contraceptive pills:

a) undiagnosed vaginal bleeding
b) a hepatoma of the liver
c) suspected history of transient ischemic attacks (TIAs)
d) smoking

414

A 20-year-old Hispanic male complains of right knee pain after twisting it while playing soccer. The patient anxiously tells the nurse practitioner that the injured knee sometimes locks up when he walks or attempts to straighten the leg. This best describes:

a) injury to the meniscus of the right knee
b) injury to the patella of the right knee
c) injury to the ligaments of the right knee
d) rupture of the quadriceps tendon

415

Which of the following is the best course of treatment for this patient:

a) refer him to an orthopedic specialist
b) refer him to a chiropractor
c) advise him that the clicking noise will resolve within 2 to 4 weeks
d) advise him to use an ACE bandage wrap during the first 2 weeks for knee support and to see you again for reevaluation

416

All of the following are correct statements regarding oral contraceptives except:

a) the actual failure rate of oral contraceptives is 3%
b) desogestrel belongs to the progesterone family of drugs
c) the newer low-dose birth control pills don't require back-up during the first 2 weeks of use
d) oral contraceptives are contraindicated for women 35 years of age or older who smoke

417

Which of the following hormones induces ovulation:

a) follide-stimulating hormone (FSH)
b) luteinizing hormone (LH)
c) estradiol
d) progesterone

418

A cauliflower-like growth with foul smelling discharge is seen during an otoscopic exam inside the middle ear of a new patient with a history of chronic otitis media infection. No tympanic membrane is visible and the patient reports hearing loss in the affected ear. Which of the following conditions is most likely:

a) chronic perforation of the tympanic member with secondary bacterial infection
b) chronic mastoiditis
c) cholesteatoma
d) cancer of the middle ear

419

All of the following are considered as ethical concepts except:

a) beneficence
b) nonmalfeasance
c) honesty
d) advocacy

420

The best form of aerobic exercise for a patient with severe rheumatoid arthritis is:

a) walking
b) swimming
c) riding a bicycle
d) passive range of motion

421

Benzodiazepines are useful in treating all of the following conditions except:

a) acute alcohol withdrawal/delirium tremens
b) status epilepticus
c) insomnia
d) mood disorders

422

All of the following patients are at higher risk of active tuberculosis disease except:

a) diabetic patients
b) a healthy nurse whose PPD test becomes positive after a history of negative tests and denies tuberculosis signs and symptoms
c) patients with acute renal failure
d) patients who are alcoholics

423

All of the following are considered emancipated minors except:

a) 15-year-old male who is married
b) 14-year-old female who is a single parent
c) 17-year-old male who is enlisted in the U.S. Army
d) 13-year-old being treated for a sexually transmitted disease

424

All of the following factors are not associated with an increased risk of osteopenia in teenage girls except:

a) drinking one glass of low-fat milk daily
b) anorexia nervosa
c) exercise
d) normal BMI (basal metabolic index)

425

A 36-year-old hospital janitor is being treated for an acute urinary tract infection (UTI) by the employee health nurse practitioner. The patient thinks that he had the same symptoms 4 months ago. Which of the following is the best intervention:

a) refer the patient to a urologist after treatment
b) prescribe the patient ofloxacin (Floxin) for 2 weeks instead of 1 week
c) advised the patient that he needs to void every 2 hours and drink more fluids
d) refer the patient to the local emergency room (ER) because he has a high risk of sepsis

426

Which of the following is a true statement regarding the beliefs of the majority of Jehovah's witness patients:

a) transfusion of blood is prohibited even in cases of emergency
b) consumption of pork products is strictly prohibited
c) transfusion of blood is allowed in certain medical conditions
d) consumptions of alcohol products is strictly prohibited

427

Which of the following is not a true statement:

a) a protocol agreement with a physician is a requirement for nurse practitioners to practice in this country
b) if a nurse practitioner is sued, the physician whom he or she has a protocol agreement with is not held liable
c) protocol agreements should be reviewed annually by both the nurse practitioner and the physician
d) protocol agreements help protect nurse practitioners from certain types of lawsuits

428

A postmenopausal female complains of intermittent vaginal bleeding for the past 6 months. Which of the following is recommended management for this condition:

a) cervical biopsy
b) Pap smear
c) colposcopy
d) endometrial biopsy

429

Which of the following findings is not a characteristic of delirium:

a) sudden onset
b) patient is coherent
c) worse in the evenings
d) it has a brief duration

430

The signs and symptoms of dementia include all of the following except:

a) personality changes
b) difficulty in verbalizing
c) difficulty in recognizing familiar objects
d) abstract thinking ability is increased

431

All of the following drugs are known to interact with theophylline either by decreasing the therapeutic blood level or by elevating it to toxic levels. All of the following drugs are known to interact with theophylline except:

a) clarithromycin (Biaxin)
b) carbamazepine (Tegretol)
c) captopril (Capoten)
d) ciprofloxacin (Cipro)

432

A women's health nurse practitioner is performing a pelvic exam on a middle-aged woman who recently became sexually active. On examination of the external vagina, a tender and warm cystic mass is found on the lower edge of the left labia majora. According to the patient, she does not use condoms because she is now on birth control pills. Which of the following is most likely:

a) Skene's gland cyst
b) cystocele
c) lymphogranuloma venereum
d) Bartholin's gland abscess

433

A 17-year-old high school student visits the local Planned Parenthood clinic. She tells the nurse practitioner who is evaluating her that she wants to be on birth control pills because she recently became sexually active with her boyfriend. Which of the following is a true statement:

a) the nurse practitioner can examine and prescribe birth control pills to minors because there is no legal requirement for parental consent in cases concerning sexual activity and pregnancy
b) patients who are minors must obtain a signed consent from a parent before being examined or treated for possible pregnancy
c) some visits to a health care provider are allowed without parental consent as long as the patient is informed fully about the treatment options
d) Planned Parenthood clinics are exempted from the consent rule as a result of a ruling from the landmark case of Roe v. Wade

434

A patient diagnosed with bacterial vaginosis should be advised that her sexual partner be treated with:

a) ceftriaxone (Rocephin) 250 mg IM with doxycycline 100 mg BID for 14 days
b) metronidazole (Flagyl) 500 mg po twice a day for 7 days and one dose of azithromycin (Zithromax)
c) her partner does not need treatment
d) clotrimazole cream (Lotrimin) on his penis BID for 1 to 2 weeks

435

All of the following are correct statements regarding physiologic changes found in the elderly except:

a) there is an increase of the fat-to-lean body ratio
b) the metabolism of drugs by the liver decreases
c) there is an increase in the production of cholesterol by the liver
d) there is a loss of low-frequency hearing secondary to presbycusis

436

The following clinical signs are seen in patients with advanced Parkinson's disease except:

a) pill-rolling tremor
b) difficulty initiating involuntary movement
c) shuffling gait
d) increased facial movements

437

When a patient is instructed to smell a small amount of coffee grounds or a lemon, which of the following cranial nerves is being evaluated:

a) CN 1
b) CN 2
c) CN 3
d) CN 4

438

A possible complication from Bell's palsy is:

a) corneal ulceration
b) acute glaucoma
c) inability to swallow
d) loss of sensation in the affected side

439

Which of the following is least likely to cause delirium:

a) severe dehydration
b) multiple brain infarcts
c) metabolic derangements
d) adverse drug reactions

440

A 38-year-old sexually active Asian woman with a history of infertility treatment and severe endometriosis complains to the nurse practitioner in the emergency room that she has right-sided pelvic pain that is steadily getting worse. She has also noticed small amounts of yellow-colored vaginal discharge on her underwear for at least 1 week. The patient reports that she is expecting her period, which has not appeared for the last 2 months. Which of the following evaluations is best performed initially:

a) follicle-stimulating hormone (FSH) and a culture with sensitivity testing of the vaginal discharge
b) serum quantitative pregnancy test and cervical Gen-Probe testing
c) pelvic ultrasound and serum quantitative pregnancy test
d) microscopy of the vaginal discharge and CBC (complete blood count) with white cell differential

441

Regarding the above question, which of the following conditions are the most important differential diagnoses to consider in this patient:

a) tubal ectopic pregnancy and PID (pelvic inflammatory disease)
b) mucopurulent cervicitis and tubal ectopic pregnancy
c) human papilloma virus infection of the cervix and PID (pelvic inflammatory disease)
d) ovarian cysts and severe endometriosis

442

Which of the following effects are seen in every woman using Depo-Provera (medroxyprogesterone injection) for more than 4 years:

a) melasma
b) amenorrhea
c) weight loss
d) headaches

443

The following are useful for treating migraine headache. Which one of the following is not considered as effective therapy:

a) propranolol (Inderal) prophylaxis
b) cold packs to the forehead
c) trimethobenzamide (Tigan) suppositories for nausea
d) sodium restriction to decrease water retention

444

Which of the following groups of patients should avoid handling crushed or broken tablets of finasteride (Proscar) tablets directly:

a) adult males
b) elderly males
c) elderly females
d) reproductive-aged females

445

The gag reflex is a function of which cranial nerve:

a) CN9
b) CN10
c) CN11
d) CN12

446

A 75-year-old hypertensive male reports a history of an upper respiratory viral infection 4 weeks ago. He is currently complaining of a gradual onset of shortness of breath accompanied by very sharp midchest pain that increases in intensity when he lies down in a supine position. During the physical exam, a precordial rub is auscultated along with a soft S4. The most likely diagnosis would be:

a) pulmonary embolism
b) a dissecting aneurysm
c) acute pericarditis
d) esophageal reflex

447

Which type of exercise is recommended for a 65-year-old arthritic patient who complains of new onset of a painful and swollen left knee due to overworking in his garden for 3 days:

a) quadriceps strengthening exercises of the left knee followed by cold packs for 30 minutes on the swollen knee three times a day
b) rest and elevation of the knee with intermittent application of cold packs × 15 minutes four times a day for the next 48 hours
c) passive range of motion exercises after a warm tub bath
d) warm showers to relax the quadriceps muscle followed by cold packs for the swelling

448

Irritable bowel syndrome (IBS) is most commonly seen in young women. These patients usually report a recent history of a stressful event in their life as a precipitating factor for an acute exacerbation. Most complain of the following symptoms except:

a) abdominal pain
b) diarrhea or constipation
c) relief of abdominal cramping after defecation
d) severe vomiting

449

Peak expiratory flow (PEF) meters are useful for monitoring the progress or worsening of patients with asthma. The patients are instructed to try blowing as hard as they can at least three times. The personal best or highest volumes are recorded in a diary. All of the following factors are used to determine the PEF except:

a) age
b) gender
c) height
d) weight

450

A high school student presents to the nurse practitioner complaining of an acute onset of an itchy rash on the back of her neck. During the physical exam, the nurse practitioner notes a bright red maculopapular rash in a linear pattern on the back of the patient's neck. The student is wearing several pieces of jewelry. Which of the following is most likely:

a) contact dermatitis
b) erythema migrans
c) atopic dermatitis
d) scabies

451

All of the following are considered risk factors for urinary tract infections in women except:

a) diabetes mellitus
b) diaphragms and spermicide use
c) pregnancy
d) IUD (intrauterine device)

SECTION J

452

A serious sign to look for while performing a physical exam are enlarged sentinel nodes (Virchow's nodes). The sentinel nodes are located in which area of the body:

a) right axillary area
b) left supraclavicular area
c) posterior cervical chain
d) submandibular chain

453

Pete, a 30-year-old White male, is being seen for a physical exam by the nurse practitioner. He complains of pruritic macerated areas on his groin that are slowly getting larger. Which of the following is the most likely:

a) tinea cruris
b) tinea corporis
c) tinea capitis
d) tinea pedis

454

Cluster headaches are most often seen in:

a) adolescent females
b) middle-aged men
c) elderly men
d) postmenopausal women

455

A middle-aged female with a history of hypertension and osteoarthritis reports to the nurse practitioner that she is taking vitamin C for her common cold. She is currently taking a dose of 500 mg twice a day. Which of the following is a true statement:

a) the patient should continue taking the Vitamin C at the same doses
b) the patient should increase the dose of the Vitamin C to 1,000 mg twice a day
c) it does not matter since there is no solid evidence regarding the efficacy of vitamin C for the common cold
d) the patient should continue taking the Vitamin C and combine it with a multivitamin once a day to increase its effectiveness

456

Robert, a homeless man with an extensive history of alcohol abuse, is found in the local park, confused and combative. Family members report that Robert has not consumed any alcoholic drinks for at least 2 days because of a severe case of gastroenteritis. His behavior has progressively worsened and he is getting more uncontrollable. The most likely cause for Robert's behavior is which of the following:

a) subdural hematoma
b) delirium tremens secondary to acute withdrawal of alcohol
c) thiamine intoxication
d) gastrointestinal hemorrhage

457

A middle-aged woman is complaining of feeling anxious and irritable for several months. She reports weight loss and a fine tremor in her hands even when she is at rest that bother her. She has lost weight without changing her usual diet or activity. The patient reports that her appetite has increased. Her menstrual cycles have become very irregular. Which of the following conditions is best described:

a) hyperthyroidism

b) obsessive-compulsive disorder (OCD)
c) mood disorder
d) MODY (maturity onset diabetes of the young)

458

A middle-aged Hispanic patient with type 2 diabetes mellitus, chronic bronchitis, and hypertension is currently on hydrochlorothiazide 12.5 mg daily. The patient has gained 6 pounds since the last visit. The blood pressure is currently at 140/90, the pulse is 82 beats per minute, and the respirations is at 12 breaths per minute. Which of the following agents is the best choice for this patient:

a) calcium channel blockers
b) ARB (angiotensin reuptake blockers)
c) beta blockers
d) alpha blockers

459

The cremasteric reflex is elicited by:

a) ask the patient to open his mouth and touch the back of his pharynx with a tongue blade
b) hit the biceps tendon briskly with a reflex hammer and watch the lower arm for movement
c) hit the patellar tendon briskly with a reflex hammer and watch the lower leg for movement
d) stroke the inner thigh of a male and watch the testicle on the ipsilateral side rise up toward the body

460

The nurse practitioner has diagnosed Tom, a 30-year-old farmer, with contact dermatitis on the left side of his face secondary to exposure to poison ivy. Which of the following is the best treatment plan for this patient:

a) wash the rash with antibacterial soap twice a day to reduce risk of secondary bacterial infection
b) apply hydrocortisone cream 1% BID to the rash until it is healed
c) apply clotrimazole (Lotrimin) cream BID for 2 weeks on the rash
d) use halcinonide (Halog)1% ointment BID for 2 to 4 weeks

461

Pulsus paradoxus is best described as:

a) an increase in systolic blood pressure of >5 mm Hg on inspiration
b) a decrease in the diastolic blood pressure on exhalation
c) a decrease in the systolic blood pressure of >10 mm Hg on inspiration
d) an increase in diastolic blood pressure of >15 mm Hg on expiration

462

An 18 year old sexually-active male complains of the sudden onset of an extremely painful and swollen left scrotum upon awakening that morning. On questioning, the patient denies any trauma, dysuria, and penile discharge but complains that he feels nauseated from the pain. The urine dipstick is negative for blood, leukocytes, and nitrites. On palpation, the nurse practitioner finds an extremely tender, swollen, and red-colored left scrotum. There is no penile discharge. Which of the following conditions is most likely:

a) epididymitis
b) acute gastroenteritis
c) testicular torsion
d) orchitis

463

What type of follow-up should this patient receive:

a) refer him within 48 hours to a urologist
b) refer him to the emergency room as soon as possible
c) prescribe ibuprofen (Advil) 600 mg QID for pain
d) order a testicular ultrasound for further evaluation

464

A female teenager complains to the gym instructor that she recently noticed that one of her hips is higher than the other. She denies pain or any difficulty with ambulation and physical activity. The instructor instructs the girl to bend down forward with her spine in a straight line. On closer inspection, the instructor notices that the thoracic spine has a lateral curvature of about 10 degrees and suspects scoliosis. Which of the following is a true statement:

a) the curvature is considered mild and will correct spontaneously over time as the patient continues to grow
b) the girl needs to be referred for surgical correction as soon as possible before further damage to the spine results
c) the usual clinical strategy is watchful waiting for curves of 10 degrees or less
d) the patient always needs to wear a special brace for her back during the daytime

465

Which of the following cholesterol levels is classified as borderline:

a) 180 to 199 mg/dL
b) 200 to 239 mg/dL
c) over 240 mg/dL
d) over 300 mg/dL

466

The school health nurse practitioner is performing a sports physical on a teen who belongs to the school's swim team. She documents the girl as Tanner stage II. The mother is advised that her daughter will probably start menarche within:

a) 1 to 2 years
b) $2^1/_2$ to 3 years
c) 3 to 4 years
d) it is dependent on the girl's genetic makeup

467

All of the following do not require parental consent be obtained by the nurse practitioner except:

a) 17-year-old who wants to be treated for a sexually transmitted infection
b) a 14-year-old who wants a serum pregnancy test
c) a 15-year-old who wants birth control pills
d) a 16-year-old who wants to be treated for dysmenorrhea

468

All of the following conditions fulfill the criteria for metabolic syndrome except:

a) glucose intolerance
b) microalbuminuria
c) hypertension
d) obesity

469

Transillumination is useful in helping diagnose which of the following conditions:

a) sinusitis and hydrocele
b) testicular tumor and acute otitis media
c) nasal masses and other tumors in the facial region
d) hydrocephalus and epididymitis

470

Which of the following is less likely to be found in a patient with emphysema-dominant COPD (chronic obstructive pulmonary disease):

a) exertional dyspnea
b) weight loss
c) prolonged expiration
d) a cough that is productive of large amounts of sputum

471

A split S2 is best heard at which following auscultatory area:

a) the aortic area
b) the pulmonic area
c) the tricuspid area
d) the mitral area

472

Balanitis is caused by:

a) *Staphylococcus aureus*
b) *Streptococcus pyogenes*
c) *Candida albicans*
d) diabetes

473

Which of the following is the most common type of anemia in the United States:

a) iron-deficiency anemia
b) thalassemia trait
c) folate-deficiency anemia
d) normocytic anemia

474

A newly diagnosed diabetic patient reports to the nurse practitioner that she had severe hives and swollen lips 1 year ago after taking trimethoprim/sulfamethazole (Bactrim) for a bladder infection. Which of the following statements is correct:

a) she cannot take any pills in the sulfonylurea class
b) she can take some of the pills in the sulfonylurea class
c) she can take any of the pills in the sulfonylurea class
d) none of the above

475

Which of the following is responsible for the symptoms of dysmenorrhea:

a) estrogen
b) human chorionic gonadotropin
c) prostaglandins
d) progesterone

476

Which of the following laboratory tests is the next step in working up a 55-year-old diabetic male with the following CBC results: Hgb 11 g/dL, Hct 38%, and an MCV of 102 fL:

a) serum ferritin and peripheral smear
b) hemoglobin electrophoresis

c) serum folate and B12 level
d) Schilling test

477

Auscultation of normal breath sounds of the chest will reveal:

a) bronchial breath sounds heard at the lower bases
b) high-pitched vesicular breath sounds heard over the upper lobes
c) vesicular breath sounds heard over the trachea
d) vesicular breath sounds in the lower lobe

478

The bell of the stethoscope is best used to auscultate which of the following heart sounds:

a) S3 and S4 and low-pitched tones
b) S3 and S4 only
c) S1 and S2 and high-pitched tones
d) S1 and S2 only

479

Vaginal candidiasis is best diagnosed in the primary care arena by the following method:

a) microscopy
b) Tzanck smear
c) KOH (potassium hydroxide) smear
d) clinical findings only

480

When an adolescent male's penis starts to grow in length along with the continued growth of the testicles and the scrotal sac, at which Tanner stage would this male be classified:

a) Tanner stage I
b) Tanner stage II
c) Tanner stage III
d) Tanner stage IV

481

A teenage male wants to be treated for acne. He has a large number of black and white comedones especially on the cheeks and chin. The patient has treated himself in the past few months with several types of over-the-counter benzoyl peroxide and salicylic acid products with minimal results. Which of the following agents is the best choice for this visit:

a) isotretinoin (Accutane) pulse therapy
b) tetracycline
c) Retin-A 0.25% cream
d) use a combination of benzoyl peroxide cream and topical vitamin C cream BID

482

The Romberg test is done to check which area of the central nervous system:

a) frontal lobe
b) temporal lobe
c) the midbrain
d) the cerebellum

483

All of the following vaccines are contraindicated in pregnant women except:

a) influenza vaccine injections
b) mumps
c) varicella
d) rubella

484

Females with polycystic ovary syndrome (PCOS) are at higher risk for the following:

a) heart disease, infertility, uterine cancer, diabetes, and endometrial cancer
b) fibroids and ovarian cancer
c) premature menopause and anovulation
d) oligoamenorrhea, ovarian cancer, and cervical cancer

485

Which of the following is the best measure of the size of red blood cells in a sample:

a) MCHC (mean corpuscular hemoglobin concentration)
b) MCV (mean corpuscular volume)
c) RDW (red cell distribution width)
d) hematocrit

486

A college student who is on oral contraceptives calls the nurse practitioner's office asking for advice. She has forgotten to take her pills 2 days in a row during the second week of the pill cycle. Which of the following is the best advice:

a) start a new pack of pills and dispose the old one

b) take two pills today, then two pills the next day and use condoms for the rest of the pill cycle

c) stop taking the pills right away and start a new pill cycle and use condoms

d) take one pill now and two pills the next day

487

All of the following patients should be screened for diabetes mellitus except:

a) an obese male of Asian descent

b) an overweight middle-aged African American woman whose mother has type 2 diabetes

c) a woman who delivered an infant weighing $9^1/_2$ pounds

d) a 30-year-old White female who smokes

488

A middle-aged medical assistant who is overweight complains to the nursing supervisor of a new onset of low back pain in the past 24 hours. She reports lifting some obese patients while working the previous night shift. She is advised to seek follow-up with the hospital's employee health nurse practitioner. Which of the following statements is correct:

a) medical treatment for any work-related injury is covered under an employer's worker's comp insurance

b) the injury is not covered by worker's comp because she has health insurance from the hospital

c) the patient is not allowed to sue her employer for more benefits

d) worker's comp insurance premiums are paid by the employees of the hospital

489

A sexually active 22-year-old man is asking to be screened for hepatitis B because his new girlfriend has recently been diagnosed with hepatitis B infection. His lab results are the following: anti-HBV is negative, HBsAg is positive, HBeAg is negative. Which of the following is indicated:

a) the patient is immune to the hepatitis B virus

b) the patient is not infected with hepatitis B virus

c) the patient needs hepatitis B vaccine and hepatitis B immune globulin

d) the patient needs only hepatitis B immune globulin

490

A severe case of mitral regurgitation will radiate to which of the following areas:

a) axilla

b) neck

c) the middle of the back

d) the throat

491

You would advise a patient who is on an MAOI (monoamine oxidase inhibitor) prescription to avoid the following class of drugs because of an increased potential for neuroleptic syndrome. Which of the following class of drugs can cause this serious condition:

a) benzodiazepines

b) SSRIs (selective serotonin reuptake inhibitors)

c) amphetamines

d) lithium salts

492

An elderly patient complains of pain in the middle portion of her right buttock that radiates to the thigh. She denies trauma but reports that she has recently moved to a new apartment. The patient has noticed that the pain is worse after she sits for long periods. Which of the following is best described:

a) sciatica

b) acute muscle spasm

c) cauda equina syndrome

d) acute muscle strain

493

Which bacterium is commonly found to colonize the lungs of patient diagnosed with cystic fibrosis:

a) *Streptococcus pneumoniae*

b) *Chlamydia pneumoniae*

c) *Pseudomonas aeruginosa*

d) *Staphylococcus aureus*

494

Which of the following statements is false regarding physiologic changes in the body as people age:

a) the half-life of drugs is prolonged

b) there is an increase of cholesterol production by the liver

c) there is a mild increase in renal function

d) there is a slight decrease in the activity of the immune system

495

Which of the following cephalosporins is classified as a Category C drug:

a) ceftriaxone (Rocephin)
b) clarithromycin (Biaxin)
c) azithromycin (Zithromax)
d) cefuroxime axetil (Ceftin)

496

Which of the following is secondary to chronic GERD (gastroesophageal reflux disease) and is considered a precursor to esophageal cancer:

a) Barrett's esophagus
b) esophageal varices
c) basal cell metaplasia
d) Wilson's disease

497

Which of the following is recommended as prophylactic treatment for post-herpetic neuralgia:

a) amitriptyline (Elavil)
b) sertraline (Zoloft)
c) naproxen sodium (Naprosyn)
d) alprazolam (Xanax)

498

Which of the following findings on a thyroid scan may be indicative of a possible malignancy:

a) simple cyst
b) complex cyst
c) cold nodule
d) hot nodule

499

Carpal tunnel syndrome is inflammation of the:

a) ulnar nerve
b) radial nerve
c) brachial nerve
d) median nerve

500

Which of the following is found to be a helpful adjunct in the treatment of arthritis:

a) glucosamine
b) B-complex vitamins
c) vitamin C
d) cod liver oil

Answers to Questions

SECTION A

[1]
b) DeQuervain's tenosynovitis

[2]
c) even though the nurse practitioner is no longer insured by the same insurance company, any claims made against her on the dates that her malpractice insurance was active is still eligible for coverage

[3]
a) it is the average blood glucose level during the previous 3 months

[4]
a) endocarditis prophylaxis is indicated for some dental, urologic, and gastrointestinal invasive procedures

[5]
c) nursing home care

[6]
b) acute appendicitis

[7]
b) it is an increase in the blood glucose levels early in the morning due to the physiologic spike of growth hormone

[8]
b) meningococcemia

[9]
b) mycoplasma pneumonia

[10]
c) beta blockers

[11]
c) give an injection of epinephrine 1:1,000 intramuscularly immediately

[12]
b) testicular torsion

[13]
a) spoon-shaped nails and pica

[14]
b) advise the patient to check his blood glucose QID daily and return to the clinic for a follow-up in 48 hours

[15]
d) supplementing with fiber such as psyllium is never recommended

[16]
b) chlamydia trachomatis

[17]
a) educate the patient about Kegel exercises

[18]
b) higher than normal

[19]
a) calcium channel blockers

[20]
a) instability of the knee due to anterior cruciate ligament damage

[21]
b) Tanner stage III

[22]
d) start exercising vigorously as soon as possible so that the circulation in the affected lower extremitiy improves

[23]
a) laryngeal cancer

[24]
c) osteoarthritis

[25]
b) instability of the knee

[26]
b) the force is being directed away from the body

[27]
d) sexual abstinence

[28]
b) creatinine

[29]
a) chronic intake of nonsteroidal analgesics (NSAIDs) can cause the disorder

[30]
d) apraxia

[31]
a) on deep inspiration by the patient, palpate firmly in the right upper quadrant of the abdomen below the costovertebral angle

[32]
b) acetaminophen (Tylenol)

[33]
a) middle-aged to older women

[34]
c) severe vaginal atrophic changes

[35]
b) hepatomegaly, AV (arteriovenous) nicking, bibasilar crackles

[36]
c) tinea cruris

[37]
b) bacterial vaginosis

[38]
a) call the patient to return to the clinic so she can get tested for a possible cervical infection

[39]
b) lichen sclerosus

[40]
b) closure of the semilunar valves

[41]
a) lower limb amputations

[42]
d) anesthesiologists' services

[43]
d) a grandmother who has recently been diagnosed with both hypertension and hypothyroidism

[44]
d) subconjunctival hemorrhage

[45]
c) advise the patient that it is a benign condition and will resolve spontaneously

[46]
a) urine for culture and sensitivity

[47]
b) they affect the kidneys and can elevate blood pressure

[48]
b) bupropion (Zyban)

[49]
b) tick

[50]
b) it does not have a linear distribution

SECTION B

[51]
a) varicella zoster virus infection of the cornea

[52]
c) pregnancy test

[53]
a) S3

[54]
b) elevation of the affected limb with episodic applications of cold packs for the next 48 hours

[55]
a) G6PD-deficiency anemia

[56]
d) recommend immediate referral to the emergency room

[57]
a) St. John's wort

[58]
b) prevent anencephaly

[59]
a) acute pyelonephritis

[60]
b) *Chlamydia trachomatis*

[61]
b) 5 mm

[62]
c) varicella and nasal flu vaccine (FluMist)

[63]
a) irritable bowel syndrome (IBS)

[64]
d) HIV test

[65]
d) during the postpartum period

[66]
d) eyeglasses and routine dental care

[67]
b) normocytic anemia

[68]
b) left heart failure

[69]
c) furosemide (Lasix)

[70]
b) avoid foods with high potassium content

[71]
b) amoxicillin 2 gm 60 minutes before the procedure

[72]
b) Koplik's spots

[73]
a) Hashimoto's disease

[74]
c) *Treponema pallidum*

[75]
d) torsion of a testicular appendage

[76]
c) acute pancreatitis

[77]
b) Western blot test

[78]
b) order a serum TSH, a digoxin level, and an electrolyte panel

[79]
b) Kernig's sign

[80]
b) claims against the nurse practitioner are covered as long as she had an active malpractice policy at the time of the incident

[81]
b) *Chlamydia trachomatis*

[82]
d) initiate CPR (cardiopulmonary resuscitation) immediately

[83]
a) cluster headache

[84]
c) apply acetic acid to the penile shaft and look for acetowhite changes

[85]
d) all of the above

[86]
a) paroxetine (Paxil CR)

[87]
b) she should not get pregnant within the next 3 months

[88]
c) obtain the history from the patient, friends, and family members

[89]
a) recheck the patient's urine during the visit and then refer her to the nephrologist

[90]
d) spinach, liver, and whole wheat bread

[91]
b) they are both tests to detect for antibodies against the HIV virus

[92]
b) gross obesity

[93]
a) alpha blockers

[94]
b) chronic obstructive lung disease

[95]
b) it is a precancerous lesion and needs to be followed up with her dermatologist

[96]
c) 9 provisions

[97]
c) MCV (mean corpuscular volume)

[98]
a) angina pectoris

[99]
b) consult with a cardiologist for further evaluation

[100]
d) transient ischemic attack (TIA)

SECTION C

[101]
a) drinking organic juice

[102]
b) dextromethorphan and guaifenesin (Robitussin DM) 1 to 2 teaspoons every 4 hours

[103]
b) mumps

[104]
a) an immune-mediated reaction precipitated by the destruction of a large number of spirochetes due to an antibiotic injection

[105]
b) tell her to return 1 week after her period so her breasts can be rechecked

[106]
c) acute myocardial infarction

[107]
c) a large number of squamous epithelial cells whose surfaces and edges are coated with large numbers of bacteria along with a few leukocytes

[108]
d) mitral valve prolapse (MVP)

[109]
d) renal artery stenosis

[110]
b) pterygium

[111]
a) discontinue his pravastatin and order a liver function profile

[112]
a) severe congestive heart failure

[113]
a) breast buds and some straight pubic hair

[114]
a) inflammation of the median nerve

[115]
d) clarithromycin (Biaxin) BID, amoxicillin BID, and omeprazole (Prilosec) QD daily

[116]
c) acute viral upper respiratory infection (URI)

[117]
d) its effects only last 2 weeks and are reversible

[118]
a) albuterol inhaler (Proventil)

[119]
c) ceftriaxone (Rocephin)

[120]
c) systemic steroids

[121]
c) Group A beta-hemolytic streptococcus

[122]
c) cauda equina syndrome

[123]
b) Rovsing's sign

[124]
b) EBV (Epstein-Barr Virus)

[125]
b) Adams forward bend test

[126]
a) treat the patient with a 7 day course of antibiotics and order a urine for culture and sensitivity (C&S) before and after treatment

[127]
d) *Chlamydia trachomatis*

[128]
c) the ICP (intracranial pressure) of the brain is increased

[129]
b) GERD (gastroesophageal reflux disease)

[130]
a) cataracts

[131]
c) Alzheimer's disease

[132]
d) leukoplakia of the tongue

[133]
a) doxycycline (Vibramycin) 100 mg po BID × 21 days

[134]
a) the Nurse Practice Act of the state where they practice

[135]
b) order a mammogram and refer the patient to a breast surgeon

[136]
d) a 22-year-old female recently diagnosed with asthma

[137]
c) this is a normal finding in some young athletes

[138]
d) four risk factors

[139]
d) gastrointestinal upset

[140]
a) atrial fibrillation

[141]
c) a 21-year-old woman who is under treatment for a sexually transmitted infection

[142]
b) congestive heart failure

[143]
a) advise the patient that she had a normal exam

[144]
a) the patient can see at 20 feet what a person with normal vision can see at 30 feet

[145]
b) Dawn phenomenon

[146]
a) HCV RNA

[147]
d) check the pedal and posterior tibial pulses

[148]
b) montelukast (Singulair)

[149]
c) mitral regurgitation

[150]
b) ciprofloxacin (Cipro)

SECTION D

[151]
b) Raynaud's disease

[152]
b) small red spots with bluish centers located by the posterior molaris

[153]
c) squamous epithelial cells and endocervical cells

[154]
a) T score of less than –2.50

[155]
a) trigeminal neuralgia

[156]
d) atypical bacterial infections

[157]
d) bupropion hydrochloride (Wellbutrin)

[158]
d) auscultation

[159]
b) gentle exercises of the lower extremities

[160]
c) Nongonococcal urethritis

[161]
a) yogurt and sardines

[162]
a) green leafy vegetables have high levels of vitamin K that can bind with the blood clotting cascade and increase bleeding time

[163]
b) order a liver function profile

[164]
d) stop taking the medicine until the lab results are available

[165]
d) ankylosing spondylitis

[166]
b) schedule the patient for a uterine ultrasound and uterine biopsy

[167]
a) anticholinergics

[168]
a) fever occurs in up to 80% of the patients

[169]
a) ACE (angiotensin converting enzyme) inhibitors

[170]
b) bacterial vaginosis

[171]
a) peripheral vision

[172]
c) acne

[173]
a) administer a booster dose of the Td vaccine

[174]
d) the left side of the sternum at the fifth ICS by the midclavicular line

[175]
b) rosacea

[176]
d) iron-deficiency anemia

[177]
b) lung cancer

[178]
c) it can be a normal variant if heard on a person aged 40 or older

[179]
b) inflammation of the sciatic nerve

[180]
a) an eye exam with an ophthalmologist

[181]
d) she needs to be evaluated by a dermatologist

[182]
b) albuterol (Ventolin) inhalers

[183]
b) degenerative joint disease

[184]
c) macrocytic and normochromic cells

[185]
b) aortic stenosis

[186]
a) hordeolum

[187]
c) propranolol (Inderal)

[188]
b) cluster headache

[189]
c) clarithromycin (Biaxin)

[190]
a) There is no delay in seeking medical treatment

[191]
a) a 50-year-old construction worker who drinks one beer nightly while watching sports programs on television

[192]
c) microcytic and hypochromic anemia

[193]
d) mitral stenosis

[194]
d) scabies

[195]
d) renal system

[196]
d) all of the above

[197]
c) CN 11

[198]
a) the patient is at higher risk for active tuberculosis disease within the next 2 years

[199]
c) tertiary prevention

[200]
b) 42-year-old obese woman taking prednisone 10 mg daily for severe asthma for 2 years

SECTION E

[201]
d) gluten

[202]
d) microaneurysms

[203]
c) migraine headache with aura

[204]
a) lung cancer

[205]
d) macrocytic and normocytic red blood cells

[206]
c) elevated

[207]
b) rheumatoid arthritis

[208]
d) Creutzfeldt-Jakob disease

[209]
c) indomethacin (Indocin)

[210]
a) loss of joint mobility and renal failure

[211]
d) international health promotion programs

[212]
a) Bouchard's node

[213]
a) diabetes mellitus

[214]
d) initiate a prescription of nicotinic acid (niacin, Niaspan)

[215]
d) the meniscus of the knee

[216]
b) an endoscopy with tissue biopsy

[217]
c) June 2001

[218]
a) HgbA1c

[219]
b) a superficial vesicle filled with serous fluid greater than 1 cm in size

[220]
b) isoniazid (INH) prophylaxis is not recommended for persons ages 30 years or older because of the higher risk of hepatic injury

[221]
b) Western blot

[222]
b) condyloma acuminata

[223]
d) Depo-Provera injections

[224]
d) ovarian cysts

[225]
d) molluscum contagiosum

[226]
c) microcytic anemia

[227]
b) pelvis

[228]
b) gout

[229]
c) grade IV

[230]
a) aortic stenosis

[231]
c) hepatitis C virus

[232]
c) CN 7

[234]
c) hepatitis B vaccination and hepatitis B immune globulin

[235]
d) pregnancy

[236]
a) apical and radial pulses at the same time, then subtracting the difference between the two

[237]
d) metronidazole (Flagyl)

[238]
a) apply candida or mumps antigen to the right forearm and the PPD on the left forearm and read results in 48 to 72 hours

[239]
b) Mini-Mental Exam

[240]
b) treatment for mild acne

[241]
b) serum creatinine and potassium level

[242]
d) the patient's spouse has a right to override the durable power of attorney's decisions

[243]
b) chronic hypertension

[244]
c) chronic coughing

[245]
d) the Board of Nursing

[246]
a) premedicate himself 20 to 30 minutes prior to starting exercise

[247]
a) it is a slow or sudden painless loss of central vision

[248]
c) acute sinusitis

[249]
c) a thyroid storm

[250]
b) fluorescein stain

SECTION F

[251]
b) inability to swallow

[252]
a) ACE (angiotensin converting enzyme) inhibitor

[253]
c) moderate persistent asthma

[254]
d) psoriasis

[255]
c) antimicrosomal antibody test

[256]
c) acute glaucoma

[257]
b) the nurse practitioner may be exempted from the lawsuit if documentation is thorough and can be verified

[258]
b) thyroid stimulating hormone (TSH)

[259]
b) Brudzinski's maneuver

[260]
a) women aged 50 years or older

[261]
b) order a 24-hour urine for microalbumin

[262]
a) the destruction of Rh-positive fetal red blood cells that are present in the mother's circulatory system

[263]
a) bacterial pneumonia

[264]
b) vesicular breath sounds

[265]
c) < 130/80

[266]
a) nedocromil sodium (Tilade)

[267]
a) a patch of leukoplakia

[268]
a) document the nurse coworker's behavior and file an incident report

[269]
b) mitral stenosis

[270]
d) a 37-year-old male biker with a concussion due to a fall who appears agitated and does not appear to understand instructions given by the medical assistant checking his vital signs

[271]
b) decreased mobility of the tympanic membrane as measured by tympanogram

[272]
c) status asthmaticus

[273]
d) varicocele

[274]
d) decreased anxiety and depression are common symptoms of the abuse in the elderly

[275]
a) closure of the atrioventricular valves

[276]
d) melanoma

[277]
d) families change over time because of the influence of environmental factors

[278]
d) elevated creatinine and BUN

[279]
a) lateralization to one ear

[280]
d) cheilosis

[281]
a) raloxifene (Evista)

[282]
d) these fractures always need surgical intervention in order to stabilize the joint

[283]
b) increase only the NPH insulin in the morning

[284]
c) her son can participate in some sports after he has been checked for cervical instability

[285]
a) erythema migrans

[286]
a) cimetidine (Tagamet), digoxin (Lanoxin), diphenhydramine (Benadryl)

[287]
a) ARBs (angiotensin receptor blockers)

[288]
d) CN 5

[289]
d) GGT (gamma glutamyl transpeptidase)

[290]
a) dry cough

[291]
a) Al-Anon is not designed for family members of alcoholics

[292]
d) McMurray's test

[293]
c) the document's objectives are applicable only to people of the United States of America

[294]
a) call the patient and tell her to return for further testing with a Gen-Probe to rule out infection by chlamydia and gonorrhea

[295]
a) advocacy for civil rights

[296]
b) basilar migraine headaches and a recent history of jaundice 6 months ago

[297]
b) lung cancer

[298]
c) cervical cancer

[299]
a) reactivation of EBV (Epstein-Barr virus) infection

[300]
b) hypertrophic cardiomyopathy

SECTION G

[301]
a) 6 to 12 cm in the right midclavicular line

[302]
a) cerebellum

[303]
c) Osgood-Schlatter disease

[304]
a) scarlatina

[305]
b) this is a normal finding

[306]
a) acute cholecystitis

[307]
d) ciprofloxacin (Cipro)

[308]
b) acute pancreatitis

[309]
b) isometric exercises

[310]
c) Pneumococcal (Pneumovax) and influenza vaccines

[311]
c) paroxysms of coughing that is dry or productive of mucoid sputum

[312]
a) arcus senilis (senile arcus)

[313]
d) gold salt injections

[314]
c) night vision

[315]
d) second-degree burns on the lower arm

[316]
b) second intercostal space, left sternal border

[317]
c) <120/80

[318]
a) a severe sunburn with blistering

[319]
b) her son's physical development is delayed and needs to be evaluated by a pediatric endocrinologist

[320]
a) temporal arteritis (giant cell arteritis)

[321]
d) *Chlamydia trachomatis*

[322]
b) CN 8 (acoustic nerve)

[323]
c) thiamine intoxication

[324]
b) oral tetracycline

[325]
b) the typical lesions are bullae

[326]
a) hidradenitis suppurativa

[327]
c) edema of the ankles and headaches

[328]
a) vigorous massage of the prostate

[329]
a) PSA (prostate specific antigen)

[330]
c) macrolides

[331]
d) neovascularization and micro-aneurysms

[332]
b) this is a normal finding due to the skeletal growth spurt in this age group

[333]
b) irrigate with normal saline and apply Silvadene cream BID

[334]
a) advise the patient that he is immune to hepatitis C and no further testing is indicated

[335]
c) atrophy of the sebaceous glands

[336]
d) it reviews information via a nongovernmental agency

[337]
a) the veins are larger than the arterioles

[338]
d) ovarian hormonal imbalance

[339]
a) gonorrhea

[340]
d) acute abdomen

[341]
b) CN 3, CN 4, and CN 6

[342]
a) hemoglobin electrophoresis

[343]
c) overweight patients

[344]
c) bacterial pneumonia

[345]
b) cefuroxime (Ceftin) TID × 10 days

[346]
b) beta blockers

[347]
d) migraine headaches

[348]
a) anticholinergic effects

[349]
a) the patient becomes very agitated, confused, and aggressive after sunset and throughout the night with resolution of symptoms in the morning

[350]
a) document in the patient's record behaviors and the action taken by the nurse

SECTION H

[351]
b) educate the mother that it is a benign finding

[352]
a) informed consent

[353]
a) reduce intake of potassium because of its cardiac effects

[354]
c) tertiary prevention

[355]
c) osteoporosis

[356]
c) Thayer-Martin culture

[357]
d) Loretta Ford, PhD

[358]
a) benign prostatic hypertrophy (BPH) and hypertension

[359]
c) basilar migraine headaches

[360]
a) the blue dot sign

[361]
a) left heart failure

[362]
d) hypertension

[363]
a) *Streptococcus pneumoniae*

[364]
b) initiate a prescription of hydrochlorothiazide 12.5 mg po daily

[365]
b) antibiotics

[366]
a) microalbuminuria and diabetes

[367]
d) CAGE test

[368]
b) initiate a prescription of metformin (Glucophage) 500 mg po BID

[369]
b) strenuous exercise is contraindicated for most type 1 diabetics because of a higher risk of hypoglycemic episodes

[370]
b) *Streptococcus pneumoniae*

[371]
c) adrenal glands

[372]
b) dial 911

[373]
c) ranitidine (Zantac)

[374]
d) furosemide (Lasix)

[375]
a) severe ulcers in the stomach or duodenum

[376]
c) ciprofloxacin (Cipro)

[377]
b) psoriasis

[378]
c) It is best heard at the apex at S1

[379]
b) acute appendicitis

[380]
c) chewing breath mints

[381]
d) repeat the Gen-Probe test for *Chlamydia trachomatis* to ensure that the previous test was not a false-negative result

[382]
c) Tanner stage IV

[383]
a) Depo-Provera injections

[384]
a) clarithromycin (Biaxin)

[385]
d) G6PD-deficiency anemia

[386]
b) paroxysmal atrial tachycardia

[387]
a) oral metronidazole (Flagyl)

[388]
c) mitral regurgitation

[389]
b) she should avoid alcoholic drinks one day before, during therapy, and a few days after therapy

[390]
c) preventative therapy for *Pneumocystis carinii* pneumonia (PCP)

[391]
a) acute appendicitis

[392]
d) testes

[393]
d) nedocromil sodium (Tilade)

[394]
a) hearing loss and tinnitus

[395]
d) stroke and coronary heart disease

[396]
a) send a urine specimen for culture and sensitivity to the laboratory and treat the patient for a urinary tract infection (UTI)

[397]
a) basal skin cancer

[398]
b) cardiac effects

[399]
d) antihistamines

[400]
d) corticosteroids

SECTION I

[401]
c) ceftriaxone sodium (Rocephin) 125 mg IM and doxycycline 100 mg two times day for 7 days

[402]
d) migraine headache without focal aura

[403]
a) fruits, vegetables, and whole grains

[404]
d) acute epididymitis

[405]
c) ofloxacin (Floxin)

[406]
d) premature menopause

[407]
c) saw palmetto is always effective in reducing symptoms

[408]
b) 4% to 5.9%

[409]
b) Tanner stage II

[410]
d) lung cancer

[411]
d) slow onset of symptoms

[412]
b) *Chlamydia trachomatis*

[413]
d) smoking

[414]
a) injury to the meniscus of the right knee

[415]
a) refer him to an orthopedic specialist

[416]
c) the newer low-dose birth control pills don't require back-up during the first 2 weeks of use

[417]
b) luteinizing hormone (LH)

[418]
c) cholesteatoma

[419]
d) advocacy

[420]
b) swimming

[421]
d) mood disorders

[422]
c) patients with acute renal failure

[423]
d) 13-year-old being treated for a sexually transmitted disease

[424]
b) anorexia nervosa

[425]
a) refer the patient to a urologist after treatment

[426]
a) transfusion of blood is prohibited even in cases of emergency

[427]
d) protocol agreements help protect nurse practitioners from certain types of lawsuits

[428]
d) endometrial biopsy

[429]
b) patient is coherent

[430]
d) abstract thinking ability is increased

[431]
c) captopril (Capoten)

[432]
d) Bartholin's gland abscess

[433]
a) the nurse practitioner can examine and prescribe birth control pills to minors because there is no legal requirement for parental consent in cases concerning sexual activity and pregnancy

[434]
c) her partner does not need treatment

[435]
d) there is a loss of low-frequency hearing secondary to presbycusis

[436]
d) increased facial movements

[437]
a) CN 1

[438]
c) inability to swallow

[439]
b) multiple brain infarcts

[440]
c) pelvic ultrasound and serum quantitative pregnancy test

[441]
a) tubal ectopic pregnancy and PID (pelvic inflammatory disease)

[442]
b) amenorrhea

[443]
d) sodium restriction to decrease water retention

[444]
d) reproductive-aged females

[445]
b) CN10 (vagus)

[446]
c) acute pericarditis

[447]
b) rest and elevation of the knee with intermittent application of cold packs × 15 minutes four times a day for the next 48 hours

[448]
d) severe vomiting

[449]
d) weight

[450]
a) contact dermatitis

[451]
d) IUD (intrauterine device)

SECTION J

[452]
b) left supraclavicular area

[453]
a) tinea cruris

[454]
b) middle-aged men

[455]
c) it does not matter since there is no solid evidence regarding the efficacy of vitamin C for the common cold

[456]
b) delirium tremens secondary to acute withdrawal of alcohol

[457]
a) hyperthyroidism

[458]
b) ARB (angiotensin reuptake blockers)

[459]
d) stroke the inner thigh of a male and watch the testicle on the ipsilateral side rise up toward the body

[460]
b) apply hydrocortisone cream 1% BID to the rash until it is healed

[461]
c) a decrease in the systolic blood pressure of >10 mm Hg on inspiration

[462]
c) testicular torsion

[463]
b) refer him to the emergency room as soon as possible

[464]
c) the usual clinical strategy is watchful waiting for curves of 10 degrees or less

[465]
b) 200 to 239 mg/dL

[466]
a) 1 to 2 years

[467]
d) a 16-year-old who wants to be treated for dysmenorrhea

[468]
b) microalbuminuria

[469]
a) sinusitis and hydrocele

[470]
d) a cough that is productive of large amounts of sputum

[471]
b) the pulmonic area

[472]
c) *Candida albicans*

[473]
a) iron-deficiency anemia

[474]
c) she can take any of the pills in the sulfonylurea class

[475]
c) prostaglandins

[476]
a) serum ferritin and peripheral smear

[477]
d) vesicular breath sounds in the lower lobe

[478]
a) S3 and S4 and low-pitched tones

[479]
a) microscopy

[480]
c) Tanner stage III

[481]
c) Retin-A 0.25% cream

[482]
d) the cerebellum

[483]
a) influenza vaccine injections

[484]
a) heart disease, infertility, uterine cancer, diabetes, and endometrial cancer

[485]
b) MCV (mean corpuscular volume)

[486]
b) take two pills today, then two pills the next day and use condoms for the rest of the pill cycle

[487]
d) a 30-year-old White female who smokes

[488]
a) medical treatment for any work-related injury is covered under an employer's worker's comp insurance

[489]
c) the patient needs hepatitis B vaccine and hepatitis B immune globulin

[490]
a) axilla

[491]
b) SSRIs (selective serotonin reuptake inhibitors)

[492]
a) sciatica

[493]
c) *Pseudomonas aeruginosa*

[494]
d) there is a slight decrease in the activity of the immune system

[495]
b) clarithromycin (Biaxin)

[496]
a) Barrett's esophagus

[497]
a) amitriptyline (Elavil)

[498]
c) cold nodule

[499]
d) median nerve

[500]
a) glucosamine

References

American Cancer Society. (2006). Estimated cancer deaths for selected cancer sites by state, US, 2006. American Cancer Society. Atlanta, GA: American Cancer Society.

American Cancer Society. (2006). Estimated new cancer cases and deaths by sex for all sites, US, 2006. American Cancer Society. Atlanta, GA: American Cancer Society.

American Diabetes Association. (2006). Standards of medical care in diabetes. 2006. *Diabetes Care, 29*, S4–S42.

Anderson, B. C. (1995). *Office orthopedics for primary care*. Philadelphia: Saunders.

Bates, B., Bickley, L. S., & Hoekelmann, R. A. (1995). *A pocket guide to physical examination and history taking* (2nd ed.). Philadelphia: Lippincott.

Beers, M. H., & Berkow, R. (Eds.). (1999). *The Merck manual of diagnosis and therapy* (centennial ed.). Philadelphia: Saunders.

Bosker, G. (Editor-in-Chief) Textbook of Adult and Pediatric Emergency Medicine (2000). 1st Edition American Health Consultants, Atlanta, GA.

Brown, K. M. (2000). *Management guidelines for women's health nurse practitioners*. Philadelphia: F.A. Davis.

Centers for Disease Control and Prevention. (2006). *Sexually transmitted disease treatment guidelines*. Atlanta, GA: Author.

Chernecky, C. C., & Berger, B. J. (2004). *Laboratory tests and diagnostic procedures* (4th ed.) Philadelphia: Saunders.

Colyar, M. R., & Ehrhardt, C. R. (1999). *Ambulatory care procedures for the nurse practitioner*. Philadelphia: F. A. Davis.

Dajani, A. S., Taubert, K. A., Wilson, W., Bolger, A.F., Bayer, A., Ferrieri, P., et al. (1997). Prevention of bacterial endocarditis. Recommedations by the American Heart Association. Circulation, 96:358–366.

Dambro, M. R. (2006). *Griffith's 5-minute clinical consult*. Philadelphia: Lippincott Williams & Wilkins.

Dunphy, L. M., & Winland-Brown, J. E. (2001). *Primary care: The art and science of advanced practice nursing*. Philadelphia: F. A. Davis.

Ferri, F. F. (2004). *Ferri's clinical advisor. Instant diagnosis and treatment*. Philadelphia: Mosby.

Fishbach, F. (2000). *A manual of laboratory and diagnostic tests* (6th ed.) Philadelphia: Lippincott Williams & Wilkins.

Gilbert, D. N. (2003). *The Sanford guide to anti-microbial therapy* (33rd ed.). Hyde Park, VT: Antimicrobial Therapy.

Harruff, R. C. (1994). *Pathology facts.* Philadelphia: Lippincott.

Joint National Committee on Prevention, Detection, and Treatment of High Blood Pressure (JNC). *7th report.* Washington, DC: National Heart, Lung, and Blood Institute.

Mayo-Smith, M. F., Beecher, L. H., Fischer, T. L., Gorelick, D.A., Guillaume, J.L., Hill, A., et al. (2004). Management of alcohol withdrawal delirium. An evidence-based practice guideline. *Archives of Internal Medicine, 164*(13), 1405–1412.

McMinn, R. M. H., Hutchings, R. T., Pegington, J., & Abrahams, P. (1993). *Color atlas of human anatomy* (3rd ed). St. Louis, MO: Mosby Yearbook.

Morbidity and Mortality Weekly Report. (2005, September 30). *Updated U.S. Public Health Service guidelines for the management of occupational exposure to HIV and recommendations for postexposure prophylaxis.* Retrieved March 24, 2006, from http://www.cdc.gov/mmwr/preview/mmwrhtml/tt5409a1.htm.

Mycek, M. J., Harvey, R. A., & Champe, P. C. (2000). *Pharmacology* (2nd ed.). Philadelphia: Lippincott Williams & Wilkins.

National Asthma Education and Prevention Program. (2003). *Expert Panel report: Guidelines for the diagnosis and management of asthma.* Washington, DC: National Heart, Lung, and Blood Institute.

National Cholesterol Education Panel (2002). *Third report of the Expert Panel on Detection, Evaluation, and Treatment of High Cholesterol in Adults (Adult Treatment Panel III).* Washington, DC: National Heart, Lung, and Blood Institute.

Papadakis, M. A., & McPhee, S. J. Current Consult Medicine (2005). Lange Medical Books/McGraw-Hill. New York.

Prescribing References. (2006). *Nurse practitioners' prescribing reference.* New York: Haymarket Media.

Robbins, S. L., Cotran, R. S., Kumar, V., & Collins, T. (1999). *Robbins pathologic basis of disease* (6th ed.). Philadelphia: Saunders.

Seidel, H. (2003). *Mosby's guide to physical examination* (3rd ed.). St. Louis, MO: Mosby.

Tierney Jr., L. M., McPhee, S. J., & Papadakis, M. A. (Eds.). (2005). *Current medical diagnosis and treatment* (44th ed.). New York: Lange Medical Books/McGraw-Hill.

Tierney, L. M., Jr., Saint, S., & Whooley, M. A. (2002). *Essentials of diagnosis and treatment.* New York: Lange Medical Books/McGraw-Hill.

U.S. Department of Health and Human Services. (2003). *OCR privacy brief: Summary of the HIPAA Privacy Rule.* Washington, DC: U.S. Department of Human Services Office for Civil Rights.

U.S. Preventative Task Force. (2002). *The guide to clinical preventative services: Report of the United States Preventative Task Force* (3rd ed.). Washington, DC: International Medical Publishing.

Vennes, D. B., Biderman, A., Adler, E., Fenton, B. G., & Enright, A. D. (Eds.). (2005). *Taber's cyclopedic medical dictionary.* Philadelphia: F. A. Davis.

Watchtower. Official Web site of Jehovah's Witnesses. Retrieved August 28, 2007 at http://www.watchtower.org.

Willms, J. L., Scheiderman, H., & Algranati, P. S. (1994). *Physical diagnosis. Bedside evaluation of diagnosis and function.* Baltimore: Williams & Wilkins.

Wilson, W., Taubert, K. A., Gewitz, M., Lockhart, P. B., Baddour, L. H., Levison, M., et al. Prevention of Infective Endocarditis. Guidelines from the American Heart Association. Circulation. Released online at circ.ahajournals.org on July 30, 2007.

Index